D0538428

Assessments in
OCCUPATIONAL THERAPY
MENTAL
HEALTH

An Integrative Approach

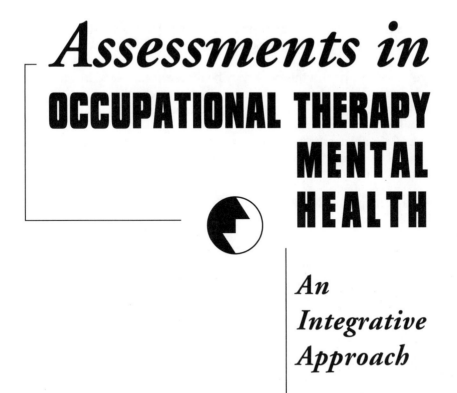

Assessments in
OCCUPATIONAL THERAPY
MENTAL
HEALTH

An
Integrative
Approach

Edited by Barbara J. Hemphill-Pearson, MS, OTR, FAOTA

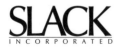

6900 Grove Road, Thorofare, NJ 08086

The work SLACK publishes is peer reviewed. Prior to publication, recognized leaders in the field, educators, and clinicians provide important feedback on the concepts and content that we publish. We welcome feedback on this work.

Assessments in occupational therapy mental health: an integrative approach/edited by Barbara J. Hemphill-Pearson.
   p. cm.
Includes bibliographical references and index.
ISBN 1-55642-266-0 (alk. paper)
   1. Occupational therapy. 2. Mentally ill--Rehabilitation.
3. Psychology, Pathological--Diagnosis. I. Hemphill-Pearson, Barbara J.
   RC487.A87   1999
   616.89′165--dc21   99-13632
                                                                                    CIP
Printed in the United States of America.

Published by: SLACK Incorporated
                      6900 Grove Road
                      Thorofare, NJ 08086-9447 USA
                      Telephone: 856-848-1000
                      Fax: 856-853-5991
                      World Wide Web: http://www.slackbooks.com

Dedication

To my husband, John, without whose support, encouragement, and unconditional love during times of challenge this book could not have been completed.

Contents

Contributors

Susan Baptiste, MHSc, OT(C)
Associate Clinical Professor
School of Rehabilitation Science
McMaster University
Hamilton, Ontario, Canada

Daniel E. Bentley, MA
Personnel Psychology Centre
Public Service Commission
Federal Government of Canada
Ottawa, Canada

Maureen M. Black, PhD, OTR/L
Professor, Department of Pediatrics
University of Maryland School of Medicine
Baltimore, Maryland

Sara J. Brayman, PhD, OTR/L, FAOTA
Assistant Professor and Graduate Coordinator
Department of Occupational Therapy
Brenau University
Gainesville, Georgia

E. Nelson Clark, MS, OTR/L, LCDR, USN, RET
Private Practice
Mental Health and Drug and Alcohol
    Counselor
Altoona, Pennsylvania

Anne E. Dickerson, PhD, OTR/L, FAOTA
Chair and Associate Professor
Department of Occupational Therapy
East Carolina University
Greenville, North Carolina

Margaret Drake, PhD, OTR/L, ATR-BC, FAOTA
Associate Professor
Department of Occupational Therapy
University of Mississippi Medical Center
Jackson, Mississippi

Marcia A. Good-Ellis, MS, OTR
Assistant Professor
Touro College
Dix Hills, New York
Private Practice
New York Institute for Special Education
Bronx, New York

Jeanne Gordon, MA
Department of Psychology
University of Maryland Baltimore County
Baltimore, Maryland

Carol Leonardelli Haertlein, PhD, OT, FAOTA
Associate Professor, Occupational Therapy
    Program
Chairperson, Department of Health Sciences
University of Wisconsin-Milwaukee
Milwaukee, Wisconsin

Barbara J. Hemphill-Pearson, MS, OTR, FAOTA
Associate Professor
Department of Occupational Therapy
Western Michigan University
Kalamazoo, Michigan

Alexis D. Henry, ScD, OTR/L, FAOTA
Research Assistant Professor of Psychiatry
Center for Research on Mental Health
University of Massachusetts Medical School
Worcester, Massachusetts

Renee Hinson, MS, OTR
Senior Occupational Therapist
Intensive Rehabilitation Unit
Holy Cross Hospital
Fort Lauderdale, Florida

Margo B. Holm, PhD, OTR/L, FAOTA, ABDA
Professor of Occupational Therapy
School of Health and Rehabilitation Sciences
University of Pittsburgh
Pittsburgh, Pennsylvania

Margaret L. Hunter, MS, OTR, MA, LLP
Team Supervisor
ACT of Kalamazoo
Kalamazoo, Michigan

Karen R. Kunz, OTR
Team Coordinator
Occupational Therapy Department
The University of Texas Medical Branch
Galveston, Texas

James P. Klyczek, PhD, OTR
Dean, School of Health and Human Services
Director of Graduate Studies
Associate Professor of Occupational Therapy
D'Youville College
Buffalo, New York

M. Jeanne Madigan, EdD, OTR, FAOTA
Professor Emerita
Department of Occupational Therapy
Virginia Commonwealth University
Medical College of Virginia
Richmond, Virginia

Trudy Mallinson, MS, OTR/L, NZROT
Department of Occupational Therapy
University of Illinois at Chicago
Chicago, Illinois

Gladys N. Masagatani, MEd, OTR/L, FAOTA
Professor
Department of Occupational Therapy
Eastern Kentucky University
Richmond, Kentucky

Patricia M. McGuigan, MS, OTR/L
Senior Occupational Therapist
Department of Occupational and Physical Therapy
University of Pennsylvania Medical Center
Philadelphia, Pennsylvania

Michael Natz, MS, BFA, OTR/L
Occupational Therapist
Baylor BioMedical Services
Dallas, Texas

Sandra M. Newman, MS, OTR
Supervisor, Outpatient Therapy
John Randolph Medical Center
Hopewell, Virginia

Marilyn Page, MA, OTR/L
Assistant Professor, College of Medicine
School of Allied Medical Professions
Occupational Therapy Division
Ohio State University
Columbus, Ohio

Nancy J. Powell, PhD, OTR, FAOTA
Associate Professor
Department of Occupational Therapy
College of Pharmacy and Allied Health Professions
Wayne State University
Detroit, Michigan

Sarah Rochon, MSc(T), OT(C)
Assistant Clinical Professor
School of Rehabilitation Science
McMaster University
Hamilton, Ontario, Canada

Joan C. Rogers, PhD, OTR/L, FAOTA
Professor and Chair of Occupational Therapy
School of Health and Rehabilitation Sciences
Professor of Psychiatry
School of Medicine at the University of Pittsburgh
Pittsburgh, Pennsylvania

John Santelli, MD, MPH
Department of Maternal and Child Health
Johns Hopkins School of Hygiene and Public Health
Baltimore, Maryland

Roger O. Smith, PhD, OT, FAOTA
Associate Professor and Director of Occupational Therapy
Department of Health Sciences
University of Wisconsin-Milwaukee
Milwaukee, Wisconsin

Franklin Stein, PhD, OTR/L, FAOTA
Professor of Occupational Therapy
Department of Occupational Therapy
Division of Health Sciences
University of South Dakota
Vermillion, South Dakota

Linda Kohlman Thomson, MOT, OT(C), FAOTA
Director of Rehabilitation Services
St. Joseph Hospital
Bellingham, Washington

Janet Hawkins Watts, PhD, OTR
Associate Professor
Director of Graduate Studies
Department of Occupational Therapy
School of Allied Health Professions
Virginia Commonwealth University
Richmond, Virginia

Foreword

A mere 17 years ago in 1982, the editor of this text published *The Evaluative Process in Psychiatric Occupational Therapy*. This work was a milestone for the profession of occupational therapy. For the first time, it brought together in one place assessments that had been developed and used by occupational therapists over the years for their work in psychiatry. To add to its value and usefulness, descriptive analysis and guidelines for its use accompanied each assessment. It is interesting to note in the editor's second compilation, *Mental Health Assessment in Occupational Therapy*, published in 1988, the refinements that had been made to the assessments included in the 1982 publication and the development of new ones, and now to examine those included in this current publication.

As measurement instruments develop within a profession, they become more sophisticated, and the profession itself is enhanced. Such instruments that are normed or standardized make it possible for occupational therapy clinicians to obtain a more discrete profile of an individual's abilities and limitations. The data collected is only a part of the total evaluative process, but an essential one. It forms the base for improved treatment outcome and the ability to conduct research that demonstrates the efficacy and efficiency (or lack thereof) of occupational therapy treatment. In other words, the performance-improvement process for the patient, the program, and the profession can then be measured, and, in doing so, what constitutes that occupational therapy treatment can be measured. Using initial assessments as a baseline measurement of functional performance level permits additional measurements at specified intervals during treatment to answer questions, such as those related to optimum timing, type, and process of interventions.

In the current health care environment, with its focus on tighter controls through managed care and rigorous cost containment, the development and implementation of critical pathways and subsequent outcome studies is more important today than ever before. With the percentage of occupational therapy personnel practicing in the mental health arena continuing to decrease, nowhere is the need for outcome studies more critical than in this area of practice. This third textbook also edited by Barbara J. Hemphill-Pearson, that includes updates and new material, in addition to assessments that have been in use over the years, is making a major contribution to the movement to strengthen the presence of occupational therapy in mental health. Through her efforts and those of the contributing authors, students, educators, and practitioners can readily link appropriate assessments with the theories and frames of reference from which they are derived, thereby congruently integrating these components of the evaluative process.

We are indeed indebted to all those who contributed directly or indirectly to this publication. Over time, efforts such as these give us more than we may realize when first studied.

Elizabeth B. Devereaux, MSW, ACSW, OTR/L, FAOTA
Associate Professor, Department of Psychiatry
Director, Division of Occupational Therapy (Retired)
Marshall University School of Medicine
Huntington, West Virginia

Preface

This book is the third in a series of textbooks that provide current information about assessments used in occupational therapy mental health. The first, *The Evaluative Process in Psychiatric Occupational Therapy*, presented a historical tribute to assessments that were developed and used at the time of publication. The second text, *Mental Health Assessment in Occupational Therapy*, discussed assessments in occupational behavior and skill acquisition theory that were not included in the first work. This third textbook, *Assessments in Occupational Therapy Mental Health: An Integrative Approach*, provides the occupational therapy practitioner with current information that is relevant to the mental health practice area. It presents a broader perspective in mental health assessment. Although this text can stand alone in its presentation, it can also be considered the third in a series of works about assessments compiled by this editor.

The assessments were selected, in part, from survey research completed by the editor. The purpose of the research was to ascertain which mental health assessments were taught by occupational therapy faculty in the professional programs. One hundred eighty-one surveys were sent to 71 occupational therapy professional schools. Eighty-one surveys were returned, a 45% return rate. Forty-seven schools participated.

The 10 most important assessments taught were: 1) Interest Checklist, 2) Bay Area Functional Performance Evaluation, 3) Role Checklist, 4) Allen Cognitive Level, 5) Comprehensive OT Evaluation, 6) Occupational Role History, 7) The Milwaukee Evaluation of Daily Living Skills, 8) Adolescent Role Assessment, 9) Magazine Picture Collage, and 10) Scorable Self-Care Evaluation.

The educators then were asked to rank those assessments that, in their opinion, were the most important to be taught in occupational therapy professional curricula. They were: 1) Kohlman Evaluation of Living Skills, 2) Allen Cognitive Level, 3) Role Checklist, 4) Bay Area Functional Performance Evaluation, 5) Interest Checklist, 6) Comprehensive OT Evaluation, 7) Occupational Role History, 8) Milwaukee Evaluation of Daily Living Skills, 9) Adolescent Role Assessment, and 10) Scorable Self-Care Evaluation.

Even though there is a discrepancy between what was taught and what was considered important, the assessments were either included in the editor's previous work or in this book.

Assessments in Occupational Therapy Mental Health: An Integrative Approach is organized into nine parts. Part I explains the author's concepts of client assessment from a holistic perspective, and it further explores the methodology for using the integrative approach to assess patients. Its relationship to goal writing and research is discussed.

Part II expands on interviewing as an important and integral part of the evaluative process by including four chapters on this topic. Three of these chapters deal with assessments in which interviewing is the primary method of client evaluation.

Part III presents three assessments. One is the performance assessment of self-care skills, another an update on vocational work assessments, while the third, the Bay Area Functional Performance Evaluation, offers research not published in the editor's first work. The purpose of these chapter is to give the clinician a summary and current information about the use of these assessments.

Part IV continues the tradition of including assessments that either were developed during the early development of occupational therapy or that stem from the earlier theory base of occupational therapy. The first chapter presents an overview of the use of projective testing; the second chapter presents information on the BH Battery; and the third chapter presents information on the Build a City. All three chapters discuss the object relations theory as the basis for assessment.

The assessments in Part V are based on the Model of Human Occupation. This part includes three chapters—two are updates on previous assessments presented in earlier textbooks, and one is new.

Part VI includes discussion of three previously published assessments. These were written to update the clinician on current research and administration changes, and are all based on the skill acquisitional theory.

Part VII has one chapter on assessment based on the biological theory. This chapter presents a method of assessing patients' cognitive skills. The assessment of cognitive skills has become important to the delivery of successful treatment of patients whose recovery depends on cognitive ability.

Part VIII presents three chapters on computerized assessments used in mental health, a new topic to the field of occupational therapy that is introduced in this textbook. This discussion is included because more assessments are being adapted to computer use. It is important that clinicians and students be aware of computerized assessments, so they can have a broader knowledge of various assessment methods.

Part IX, the last section, presents research methods that are employed in the development of evaluation instruments. Occupational therapy assessments are used as examples to illustrate the use of the research method. This section is faithful to the tradition of presenting information to clinicians and students about research methodology used to develop or improve assessment tools.

In keeping with the common thread of research, chapters written by the original assessment developers for the three textbooks are not intended to present or endorse a particular theoretical frame of reference or theory. The authors do not impose criteria for the assessments' usefulness or research development, because they believe that it is the practitioner who determines the credibility of an instrument and adds fuel for student research. Therefore, this is a compilation of assessments that have been developed, and then reported in occupational therapy journals, at workshops and conferences, and in unpublished manuscripts. This textbook, like the other two, brings together current information about assessments that were developed by occupational therapists for clinical use. Thus, it represents a collaborative effort by the originators of appropriate occupational therapy assessments. Sixteen chapters were written by the authors of original assessments.

Many of the assessments are underdeveloped, and I hope that I have provided the reader with the impetus to further develop the assessment tools used in occupational therapy mental health. Many of the assessments in this text and in the previous texts are in the beginning stages of research. Several have been researched and need further validating. By compiling these assessments, the editor hopes to provide therapists with a repertoire for assessing mental health patients, and offer students with the research skills and the incentive to further develop assessments presented in this textbook.

Because of the controversy in the medical field over the use of the terms "client" and "patient," patient is used in this textbook. The use of patient seems to be more universal and understood than client. In Chapter 3, however, the content refers to client-centered evaluation. It seems inappropriate, therefore, to use patient, as the evaluation is recognized as client-centered.

The editor wishes to acknowledge Pat Pangburn, owner of Public Relations Services, for her expertise in computer language and her ability to code the manuscript to meet the requirements of SLACK Incorporated. The editor also is grateful for her editorial knowledge about various writing styles. During the writing of this textbook, her ability to learn and understand the occupational therapy profession was outstanding.

Barbara J. Hemphill-Pearson, MS, OTR, FAOTA
Editor

PART I:
INTRODUCTION

An Introduction to the Integrative
Approach to Mental Health Assessment

Barbara J. Hemphill-Pearson, MS, OTR, FAOTA

The use of occupational therapy assessments in mental health continues to proliferate. As managed care becomes a way of life, functional assessments are becoming increasingly important in the clinical setting. Third-party payors want to know about patient progress, and progress is measured by assessments that demonstrate improvement.

Each time an assessment instrument is published in the occupational therapy literature, it seems to be in the early stages of development. As more assessment instruments are developed, it becomes difficult to know what is available and how to select an appropriate instrument.

A therapist selects an assessment instrument for a variety of reasons. Among these reasons are cost; administration difficulty; length; patient population; the therapist's educational experiences, expertise, and theoretical preference; as well as assessment research results, including reliability and validity studies.

The purpose of this chapter is to describe a structure for selecting assessments, based on their ability to identify patient dysfunction and progress. This structure allows the therapist to select and use assessments from a broad repertoire to achieve an integrative view of patients with emotional disorders.

The chapter first presents assumptions about the integrative approach, followed by a discussion of specific aspects of the approach. The integrative approach embodies the concept of the holistic view of the human being and will be presented in detail. Two case examples are also included to illustrate application of the integrative approach to patient assessment.

Several assumptions about the integrative approach are made. First, it is assumed that more than one assessment from different theoretical premises can be used to obtain an integrative view of patient dysfunction.

When using a particular instrument, the therapist is practicing the theory upon which the instrument is based. For example, the Bay Area Functional Assessment is based on the model of human occupation. If the therapist is using that instrument, he or she is practicing from the human occupation model. It is assumed, that if the therapist is using an instrument from the human occupation model, he or she will also use that theory for intervention. However, when one or more assessments are used from the same theoretical base, the patient's problem appears to stem from one theory only. It is then easy to overlook other patient problems because that one instrument is developed from a set of concepts that are based on a single theory. Furthermore, the practice of employing one instrument and using that same instrument for every patient who comes into the clinic is dangerous, in that goals and intervention end up being the same for everyone. As individual differences are not considered and because the same instrument is used, other patient needs may be overlooked.

The integrative approach rejects the practice of using one instrument or group of instruments from one theory to assess patients. The integrative approach, therefore, assumes that more than one instrument, based on more than one theory, can be used to assess patient dysfunction, which leads to the use of more than one theory to treat patients with mental disorders.

The idea of using several assessments is not new. In fact, the use of a variety of assessments, based on a variety of theories, is supported in the occupational therapy literature. Educators and therapists have long recognized the need for a system that integrates numerous bodies of knowledge into occupational therapy. Dunning[1] suggested that there were three modes that interacted simultaneously to reflect areas of human function. These areas reflected the psychological, social, and biological theories of human function.

The psychological perspective included theories about the psychic aspects of the individual; the social, about the influence of the environment and skill learning of the individual; and the biological, the physical aspects of the individual.

In 1970, three frames of reference—the analytical, the developmental, and the acquisitional—were proposed as the way to use more than one theory in clinical practice. Mosey[2] suggested that the selection of each theory's principles could be determined by whatever seemed best. This notion encouraged an eclectic, rather than an integrative, approach.

Furthermore, it generally is agreed that more than one theoretical approach to patient treatment should be used. Mosey states that "in the process of intervention with a patient, more than one frame of reference is often used to guide practice."[2] This is particularly true when the individual has multiple areas of dysfunction.

Clark attempted to organize the practice of occupational therapy into four theoretical approaches—adaptive performance, biodevelopmental, facilitating growth, and development and occupational behavior.[3] The author did not suggest a method for integrating these approaches into practice. However, the author did state, "no one theory can be expected to guide professional action. Instead, a therapist must knowledgeably select and use those theories appropriate to a specific practice situation."[3]

Other authors have attempted to provide a method for integrating conflicting theories. None has successfully provided a way to apply the conflicting theories that seem to characterize occupational therapy practice. Employing several theories and techniques to assess the mental health patient leads to the second assumption about the integrative approach.

The second assumption is that the patient is viewed from a holistic perspective. Practitioners recognize the interdependence of body, mind, emotion, spirit, and environment, and work toward the health of those parts simultaneously with the patient. The literature mentions holism as a value and a significant concept in the philosophy of occupational therapy.[1,4-5] The philosophical assumption appears to be consistent with the concept of treating the whole person. Occupational therapists view health as the total condition—one that cannot be divided into physical, mental, or social health—of a biopsychosocial being. If the initial or major health problem occurs in one area, other areas will be impacted as well.[5] In a profession in which therapists believe that major physical health problems impact mental health and social functioning, it seems reasonable to assume that such a belief would be reflected in patient assessment and treatment.

Therapists gradually have become aware that patients are searching for expanded treatment options—options that incorporate new and innovative approaches. Recently, for example, health care has begun to consider the spiritual aspect of the human health experience, which had been neglected in the past.

Spirituality has been recognized as important in the treatment of alcoholism,[6] depression,[7] and AIDS.[8] "Spirituality deals with the life principles that pervade and animate a person's entire being, including emotional and volitional aspects of life."[9] It has been stated that spiritual concerns are a part of the concern for health and cannot be ignored by any professional in health care,[9] including occupational therapy. Spirituality, therefore, should be included in the assessment process.

The occupational therapy literature, therefore, supports the view that more than one assessment, based on different theories, should be used to guide practice if the therapist is to serve the patient holistically. Authors agree that a system for integrating conflicting theories is needed for practice.

Therapists are faced with patients who have multiple areas of dysfunction, ranging from physical, social, and psychological to spiritual. The integrative approach to patient assessment provides a structure for recognizing the areas of human function, as described by Dunning.[1] It is a method that permits the use of more than one assessment instrument (based on individual need), along with their corresponding theories, for intervention in mental health practice.

The integrative approach recognizes four areas of human function—psychological, behavioral, learning, and biological. The social area described by Dunning was expanded to include behavioral and learning.[1]

AREAS OF HUMAN FUNCTION

Psychological

The psychological function "is the ability to process information from past events and information currently available ... to view one's self, others, and one's life situation realistically. The psychological functions are influenced by and derived from the emotional, feeling part of the human experience."[10] The psychological area of human function is described in the theories of Freud, Jung, Rogers, Maslow, May, and Perls.[11-16] In occupational therapy, the theories of Azima, Fidler, and Mosey[2,17-18] are also included.

Mosey coined the term "object relations" to describe a person's relationship to people and activity—the person's ego function.[2] This part of the patient's psyche helps therapists identify, for example, patient needs and body image, and achieve insight into the use of defense mechanisms.

Occupational therapists use unstructured and structured activities to allow patients to project their intrapsychic needs into the media. Projective tests, such as the Azima and Fidler Batteries, BH Battery, Shoemyen Battery, Goodman Battery, and the Magazine Picture Collage evaluate the patient from the psychological perspective.[17-22]

Behavioral

The second area is behavioral, which is the first mode Dunning identifies under social.[1] The approaches used in the behavioral area of human function come from the principles of conditioned learning—cognitive theory, social theory, and operant learning theory. Such techniques as reinforcement, modeling, token economies, desensitization, biofeedback, and stress management are used as treatment principles. Theorists such as Skinner, Bandura, and Dollard and Miller describe the behavioral area of human function.[23-25]

The body of knowledge that supports behavioral therapies comes from the writings of Reilly, Fidler, and Kielhofner.[18,26-27] In the behavioral area of human function, the therapist is concerned about the role environment plays in the acquisition of maladaptive behaviors for occupational performances.

The patient's environment (life space) and the patient's lifestyle are analyzed. The patient's life space includes the expected environment. For example, it is important to know if the patient is homeless, comes from the inner city, lives in a rural area, or comes from a middle-class neighborhood.

The patient's lifestyle (race, ethnic background, value system) influences the assessment. The patient's lifestyle also can influence the acquisition of a behavior repertoire.

This social area additionally includes the social interaction process, based on the principle that socialization is a developmental process that results from classical conditioning. Social skills, such as communication and group interaction, are attributes evaluated in this area of human function.

Such assessments as the Interest Checklist,[28] Occupational Role History,[29] Life Style Performance Profile,[30] Activity Configuration,[31] Adolescent Role Assessment,[32] Bay Area Functional Performance Evaluation,[33] History Interview,[34] Role Checklist,[35] and Revised COTE[36] are used to assess the social area of human function.

Learning

The third area of human function is learning. It is the second area of human function included in Dunning's social mode.[1] Educational theories, such as those as Harlow and Bloom[37-38] are used in assessment development.

Mosey's teaching-learning process is based on learning theory.[10] The learning area is concerned with acquisition of skills in occupational performance, not with how the patient did or did not acquire the skill.

There are two differences between the behavioral and learning areas of human function. One difference is that behavioral area assessments are administered by interview only, or by interview and task performance. Learning assessments, however, are administered by task only. The patient actually performs the skill. The second difference is that learning assessments use scales or some other form of measurement to compare patient scores, while behavioral assessments do not.

Two factors the therapist must be concerned with when using a learning assessment are the patient's cognitive function and level of skill development.

Cognitive functions, including attention, memory, orientation, thought conceptualization, intellect, and problem solving, have a direct bearing on patient performance. The patient's performance is not a measure of skill learning, but rather a measure of cognition, which is a biological function. Assessments based on learning theory do not measure cognition. The patient's developmental level must be related to the assessment or the task being performed. For a therapist to ask a 2-year-old child to tie his or her shoe would be inappropriate, because a 2-year-old is not developmentally ready to tie a shoe.

The functions associated with the learning area of human function are work skills, ADL, leisure, and social. It is most important that the assessment involve a task that simulates a life skill. Even though the same functions are assessed in the behavioral area, learning-area functions are assessed by actually performing or simulating the skill. Kohlman Basic Living Skills Evaluation, Milwaukee Evaluation of Daily Living Skills, Work Capacity Evaluation, and the Paracheck are examples of learning-area assessments.[39-42]

Biological

The fourth area of human function to be discussed is the biological. In psychological literature, it is referred to as the biomedical model. It asserts that "abnormality is an illness of the body." The assessments used measure neurological, physiological, and anatomical constructs. Occupational therapy theories, such as those of Rood, Brunstrum, Ayres, King, and Allen are used.[43-47]

King's research on the assessment and treatment of the schizophrenic is recognized.[46] The recent development of the Allen Cognitive Level (ACL) assessment,[47] which measures cognitive functioning by using a leather lacing project, has been rigorously examined to determine its reliability and validity. The ACL is particularly useful to measure functioning in depressed and demented patients.[48]

Masagatani also recently developed an assessment to identify thought processes in patients engaged in the performance of a task. The Cognitive Adaptive Skills Evaluation measures: 1) the ability to engage imitative and circular reactions; 2) the ability to use object permanence, time concepts, language, images classifications, and relational and number skills; and 3) the ability to use judgment.[49]

THE INTEGRATIVE APPROACH

The Evaluative Process

The evaluative process uses the commonly published occupational therapy process for evaluation and treatment. This process is ongoing during the treatment of mental health patients.

Figure 1-1 illustrates the integrative process that should be implemented to assess and plan treatment for a patient in a psychosocial setting. The following steps are included: 1) acquisition of the referral; 2) data gathering, including chart review, interview, and testing procedures; 3) analysis of data; 4) treatment plan; 5) evaluation of results; and 6) continuation of the process.

The data-gathering process is designed to obtain information that is relevant to human-function areas. The collected information is categorized according to the specific area of human function and the results used to determine patient needs.

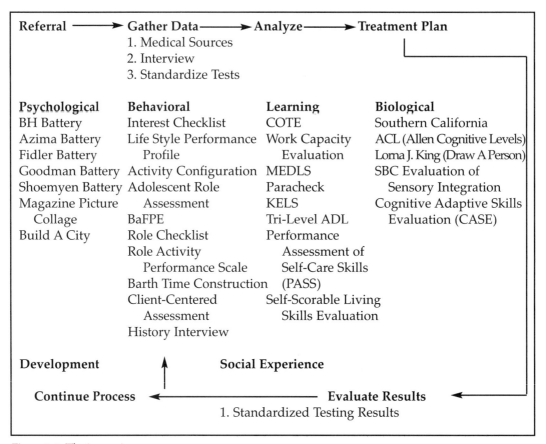

Figure 1-1. The integrative process.

The next step is to develop a treatment plan that spells out human-function goals. Reevaluation, using the same testing procedures as used initially, will determine if the goals have been met. Thus, the circle is complete, and the evaluation continues.

Additional assessments may be used and the treatment plan changed, depending on testing results, whether treatment goals have been reached, or if treatment has ended.

The client's developmental level and social level influences the selection of assessments. The therapist should select an instrument that is population-specific. In other words, if an assessment instrument is standardized for a specific population, then that instrument should be used only for that population. The social influence in assessment selection considers the patient's lifestyle and life space. Occupational therapy assessments may or may not be culture-free, which can affect assessment results. Considerations include the role culture plays in patient experience, the beliefs brought to the evaluative process, holistic orientation, the assessment itself, and the occupational therapy process.

Figure 1-1 shows all necessary steps in the occupational therapy process. It also includes the data-gathering process and the assessments, categorized within the four areas of human function.

More detailed discussion of the evaluative process is available in the earlier works in the Hemphill series.[50-51]

Selection Process

The selection of assessments begins by gathering data from the patient's chart and through interview. Information at this stage is categorized within the human-function areas.

In the interview, questions are asked that involve an area of human function or that will elicit an answer that can be categorized within one of the human-function areas. Listening is an important interview-process element that helps the therapist recognize, through the patient's response, the human function that the patient is describing. A careful listener can identify answers that act as transitions from one subject to another, and from one area of human function to another.

Through chart review and interview, the therapist is able to identify the human-function areas that need to be formally assessed, thus leading to appropriate assessment selection and goal setting. This is illustrated in the case example below.

Case Example A

Chart Review

This is the first admission for this 20-year-old female with a diagnosis of anorexia nervosa. Ms. M was admitted to an acute care setting after attempting suicide by overdosing on aspirin and Excedrin™. She complained of depression, suicidal thoughts, and inability to communicate with her family. These feelings worsened after the death of her uncle 5 weeks prior to this admission.

The psychiatrist reported that the patient had experienced eating problems since the age of 16. These eating problems included bouts of overeating, followed by forced emesis. Previous suicidal thoughts included driving a car over a cliff. The patient reported that she was afraid of dying. The patient expressed feelings of guilt about overeating and stealing food and money from her roommate at school, as well as guilt about bad feelings toward her family.

Ms. M felt that people were criticizing her looks and dress and laughing at her, although she could not hear them. She reported feeling tense, anxious, and depressed. It was felt that she had low self-esteem. A neurological exam was negative.

Psychological tests demonstrated that she had a personality common to those who have anorexia nervosa. It was shown that she had problems with impulse control, immaturity, egocentricity, low frustration tolerance, and a lack of future orientation. A high degree of anger was seen underlying a surface appearance of decreased initiative and assertiveness, passive compliance, and dependency. Her inner feelings were resentfulness, irritability, moodiness, and argumentativeness. It was concluded that she could not deal with anger directly or sublimate anger. Her investment in her mother included dependency and regressive longings, along with rage and contempt. Social withdrawal, distrust, and paranoidal ideations were evident.

Interview

Psychological Area

Ms. M reported that she had been looking for help for 2 years, having seen eight counselors. She appears to have gained some insight into her problem from reading several books on the subject. She was asked about her feelings at the time of admission, and she reported that she had felt anxious and guilty about overeating and was in pain all the time from vomiting. Ms. M stated that she was a good student in school, but that grades were no longer important to her because she was a good person, and good grades were not relevant. Ms. M appeared angry when talking about school, suddenly changing posture. She reported having a good relationship with her father but not with her mother.

Behavioral

Ms. M reported having a number of jobs, including working in a restaurant and as a tour guide. She liked being a tour guide because she knew what to say after she memorized a 12-page script. She is a good student and is on the dean's list at school. She does not want to return to her previous school because "I have too many problems there." Her favorite activity is fine, detailed, structured tasks, like needlepoint. She mostly prefers solitary leisure activities—reading, taking walks, and needlepoint.

Learning

Ms. M is dressed neatly and didn't seem to have problems with academic skills. She expressed the need to spend more time in social activities when she returned to school. She didn't report any difficulties in the work area.

Biological

At this time, Ms. M reported no problems with her health—she feels fine. The pain she experienced earlier is better, although an antidepressant she is taking causes dry mouth.

Assessment

The Comprehensive Occupational Therapy Evaluation (COTE) was administered to identify behaviors that could be treated in a short-term acute care psychiatric occupational therapy clinic. This assessment examines a variety of interpersonal behaviors. The results showed that the patient's behavior was normal in most areas. She demonstrated needs in the area of social skills, assertiveness, self-esteem, expression of emotion, and dependency.

Patient Goals

1. Increase socialization skills by participating in group activities that require interaction.
2. Increase self-assertion by providing opportunities to be self-assertive by choosing and following through on tasks and feedback.
3. Increase self-esteem and personal identity through unstructured creative activities, like ceramics.
4. Increase appropriate expression of anger through such activities as wedging and throwing clay.

Summary of Case Example A

The psychological area of human-function attributes in Case Example A are found in the following description: "anxiety, anger, depression, self-esteem, dependency, insight and suicide." The behavioral area is represented by the comments "self-assertion and leisure." The point to remember here is that the therapist is looking at the patient's environment and identifying its influence on the patient behaviorally. There does not appear to be any learning deficits. She has strengths in work and academic skills. In the behavioral area, she is experiencing pain from vomiting, but appears to be in good health.

This case example illustrates two factors. First, the integrative approach is a dynamic and flexible structure for gathering data; and second, the danger in using one assessment.

The case example suggests that Ms. M needs to improve social skills. This problem could stem from insufficient opportunities to socialize (behavioral) or from the lack of having learned social skills (learning). If the patient's environment did not provide opportunities for socialization, the therapist's treatment plan would be based on behavioral theories. If the patient did not have social skills, the plan would be based on learning theories.

By interviewing the patient and obtaining a social history, the type of treatment can be determined. In assessment, the patient would demonstrate social skills but not engage in social interaction, not because of lack of skill but because of lack of opportunity. If, however, the social history showed that the patient previously engaged in social interaction but now showed a lack of skills, that lack of social skills would be from not having the skills, rather than from not having the opportunity. It is important to determine in which area of human function the deficit lies to determine the appropriate type of intervention.

This case example also demonstrates the danger in using only one assessment. The comprehensive occupational therapy evaluation evaluates the behavioral area of human function. By using only one assessment, the therapist must rely on the chart review and the interview to determine deficits in other areas of human function.

The goals in the psychological area of human function are numbers 3 and 4; in the behavioral area, number 1, and in the learning area, number 2. In this case, there are no goals involving the biological area of human function.

Case Example B

Chart Review

Tom is a 30-year-old male patient with a diagnosis of major depression. This is the patient's second admission. The medical chart reported that Tom experiences stress, anxiety, and depression. According to the social worker's report, the patient had become shy and withdrawn. The parents reported that Tom's personality was outgoing and friendly but that he didn't talk a lot. There is a close relationship between Tom and his brother. Tom feels that his parents, with whom he lives, expect too much. The patient attended college, taking business courses, and was an average student.

According to the nurse's notes, the patient is concerned about sexual identity. He worries about homosexuality and is fearful he is gay, but denies any homosexual tendencies.

The patient's doctor reported that Tom is tense and anxious. Paranoid delusions were noted. Because people avoided him, Tom was afraid he had body odor. Tom felt that people at his previous job made fun of him, so he quit the job. The patient had suicidal ideations, poor concentration, and feelings of being unable to "handle himself." No organic problems were noted, except for a hearing problem.

The mental-status report showed that the patient was coherent in speech and oriented to time, place, and person. He demonstrated no delusions or hallucinations and seemed to be in contact with reality. Tom believes he has good insight into his problems.

Interview

The patient was cooperative and expressed the desire to get well. When asked why he was in the hospital, he said he had felt "strange feelings" for the past 2 years and hoped the doctor would identify the problem. Tom lives with his parents and expressed the need to find out how they felt about him. The patient reported that he does not have a job at the present time. He did not mention that he had been fired from his previous job. When asked about his typical day, he stated that it consisted of work, watching television, and taking long drives. He did not mention having any social contacts. Tom reported that he handled his anger by keeping it inside until it went away. He expressed some insight into how his anger affected him emotionally.

The patient saw his strengths as getting along with people but admitted feeling uncomfortable in groups. Tom's problems are seen as failure to be assertive, being dependent, worrying that people don't like him, and low self-concept. Tom indicated that he needs to feel proud of his accomplishments and to increase his self-worth. The patient's goals are to live independently, find a good job, and get involved in social activities.

Assessments

Three assessments were administered:

1. *Kohlman Evaluation of Living Skills (KELS)*. This was given because of the patient's expressed goal of living independently. The KELS is designed to determine a person's ability to perform basic living skills. The results indicated independence in all areas of living skills. There was no deficit in safety or work skills. Even though there was no problem, the patient expressed the need for assistance in budgeting, leisure skills, and work.

2. *Interest Checklist*. This was administered to identify activities that would interest the patient as possible leisure pursuits and would help motivate the patient during treatment. Tom showed interest in sports, music, and dating.

3. *BH Battery*. This projective test was used to evaluate task skills and psychological functioning. The patient was able to follow directions, make decisions, and follow through on tasks in a sequential manner. No task problems were observed. He is not psychotic and is in contact with reality. There was no obvious expression of anger or depression during the assessment process.

The assessment process indicated that Tom has low self-concept, poor assertive skills, poor group-interaction skills, a problem expressing anger appropriately, and a need for independent living skills.

Patient Goals

1. Improve self-concept by providing short-term, structured activities with immediate gratification.
2. Increase social interaction skills by reinforcing initiation of conversation in a group setting.
3. Increase expression of emotions, such as anger, by participating in high-stress role-playing situations.
4. Increase independence by providing activities that require budgeting skills.
5. Increase ability to contact appropriate agencies for assistance, when needed, by providing community resources information.

Summary of Case Example B

This case example illustrates the use of three assessments. The Kohlman Evaluation of Living Skills is an assessment of the learning area of human function. The Interest Checklist is from the behavioral area of human function, and the BH Battery is from the psychological area of human function. Information from the biological area about the patient's hearing deficit was obtained from the chart review.

Goals in the behavioral area of human function are 2, 3 and 5. A goal in the learning area of human function is number 4, and a goal in the psychological area of human function is number 1.

SUMMARY

Each of these case studies illustrates the use of the integrative approach to the selection of assessments in mental health. Each step of the data-gathering process—chart review, interview, and assessment—is designed to obtain information in the four areas of human function that will lead to identification of patient needs. The goals are expressed in terms of the area of human function that corresponds to the theory. Treatment techniques and principles from the corresponding theories are used to accomplish each goal, thus illustrating that more than one theory is used in treatment.

In Case Example A, goals 3 and 4 can be treated from the analytical theory, goal 1 from behavioral theory, and goal 2 from learning theories. The same can be said for Case Study B. The therapist justifies the goals that are written because they can be traced back to the chart review, interview, and assessment results. The criteria for selecting assessments can be further reviewed in Hemphill's second book in this series.[51]

The need to develop current assessment instruments cannot be overemphasized. Many assessments are in the developmental stage and need to be examined for reliability and validity. The need for research is an important thread that runs throughout this text. The last chapter is devoted to explaining research concepts that are used to further develop assessments in mental health. The integrative approach can be used to generate research from the data-gathering process all the way to treatment intervention. Research questions that examine various methods of intervention can be addressed.

This chapter described in detail a method for categorizing patient information. This method is referred to as the integrative approach to patient intervention. It uses the concept that more than one theory can be used in treatment to achieve a holistic approach. The selection of assessments is influenced by the patient's development, lifestyle, life space, and spiritual experiences. The assessments cited cover the four areas of human function—psychological, behavioral, learning and biological—which correspond to occupational therapy theory. These areas include human functions that interact and interrelate simultaneously. Good health is a condition in which all four are operating harmoniously to achieve competence in occupational performances.

REFERENCES

1. Dunning RE. Philosophy and occupational therapy. *Am J Occup Ther*. 1973;27:18.
2. Mosey AC. *Psychosocial Components of Occupational Therapy. Three Frames of References for Mental Health*. New York, NY: Raven Press; 1996:5,12-15.

3.   Clark PN. Human development through occupation: Theoretical frameworks in contemporary occupational therapy practice. (Pt 1) *Am J Occup Ther*. 1979;33:505.

4.   Meyer A. Philosophy of occupation therapy. *Archives of Occupational Therapy*. 1922;1:1-10.

5.   Reed K. *Models of Practice in Occupational Therapy*. Baltimore, Md: Williams and Wilkins; 1984:65.

6.   Grof S. Spirituality, addiction, and western science. *Revision 10*. 1987:(2)5-18.

7.   Prezioso F. Spirituality in the recovery process. *J Subst Abuse Treat*. 1987;4:233-238.

8.   Sullivan W. The role of spirituality among the mentally challenged. *Psychosocial Rehabilitation Journal*. 1993;16(3):125-134.

9.   Dombeck M, Karl J. Spiritual issues in mental health care. *Journal of Religion and Health*. 1987;26(3):183-197.

10.   Mosey AC. *Psychosocial Components of Occupational Therapy*. New York, NY: Raven Press; 1986.

11.   Freud S. Psychical (or mental) treatment. In Starchey J, ed-trans. *The Complete Psychological Work*, vol 7. New York, NY: Norton; 1976.

12.   Jung C. *Man and His Symbols*. Garden City, NY: Doubleday & Co Inc; 1979.

13.   Rogers C. *Client-Centered Therapy*. Boston, Mass: Houghton-Mifflin; 1951.

14.   Maslow AH. *Motivation and Personality*. New York, NY: Harper & Row; 1954.

15.   May R. *Man's Search for Himself*. New York, NY: Norton; 1953.

16.   Perls F. *Gestalt Verbatim*. Moab, Utah: Real People Press; 1969.

17.   Azima H, Azima F. Outline of a dynamic theory of occupational therapy. *Am J Occup Ther*. 1958;8(5):215.

18.   Fidler G, Fidler J. *Occupational Therapy: A Communication Process in Psychiatry*. New York, NY: Macmillan Co; 1963.

19.   Hemphill B. *Training Manual for the BH Battery*. Thorofare, NJ: SLACK Incorporated; 1982.

20.   Shoemyen C. The Shoemyen Battery. In Hemphill B, ed. *The Evaluative Process in Psychiatric Occupational Therapy*. Thorofare, NJ: SLACK Incorporated; 1982.

21.   Evaskus M. The Goodman Battery. In Hemphill B, ed. *The Evaluative Process in Psychiatric Occupational Therapy*. Thorofare, NJ: SLACK Incorporated; 1982.

22.   Lerner C. The magazine picture college. In Hemphill B, ed. *The Evaluative Process in Psychiatric Occupational Therapy*. Thorofare, NJ: SLACK Incorporated; 1982.

23.   Skinner BF. *Beyond Freedom and Dignity*. New York, NY: Knopf; 1971.

24.   Bandura, A. *Social Learning Theory*, 2nd ed. Englewood Cliffs, NJ: Prentice-Hall; 1977.

25.   Dollard J, Miller N. *Personality and Psychotherapy*. New York, NY: McGraw-Hill Book Co; 1966.

26.   Reilly M. Occupational therapy: A historical perspective: The moderation of occupational therapy. *Am J Occup Ther*. 1971;25(5):243.

27.   Kielhofner G. *A Model of Human Occupation*. Baltimore, Md: Williams & Wilkins; 1995.

28.   Matsutsuyu J. The interest checklist. *Am J Occup Ther*. 1983;23:323-328.

29.   Florey L, Michelman SM. The occupational role history: A screening tool for psychiatric occupational therapy. *Am J Occup Ther*. 1982;36(5).

30.   Fidler G. The lifestyle performance profile: an organizational frame. In Hemphill B, ed. *The Evaluative Process in Psychiatric Occupational Therapy*. Thorofare, NJ: SLACK Incorporated; 1982.

31.   Spahn R. *The Patient Gets Busy: Change or Process*. Paper presented at March 1965 meeting of the American Orthopsychiatric Society. New York.

32.   Black M. Adolescent role assessment. *Am J Occup Ther*. 1976;30:73-79.

33.   Houston D, Williams SL, Bloomer J, Mann WC. The Bay Area Functional Performance Evaluation: Development and standardization. *Am J Occup Ther*. 1979;43(3):170.

34.   Moorhead L. The occupational history. *Am J Occup Ther*. 1969;23:329-334.

35.   Oakley F, Kielhofner G, Barris R, Reichler RK. The role checklist: Development and empirical assessment of reliability. *Occupational Therapy Journal of Research*. 1986;6(3):157-169.

36. Kunz K, Brayman S. The comprehensive occupational therapy evaluation. In Hemphill-Pearson BJ (ed). *Assessments in Occupational Therapy Mental Health: An Integrative Approach.* Thorofare, NJ: SLACK Incorporated; 1999.

37. Harlow NJ. *Taxonomy of Psychomotor Domain.* New York, NY: David McKay; 1971.

38. Bloom BS et al. *Taxonomy of Educational Objectives Handbook I: Cognitive Domain.* New York, NY: David McKay; 1956.

39. Thomson LK. *Kohlman Basic Living Skills Evaluation.* Bethesda, Md: The American Occupational Therapy Association; 1992.

40. Leonardelli CA. *The Milwaukee Evaluation of Daily Living Skills: Evaluation in Long-term Psychiatric Care.* Thorofare, NJ: SLACK Incorporated; 1988.

41. Matheson L, Ogden L. *Work Capacity Evaluation.* Anaheim, Calif: Employment and Rehabilitation Institute of Southern California; 1987.

42. Parachek J, King L. *Parachek Geriatric Rating Scale,* 3rd ed. Center for Neuro-developmental Studies: Glendale, Ariz; 1986.

43. Pedretti L. *Occupational Therapy: Practice Skills for Physical Dysfunction,* 4th ed. CV Mosby Co; 1996.

44. Trombly C. *Occupational Therapy for Physical Dysfunction.* Baltimore, Md: Williams & Wilkins; 1996.

45. Ayres A. *Sensory Integration and Learning Disorders.* Los Angeles, Calif: Western Psychological Services; 1972.

46. King LJ. A sensory-integrative approach to schizophrenia. *Am J Occup Ther.* 1974;28:529.

47. Allen C, Kehrberg K, Burns T. Evaluation instruments. In Allen KA, Earhart CA, Blue T, eds. *Occupational Therapy Treatment Goals for the Physically and Cognitively Disabled.* Rockville, Md: The American Occupational Therapy Association Inc; 1992.

48. Allen CK. *Occupational Therapy for Psychiatric Diseases: Measurement and Management of Cognitive Disabilities.* Boston, Mass: Little, Brown; 1985.

49. Masagatani G et al. *Cognitive Adaptive Skills Evaluation Manual.* New York, NY: Haworth Press; 1981.

50. Hemphill B, ed. *The Evaluative Process in Psychiatric Occupational Therapy.* Thorofare, NJ: SLACK Incorporated; 1982.

51. Hemphill B, ed. *Mental Health Assessment in Occupational Therapy: An Integrative Approach to the Evaluative Process.* Thorofare, NJ: SLACK Incorporated; 1988.

PART II:
THE INTERVIEWING PROCESS

2

Interviewing as an Assessment Tool in Occupational Therapy

Marilyn Page, MA, OTR/L

The objective of this chapter is to give therapists the knowledge and understanding needed to use an interview as an assessment tool. The information includes the definition and purpose of interviewing; the knowledge, skills and attitudes required of an interviewer; the stages of an interview; and the management of different patient responses. Documenting the interview data is discussed briefly. The reader will know the specific skills, knowledge, and process for planning and carrying out a successful interview.

INTRODUCTION

An interview is one of four methods occupational therapists use to gather information for a complete evaluation of a person's ability to function. The other categories of assessment tools are observation, testing, and the case history.[1,2] These methods, including the interview, provide a systematic process for the collection of clinical data. The use of different assessment tools may depend upon which specific area of function therapists need to measure, or therapists may select the tools that match the ability of the patients to participate in the evaluation process. If patients have poor cognitive abilities, poor motivation, poor sensorimotor skills, or are too frightened to participate, therapists choose those assessment tools that encourage patient participation and are likely to obtain the most accurate functional results. A therapist's frame of reference provides guidelines for the use of specific assessment tools. The guidelines enable therapists to be consistent throughout the assessment, interpretation, and treatment process. Thus, therapists have to choose assessment tools that are consistent with the frame of reference, match the ability of the patients, promote the patient-therapist relationship, and are effective in collecting the data needed.

DEFINITION OF AN INTERVIEW

The interview is a technique many disciplines use in a variety of settings, including business, education, and health care. As an assessment tool in treatment settings, it has a specific purpose, process, and content. There is no one definition of an interview. Downs provides a general definition, stating it is a specialized communication pattern that has a specific reason for initiating an interaction and has specific content areas to be explored.[3] Shipley is more specific, "An interview is a serious conversation between someone with specific knowledge or expertise and someone who may benefit from that expertise."[4] Morrison defines a clinical interview as helping people to talk about themselves.[5] Lukas supports that idea, stating it is a time to allow patients to tell their stories in their own words.[6] Purtillo describes an interview as a time of planned, structured verbal interaction.[7] Occupational therapists employ all of these definitions. An interview as an assessment tool is planned oral communication that has a clear purpose, specific content, and a format that allows patients to tell their stories.[8] This enables therapists to understand the patient's perspective, the level of the patient's current occupational performance, whether further functional assessment is required, and to determine how occupational therapy will benefit the patient.

THE INTERVIEW AS A SCREENING TOOL

The first step of an evaluation process is called screening. This is the first meeting with the patient after the therapist has received a referral. The therapist sees the patient to learn whether intervention or further evaluation is necessary and to identify dysfunctions in the patient's occupational performance.[9] The interview is often the method chosen to gather this information. It is the one tool occupational therapists use that is based on oral interaction and does not require that the person engage in a doing process. To talk about one's performance is often less threatening than proving what one can do. Thus, many patients respond favorably to an initial interview. To use an interview requires that the therapist know how to engage the patient to establish rapport and trust enough to discuss topics that will reveal the patient's assets and limitations in occupational performance behavior.

During the screening process, it is not just the therapist who is making an initial assessment. The patient is gaining an impression of the therapist. If further intervention is warranted, it means that this interaction is the beginning of the therapeutic relationship. The quality of this brief interaction can make the difference in the patient's cooperation or resistance.

THE INTERVIEW AS AN ASSESSMENT TOOL

Most treatment approaches include an interview as one method to develop a comprehensive evaluation.[2,8,10] According to the Occupational Therapy standards of practice, a therapist is to "select assessments to determine the individual's functional abilities and problems as related to occupational performance areas: occupational performance components; physical, social, and cultural environments; performance safety; and prevention of a dysfunction."[9]

Mosey adds that evaluation is a collaborative process in which the patient and the therapist work together to identify the patient's assets and limitations.[8] An interview early in the evaluation process provides a format in which the therapist and the patient work together to determine the patient's needs and how occupational therapy can help. As mentioned earlier, an interview does not require that a person show functional abilities or limitations. Those patients for whom doing is difficult and threatening may initially save face by using their verbal skills. They may focus on their education, intelligence, or what they perceive to be assets in their functional performance. A sensitive interviewer supports this behavior as part of rapport building in the relationship. After using the interview to gain an initial understanding of the patient, occupational therapists should plan to use active assessment tools to complete the evaluation. The therapist informs the patient that the interview is the first step and that further functional assessment will be needed.

As the interview method is used by several team members, occupational therapists need to have a clear focus about the content of their interviews. A common complaint of patients is that they have to tell their story repeatedly to the varied health professionals. To avoid this problem, occupational therapists need to structure interviews so that patients will value and discuss their occupational performance.

Fidler provides guidelines on determining the purview of occupational therapy. The focus of occupational therapy is on patient performance. The emphasis is on patients' ability to do those roles and daily living tasks that are age-appropriate, relevant to their sociocultural norms and interests, and to the requirements of the social structure in which they live.[11] Following this overview, Fidler states that assessment and intervention will address four basic questions:

1. What must the patient be able to do? What specific performance skills are essential for the patient at this time?
2. What can the patient do? What are the strengths, abilities, and interests of the patient, and does the social structure support these?
3. What can the patient not do? What are the internal and external factors that limit performance?
4. What intervention, what specific purposeful activity, and in what priority, needs to be taken to enable the patient to develop the needed skills and performances?[11]

Throughout the interview, some information needed by the occupational therapists overlaps with that of other team members, but the specific focus on occupational performance needs to be clear. The interpretation of the functional status of the patient will be determined by the theoretical treatment approach used by the therapist, by the team's concerns, and by the clinical setting. Obviously, a therapist does not immediately confront patients with these specific questions. The attitudes and skills described in this chapter will need to be applied if therapists are to gain accurate assessments of the patients' performance levels.

Although observation is identified as a separate type of evaluation, as stated earlier, it is an integral part of every assessment procedure.[2] To observe is to use one's senses to attend to the behavior of a patient. Mosey states that it is to watch, to listen carefully, with alertness, taking particular note of detail.[8] This includes the odors or aromas that may be present; the temperature, tone, and color of the patient's skin; and the individual's posture, gestures, speech patterns, use of eye contact, manner of dress and grooming, and response to the present situation. It will be the decision of the therapist whether or not to reflect on these observations during the interview. When a therapist points out a patient's contradiction or limitation too soon in the relationship, the patient may perceive it as confrontation and become defensive. Whether the observations are discussed or not, they need to be understood as part of the total information gained from the interview. Later when the relationship is more established and a treatment plan implemented, the therapist can return to these issues for clarification.

The interview is a vital tool that is available at any time or place, does not require equipment, pencil or paper, and includes observed data. Throughout an interview, the therapist is able to observe and discuss specific events, behaviors, and goals with patients, and to identify and understand the cultural, economic and social aspects of their performance and environments. This understanding is vital to the planning of effective treatment, but it also provides guidance to therapists, as they interpret other performance-based assessments.

THE THERAPIST AS AN INTERVIEWER

A skilled clinical interviewer will need the specific skills, attitudes, and knowledge needed to establish rapport with people who experience a variety of problems. A good communicator has enough skills to adapt to the style of the patient. Therapists need to have varied skills, so they can be more flexible than their clients.[12] "A good interviewer must know how to work with a range of different personalities and problems; give a free reign to the informative patient, to guide the rambling one, to encourage the silent one, and to mollify the hostile one."[5]

The therapist cannot organize an interview in a rigid framework or think of it as a formula.[7] This initial interaction between the therapist and patient sets the tone for the entire relationship. Thus, a therapist must have integrated basic attitudes and have learned a variety of strategies and techniques that can be used as the need arises. The combination of identified attitudes, knowledge, and skills enables the therapist to respect and relate to the uniqueness of each patient. This, in turn, enables the patient to share vital information and feel a sense of positive relatedness to the therapist.

The Interviewer's Attitudes

A vital attitude in a therapist is to be open and accepting, to be *non-judgmental* in response to a patient's revelations. A therapist's own subjective, personal feelings cannot be permitted expression.[13] To develop emotional objectivity is more of a journey than an accomplished goal. It means that therapists have their subjective feelings, thoughts, and values under control, so they can focus totally on the patient's needs, values, and perspectives.[5] If a therapist keeps the focus on understanding the patient, it becomes easier to put one's personal perspective aside. The attitude of *respect* for the patient is a given, as stated in the *Occupational Therapy Code of Ethics*.[13] Yet therapists may be challenged when confronted with patients' unexpected or unusual behaviors. The therapists must have integrated a deep respect for all people, no matter their behavior or the condition in which they now find themselves. This requires therapists to look beyond the obvious and believe in each person's basic value, ie, value that is not based on age, job, education, or economics, but on the premise that the person is a human being and, for that reason alone, deserves respect. Therapists need instill in themselves the attitude of *hope* and a belief in a person's ability to change. The change process may be through learning, self-discovery, or environmental compensation, but therapists need to believe that patients can improve their functional levels. *Compassion* is required in therapists so that they can easily and genuinely express their concern for patients. Therapists can actively engage patients in sharing their emotional reactions, without becoming defensive or developing pity.[14] With the integration of these attitudes and the use of communication techniques, therapists can experience *empathy* for the patients. When these attitudes are an authentic part of the interview relationship, therapists can establish trustworthy environments in which patients feel safe, respected, and able to develop hope and the courage to change behavior or circumstances.[15]

Therapists need to be willing to seek *self-awareness*. They need to know the thoughts and feelings that their culture and experiences have developed in them. Therapists may need to examine their assumptions about a patient's ethnicity, age, diagnosis, language, cognition, size, religion, clothing, or any other difference. Therapists need to acknowledge that they, like other people, are reared within a cultural context that may include stereotypes and misinformation about other groups. Therapists are responsible for monitoring their own personal reactions and any influence those responses may have on clinical judgments. Therapists need to continually strive to keep assumptions about people from skewing their understanding of patients.[16]

To be culturally sensitive, therapists need to know and accept cultural diversity. Pedersen and Ivey believe that the concept of culture, broadly defined, includes the ethnography, demographics, status, and affiliations that have given each person a framework of assumptions.[17] Culture is not something outside us, rather it is an internal perspective that comes from what we have learned from life events and those things about which we have read or heard.[17] Therapists need to start by identifying their own cultural assumptions and clarifying their assumptions about the meaning and motivation of different behavior. Once that self-knowledge is gained, therapists will find it easier to accept that differences in world views are an important aspect of understanding people. Self-knowledge also enables therapists to be more secure in their own ways of behaving, which in turn allows them to be open to differences in others. Rogers, in his client-centered approach, believed that one reason counselors had difficulty perceiving the patient's point of view was a hidden fear that one's own values might be vulnerable to change.[19]

Therapists may not know the specific beliefs and behaviors of various cultural groups; however, they can be aware of differences and open to exploring and understanding them. It is essential that therapists learn and acknowledge the perceptions, values, beliefs, and behaviors present in the majority cultures represented by the patients. Taylor presents a list of cultural aspects to which therapists need to be sensitive. Some cultural aspects include family structure; roles; important life events; standards for health and hygiene; dress; appearance; perceptions of work, play, time, and space; and life expectations.[20] Especially important to communication are assumptions about the meaning of verbal and non-verbal behavior. Cultural differences will influence what people will say, how they will express themselves, what they are willing to tell to a stranger, which specific language skills are used, and the style and meaning of body movements.[20]

With education and experience, an occupational therapist learns to speak within a professional or scientific context, rather than from a lay person's perspective. As stated earlier in this chapter, the frames of reference used by therapists provide guidelines, not only in selecting assessment tools, but also in interpreting and identifying the meaning of raw data. When therapists can articulate the theoretical constructs they use to interpret interview content, they will more readily identify false assumptions. Using a theoretical base keeps therapists consistent, focused, and objective by providing scientific guidelines for the selection and interpretation of assessment tools. Knowledge of the different psychiatric and behavioral disorders is a needed foundation for therapists to accurately understand patient behaviors.

Besides personal and professional knowledge, therapists need to know how the dynamics within their patient care settings can skew their conclusions about the patients' abilities. Typical influences are time pressures, team dynamics, colleagues' opinions, and reimbursement criteria. Therapists may draw conclusions with too little information or may misinterpret patients' behaviors that are in response to their coping with the present situation. In addition, therapists may be focused on meeting the expectations of the health care setting, rather than on the needs of patients. Along with these attitudes and knowledge, therapists who are competent in basic communication skills will be able to focus on gathering authentic information from patients, so accurate interpretations and intervention plans can be developed.

The Interviewer's Communication Skills

To be able to plan and execute an effective interview, one must know the basics of communication and some criteria to determine its effectiveness. To communicate is to send and receive messages in a way that the sender feels understood. Every communication interchange consists of a sender, a receiver, and the channel through which the message is sent. The sender and receiver are encased within their own respective world views (context) that incorporate their culture, age, life experiences, feelings, and thoughts.[21] Communication has been identified as the largest single factor determining which kinds of relationships a person will make with others.[5,21] A therapist needs to respect the power of communication and how it may affect the patients and their treatment. It is the gauge that each participant uses to measure the other person.[21] Good human relations require that people know each other's meaning, despite the words used.[21] Using language that is comfortable and tailored to the wording, pace, and level of the patient is important. It is best to avoid medical jargon.[12] The therapist must approach the interview as a listener, ready to adjust to the patient, the environment, and the topics discussed, if the interview is to be effective.

The Art of Asking Questions

If an interview only involved the patient's answering questions, we could assign the task to a computer.[5] When a therapist uses a series of short, rapid questions it prevents the patient from telling his story.[5] An interviewer needs to adapt the pace, the type of questions, and the length of an interview to help the patient share pertinent information. It is often recommended to begin the body of an interview with an open-ended question, one that cannot be answered in one or two words, and one that requires that the person contribute information. "How do you like to spend your time?" "Which activities have you enjoyed doing in the past month?" Another variation is to use statements rather than questions. "It would be helpful if you would describe what a typical day is like for you." "Please tell me what kind of work you have done in the past year." Whichever approach is used, encourage patients to tell their stories about a given topic in their own way. These techniques encourage people to respond with the information that is most important to them or that they feel safe revealing. Avoid asking *why* questions. A *why* question puts the patient on the defensive, as its use implies disapproval.[13]

As patients begin their stories, the therapist needs to be able to guide them into telling about their occupational performance. Closed-ended questions are used to clarify or to request specific information. These questions require a specific answer. "Did you say you had one or two jobs last year?" "Did you enjoy the job of filing papers?" A word of caution is needed about the therapist's using closed-ended questions too soon or too frequently. If the patients begin to feel that the therapist only wants specific information and does not want to hear what is important to them, they will no longer share information, but will wait for the list of questions that satisfies the therapist.[13] Keeping the use of closed-ended questions to a minimum and asking only those specific questions that will provide the data needed for the assessment is critical. A good interviewer lets people tell their stories in their style, while guiding them in providing the needed information. The nervous or curious therapist may ask questions that do not relate to the stated purpose of the interview. To encourage patients to discuss irrelevant information may mislead them and lead to their focusing on topics unimportant to them or to the therapist. If therapists are not aware of this dynamic, they may inaccurately interpret the patients' concerns. Some questions, such as specific details regarding their diagnoses or medications, may cause patients to believe they are to share concerns that are outside the purview of occupational therapy. When therapists attempt to interject an occupational therapy focus by changing the topic, the patients may be left wondering why the questions were asked or if they said something wrong or displeased the therapist.[13] When the interview has wandered from its focus the therapist needs to wait for a pause, then support the patient's concerns, restate the purpose of the interview, and gently return to the occupational therapy topics. These techniques keep the focus on patients' needs and promote patient-therapist rapport.

Listening to Understand

To listen is to understand. A critical skill in the art of communication is to focus only on the verbal and non-verbal messages of the sender. A cardinal rule in interviewing is for the interviewer to listen rather than talk.[5] When unsure of what to say, be quiet! Listening is an active rather a than passive skill. The interviewer focuses all attention and energy into receiving the message. When using this skill, therapists put aside their personal concerns and clinical assumptions, and their anticipation of what the patient will say. They do not jump to conclusions about the patient's needs. When therapists are actively listening, they are not consciously aware of their thoughts, other than those concerning the patient, nor are they aware of mild physical discomfort. To listen means therapists are not interpreting or thinking of questions while patients are speaking. Their focus is on understanding the patient's unique responses to the topics. After the patient has finished a response, the therapist silently analyzes the information and forms the next step of the interview. A therapist does not agree or disagree with a patient during an assessment interview. The skill is to receive a message to understand, not to provide a critique or judgment of its value.[5] The primary aim of listening is to understand the patients' messages and assure them that the intended message was received. To listen and to understand enables the therapist to have empathy for the patient.

The Sounds of Silence

Silence is a part of communication, not the absence of communication. The sounds of silence are many. Silence may express reflection, resistance, anger, fear, discouragement, or completion. As in the previous technique, the therapist listens to the patient, totally focusing on the incoming message. When the patient has completed the response to a request, silence occurs. This pause allows time for the therapist to reflect, assimilate, and analyze the message, and then continue guiding the interview. A reflective silence may encourage the patient to add more information after thinking about what has been said. An angry or hostile silence may occur when patients believe a topic is irrelevant to their needs or believe that the interviewer is not listening, is uninterested, or is misunderstanding what they are saying. The angry silence is not the same as that of angry patients pausing in the discussion. In these cases the anger is focused on a target outside of the interview duo. When patients are expressing some level of anger or resentment toward the therapists or what they represent (loss of freedom), an angry, hostile silence will be evident. A *fear* of being judged as inadequate or as ill may motivate patients to become silent. When patients feel they are *overexposed*, that they have revealed too much of their personal concerns or have shared embarrassing or difficult information, a silence often occurs. When patients are *disoriented, forgetful,* unable to remember the topic or to sort out the jumbled thoughts or voices in their heads, they often end a topic abruptly and sit in silence. A more comfortable silence of *completion* occurs when both the patient and the therapist sense that a given topic has been covered and that a new topic is needed.

Each silence carries an emotional message. The interviewer needs to listen to the emotional message and respond to it. One response is to wait until the patient breaks the silence. What is said by the patient at the end of a silence may be helpful in identifying topics of top concern or revealing how the person handles the stress. Another response is for therapists to state their feelings or perceptions of the silence: "It seems the subject makes you sad." "You are angry about the interview." This allows patients to identify, refute, or expand upon what is important to them. The direct approach acknowledges that all feelings, even negative ones, are acceptable and do not scare or intimidate the therapist. If the silence suggests intense anxiety in the patient or if the patient has stated a fear, such as "I think I'm crazy," the therapist needs to break the silence and respond to the comment. Otherwise, the silence may suggest the therapist agrees with the patient's fear.[5] If a therapist is listening to the silence and senses it is time to move onto another topic, then asking an open-ended question on a new topic is appropriate. The dynamics of the interview, along with the needs of the patient, are used to suggest the interpretation of silences and the timing of questions.

One of the most difficult aspects of silence for new therapists is avoiding the tendency to fill silence with talk. They are uncomfortable with the silence and feel they must respond immediately. Their comments are often irrelevant or not well thought out. In this situation the lack of comfort in the therapist is what is driving the interview, rather than the need for assessment for the patient's benefit. A therapist needs to learn to be silent, to listen, and to value the silence.

An important aspect of silence is that it can connote respect and acceptance. Some patients are initially unable to express themselves orally. If pressured to verbalize they may become angry or fearful, which can aggravate their inability to cooperate in the assessment. When therapists acknowledge the patient's feelings and accept their behavior they send a powerful message of understanding. This provides a foundation for the patient-therapist relationship and enables patients to cooperate at their maximum level.

Identifying Thoughts and Feelings

Feelings are a person's responses to his or her experiences in the world. Thoughts are a person's interpretation of the response and the experiences.[22] To identify feelings means to be sensitive to the underlying emotion behind the person's content.[5] According to Egan, every core message has an experience (what happened to the person) or behavior (what action the person feels like taking), and an affect (the emotional response that accompanies the experience or behavior).[18] Egan developed a guide to help therapists respond to a core message, "You feel (affect) because of (experience/behavior)."[18] One is not to use this wording verbatim, but as a guide to identify a person's emotional response to a situation. A message might be, "I'm getting a raw deal. They say I will be going home soon, but they have not told me my diagnosis." The response might be, "You're feeling frightened that you will be sent home without treatment." The person can validate or correct the statement. A therapist need not be overly concerned with identifying the precise feeling, as the process expresses concern for the patient's well-being and encourages the more precise clarification of one's feelings.

People often discuss experiences that caused strong emotional reactions, without mentioning their feelings. It is helpful if the therapist attempts to identify the feelings that accompanied the experiences. To do so the therapist needs to observe the non-verbal behavior carefully. The tone of voice, the pressure of speech, the timing of words, along with the non-verbal use of the body, can all suggest affective reactions. In addition symbolic language can provide clues to feelings. When a patient states, "He is a pain in my neck," one can infer possible anger, sadness, or frustration. A therapist may start with a general category of feeling like *being upset*, then move to more specific feelings, such as *being frustrated*, to *being peeved*, or to *being angry*. Most beginning therapists have a limited affective vocabulary, so they may need to develop a list of feelings, including a range of intensity, that they can study to prepare them to help patients clarify their feelings.

The Use of Reflection

To reflect the content of a patient's message is more than imitating a tape recorder.

The art of reflection is stating the essence of the message in a few words and in a changed format. The sender can then hear the message from a different perspective. Reflection may help the person validate, clarify, elaborate, or refute the therapist's understanding. To be succinct and use key words stated by the patient is helpful. The temptation may be to parrot what patients have said, rather than to use reflection. If patients' words are repeated back to them, it often leads to anger and causes patients to question the therapist's competence. Reflecting so that the patient can hear the message in different words can help sort out feelings and thoughts. It may take several interactions of reflection before the specific message is understood by both the patient and the therapist. The focus is not on the technique, but on the therapist's understanding of the patient.[19]

Clarifying a Message

When patients are relating difficult information, several messages may be lumped together, either because they have not been able to sort them out or because they cannot identify which one is the most important. Clarification is the process of making a message clear.[5] This requires that the therapist listen for the different messages, then have the patient clarify different aspects until the message is clear. Therapists can identify two or three primary messages and ask the patients to elaborate on one or more of them. The therapist might say, "It sounds as though you are concerned about your job, the welfare of your family, the reason you are here, and how you will pay for it." To make an open-ended statement allows the patient to keep silent, respond to one of the topics, or to add new ones. If the patient continues to mix messages, the therapist continues to guide him or her through the sorting process until the messages are known or the lack of clarity is identified as a reason for treatment.

In relating a story, the patient may skim over a topic not believing it is important. The therapist knows the content is related to the patient's functional pattern, but needs clarity to ensure an understanding of the topic. Clarification may also be needed if the patient refers to specific topics or uses culture-specific language. It is the responsibility of the therapist to ask for clarification of the issue. The therapist is not to pretend to understand minimal or ambiguous information.[13] When asking for clarification it may help if the therapist states why the information is important to the evaluation process. It is helpful if the request is as open-ended as possible, although closed questions may be used for specific details. Open-ended requests might be, "Please tell me more about how you quit your job last week." "I am not sure I understand, please say more about losing your job." If relevance is needed, one might state, "In occupational therapy, we are concerned about how people spend their time. Please tell me more about your morning routine." Or, "In occupational therapy, we realize people sometimes do things they do not like to do. Please tell me what in your schedule you do not like to do."

Using Prompts

At times people need assistance to continue discussing their thought or topic. Communication is encouraged by using a manner, gesture, or words that do not specify the kind of information sought. Techniques that facilitate communication are called prompts. Prompts can be verbal or non-verbal. A common verbal prompt is to *highlight a word*. The patient says, "Last week when I lost my job I went shopping." The significant aspect of this statement may be the loss of the job, although the patient continues to talk about shopping. During the pause after the patient's comment, the therapist may reply, "Lost?" This will focus the patient on that part of the statement. If one word does not seem effective, then the therapist may *highlight a phrase*, "Lost your job?" This again encourages the patient to say more about the job loss. Other verbal prompts include "Please go on," "Yes, I'm listening," "I see," or "Uh-hm."

One of the most common non-verbal prompts is a *positive nod* of the head. This encourages patients to continue their train of thought. However, a nod of the head can also express agreement and a therapist needs to avoid giving incorrect messages. In some cultures, the up and down movement of the head means no. Again, therapists have to be aware of the patient's cultural context. A gentle *touch* may be used when a person is feeling sad. The therapist may put a hand on the back of the patient's hand, forearm, or at times, a shoulder. The touch must be strong enough to show caring. A light touch may trigger the autonomic system's flight or fight response, causing the patient to hit out in reflex. To pat a person is often perceived as a belittling or paternalistic expression, especially in the larger American culture. All non-verbal gestures exist within a cultural context. The therapist needs to be aware of other meanings for commonly used gestures and be alert to possible mis-understandings.

The Interviewer's Non-Verbal Communication Skills

The therapist's posture and general body language is a significant factor in the communication process. A therapist needs to be positioned at the patient's eye level This may require sitting or, in informal settings, it may require squatting. When planning the interview, arrange for both the therapist and the patient to be seated comfortably. The therapist needs to be seated with the patient in a *kitty-cornered* position, so that both of them can easily see each others' non-verbal behavior. Sitting side by side prevents both the therapist and the patient from seeing the other person's body language, especially facial reactions. To sit directly across from each other may connote the therapist's authority position and inhibit patient participation.

Once seated, it is important to communicate attention by keeping the body relaxed but alert. When the therapist leans forward slightly, it shows interest in the patient. The therapist needs to avoid sitting too far forward and holding his or her head up with his or her hands. Not only is it uncomfortable for the therapists, but it may be perceived by patients as boredom or exhaustion. To lean back in the chair may express lack of interest. A therapist who sits too rigidly may be perceived as too intense or too intrusive, which usually will limit interaction. The therapist's feet need to be kept on the floor or crossed at the ankles. Be alert to the movement of the patient's feet and hands, and his facial reactions. Many people have learned to control facial reactions, but not the way they express emotions in the rest of the body. People often are not aware of the steady kicking of their legs and feet or of playing with various materials with their hands. The use of eye contact is important in many cultures, but may be interpreted differently. In the general American culture, direct eye contact connotes respect, honesty, and concern. In other cultures, the rules of establishing eye contact depend on one's status, age, or gender. When the therapist is not familiar with the persons' culture or notes discomfort when the patient asks for clarification, information is necessary. If the therapist continues the interview without checking the reason for the discomfort, it may be perceived by the patient as disrespect or lack of concern.

Structure and Control of the Interview

The interviewer needs to structure and maintain control of the interview. To structure means to set the boundaries, identify the primary topics, develop a time frame, and provide a confidential, comfortable environment. To control means to manage and regulate the achievement of the interview. Control does not mean the therapist is to dominate and restrict the information. An efficient interview is one that the therapist has structured carefully so that the patient is the one talking and sharing critical information while rapport is being developed. It is the patient's perspective that the therapist needs to know and understand, so it is important that the structure allow that person's story to emerge. The effective use of communication techniques allows patients to have control over the information they choose to share within the structure provided by the therapist.

PREPARATION FOR AN INTERVIEW

The effectiveness of an interview is directly related to the quality of the therapist's preparation. The novice may plan extensively, whereas the experienced therapist, who is familiar with the setting and population, can probably plan and organize one in a few minutes. One part of planning is to establish the structure, set the boundaries, the topics, and the time frame. The novice may need to write down the topics and practice several open-ended questions. Practice helps establish the focus in the interviewer's mind so that when under stress, the topics will be recalled quickly. Without practice, most therapists will use closed questions and be thinking of responses while the patient is talking. The therapist needs to clearly understand the purpose of the interview, the information that is needed, and the priority of the different topics, ie, knowing which information is crucial, and what could be gotten later. Knowing other interviews this patient will have with team colleagues is helpful. As stated earlier, it is frustrating to a patient to be asked the same questions by many professionals. It is also possible that, in the multiple interactions, the patient comes to know which concerns are received favorably by staff so he or she begins to give them as responses.

Some therapists prepare by reading the patient's chart or attending the admission meeting. Other therapists prefer to meet with the patient before knowing the impressions of other colleagues. Each method has positive and negative features, so the therapists need to decide what works best in a given setting.

Choose the place of the interview carefully. It should be a place where the patient will feel physically and emotionally safe and know the conversation is private and confidential. A screening interview is often done in the patient's room, since it is one place that may be familiar and comfortable. If it is not a private room, the therapist probably will not pursue questions that infringe on the patient's desire for privacy, but often the therapist does not need this information to decide the patient's need for treatment. An in-depth interview needs a place that is quiet and that has controlled access to prevent interruptions. If a telephone or pager is in the area, the ringers should be turned off. When patients are sharing difficult personal information, they may feel disrespected if therapists respond to an incoming call. The patient may not be able or willing to return to the topic after an interruption. An interruption also may cause therapists to lose their train of thought and not return to an important topic. A room that is used for interviewing, especially if it is a clinical setting, needs to be neutral in its demand for competence. A display of many well-constructed crafts can give the message that one must perform well to be accepted. Often people who feel incompetent in their ability to function will be overwhelmed in such an environment and may refuse to participate in the interview. On the other hand, a poorly organized clinic, with poor quality activities, may imply a lack of respect for what the patient is capable of doing.[23] The clinic needs to look efficient, friendly, and like a place that promotes function.

GIVING THE INTERVIEW

There are three parts to an interview: the introduction, wherein the relationship is initiated; the body, where major information is gathered; and the closing, where the outcome of the interview is summarized and the next step stated.[7] Each part has a crucial role in creating a successful interview; therefore, a therapist cannot decide to cut out one step to save time.

Introduction

A vital part of an interview is to begin by clearly and concisely stating the therapist's name and role to the patient. This needs to be done immediately. The therapist's name is stated slowly, giving the patient time to repeat it if he or she wants. The patient has a right to know who the staff member is and why he or she has the entered their room and asked to interview him or her. Next, validating the patient's name, its pronunciation, and how the person would like to be addressed is important. To show respect, the therapist will let the patient decide the use of first or last name, or a nickname. To a staff member, the place and routine are known and comfortable; whereas the experience is most likely foreign and frightening to the patient. Explain the purpose of the interview and check the patient's understanding of it. Include how the information is important, how it is used, and how much confidentiality the patient can expect. The patient may ignore the therapist's comments and express concern about non-occupational therapy topics, such as why other staff have not seen him or her, or he or she may have a complaint that he or she needs to voice. Whatever the patient's immediate concern is, the therapist needs to listen and respond to it. This behavior shows that the therapist is focused on the patient's needs. As the therapist responds to the patient, the concern often can be addressed by clarifying procedures, agreeing to follow through with some action, or by incorporating the concern into the occupational therapy interview.

Although this introduction contains vital content and sets the tone for the interview, the time required is only a few minutes. It cannot be skipped in the name of efficiency. From the beginning, personalizing the interview is important. The patient is not just another *admit* to be seen for occupational therapy. This is a person in an emotional crisis, whether he or she can express it or not. The therapist needs to take a minute to identify something about the patient that will show that the therapist sees the patient as a unique person. It may be a picture, a flower arrangement, or a comment that the patient makes. "Is that your son (husband, etc)? Does he live at home with you?" The patient may respond about the relationship with that person. "Your flowers have the colors of the season. Do you enjoy flowers?" These comments are sometimes called *social chit chat*. The therapist needs to realize that, in fact, most conversation between strangers starts with *breaking the ice* comments. In the evaluation and treatment setting, such comments suggest an interest in the patient as a whole person, not as a disease. Patients at times may feel that the staff only see what is wrong with them and do not honor the health that remains. When patients feel that the therapist has acknowledged them as competent people who have a life outside the treatment setting, sharing it eases their fear of discussing limitations in their functioning. These social comments elicit a healthy context about the patient. Avoid statements that have a judgment of good, nice, or fun qualities, as they create the assumption that the therapist is there to judge the patient.

In this initial stage of the interview, the patient may make statements suggesting worry or concern. "I don't know if my family can manage without me. I'll lose my job if my boss knows I'm here." A therapist needs to avoid making comments that offer false reassurance, that seek to placate patients. such as "I'm sure everything will be okay" or "Don't worry; we'll have you home soon." This type of communication is based on the therapist's need to avoid difficult emotions or situations. The comments are made under the guise of helping the patient feel better, when in fact, they imply that the therapist does not respect or understand the patient's perception of the situation. Actual reassurance occurs when the therapist responds to the patient's concerns and explores them until an understanding of the patient's reactions is achieved. Then the therapist shares available information and uses communication techniques to support the patient in coping with the unknowns.

Another important part of the introduction is to establish a time frame for the interview. Stating how much time the interview will take is essential. Knowing the time frame helps patients gauge the intensity of the desired information. A 10-minute request suggests becoming acquainted, while a 30-minute request indicates a more in-depth expectation. This helps the patients set their expectations and plan accordingly. If 30 minutes is negotiated, and only 10 minutes are used, the therapist needs to clarify the reason for the change. Patients can imagine many reasons for the early end of an interview. Most often their assumptions will be that they are not liked by the therapist or that they have done something wrong. On the other hand, if the therapist needs more time than requested, the therapist needs to stop the interview momentarily, explain the need for more time, then check to see if the patient is willing. If the patient agrees, then the therapist sets a new time frame that is acceptable to the patient. If the patient does not agree to an extended time, the therapist needs to use the remaining time to cover the most critical areas and finish on time. Setting a time frame puts a boundary on how much content will be covered. Patients can sense if this is a time to share more of their turmoil or if this simply is a preliminary to other assessments. When the therapist plans to use testing methods during the interview, the patient needs to be given that information at this time. Stating the purpose and the time frame early in the interview helps patients have control over participation in the interview.

This introductory step allows the patient to gain a sense of the who, why, what, and how of the interview. With this information and respectful behavior on the therapist's part, the patient can relax a little, feel that the therapist is concerned, and form a positive emotional base for the interview. The process can be accomplished in 2 to 5 minutes and will save time, as it encourages the patient involvement in the evaluation process. Setting a time frame in the first part of the interview prepares for the end of the interview in the third step.

The Body of the Interview

The body of the interview requires the largest time block and is when the oral interactions are directed to establish a positive patient-therapist relationship and to gather desired information. The therapist follows a planned sequence of topics, yet is flexible and able to follow where the patient may take the topic. As each topic is covered, a new topic begins with another open-ended question, followed by use of appropriate communication techniques until the therapist has an understanding of the patient's functional level. At the end of each topic, the therapist needs to summarize the core message and encourage the patient to validate, elaborate, or correct any information. If the patient jumps to a different topic, the therapist is to follow along and determine what made the topic important.

The therapist begins the body of the interview with an open-ended question, such as, "What was a typical day like for you before you came into the treatment center?" After that, the therapist can narrow the discussion to a function area. "You stated you took care of the house. Please tell me more about the tasks, and the time they took." "You mentioned work. Please say more about that." If the therapist needs to make an obvious change in topics, he or she should state it so that the patient can follow the theme of the interview. For detailed data, the therapist can use probing closed-ended questions. If the patient resists the therapist control or the change in a topic, the therapist needs to summarize what has been understood and how that information is helpful in establishing treatment for the patient. This reflection of the comprehensive picture allows the patient to feel heard and clarifies any content that may be misunderstood. If the patient believes that the therapist is trying to understand, he often will cooperate as much as possible, and the relationship for further work will then be well established.

Closing the Interview

The closing of the interview begins when the therapist states the purpose and time frame at the start of the interview. The therapist needs to be aware of the time and start closing the interview by stating how much time remains. A 3- or 5-minute warning is sufficient for short interviews. If the interview is longer than 30 minutes, a 10-minute warning is best. These cues allow patients to have some control over how much more they want to reveal and to say whatever they may have been holding back, not knowing when to bring it up. At this point, the therapist needs to summarize the basic content of the total interview. Again, this allows the patient to add, change, clarify, or deny what the therapist understood to be primary information. A therapist may need to request clarification on some topics or details. It is important to not open new areas of exploration or ask open-ended questions about related areas. If the patient has difficulty stopping, giving frequent statements of the time remaining is important. "We have five more minutes. Please clarify your comments about the neighbors yelling at you." "In the remaining minute, I wonder if you have anything you'd like to ask me." Part of closing an interview is to clarify the next steps. The patient needs to know what happens to this information. With whom will it be shared? Will it go in the chart? Will it be reported to others on the team? Will friends or family members be told? In addition, the patients need to know if and when he or she will meet again with the therapist. Before leaving, the therapist thanks the patient for their time and cooperation. To complete the interview on a positive emotional level, the therapist makes warm personal comments about the patient. This personal chit chat helps the patient feel accepted and cared about.

DOCUMENTING THE INTERVIEW

The focus of the therapist throughout an interview needs to be on the patient, not on taking notes.[4] As stated earlier, the establishment of rapport and the use of conversation skills are vital to being able to gain accurate significant information. If therapists take notes, they introduce a factor that could sabotage that goal. An experienced therapist can probably listen and record significant data with little interference. A novice is apt to focus on the note taking, thus interrupting the communication process. If a therapist does choose to document while interviewing, it is best to use a clipboard, so time and focus are not lost looking for a writing surface. A check sheet or short comment sheet will allow recording of pertinent data, without having to look at the paper for an extended time. If one chooses to take notes, the patient needs to be informed in the introduction phase. The notes must be taken openly, and the patient needs to be told that they can be read anytime during the interview. If done carefully, note taking may help the patient feel that what he or she is saying is important and being taken seriously.[5]

The use of a laptop computer requires skill in recording information, while maintaining eye contact and developing rapport. To the anxious patient, a computer can be inhibiting and interfere with his or her ability to share personal information. Too frequently, the computer becomes the focus when the system does not work smoothly or the therapist makes an error. One needs to decide if the use of a computer enhances the assessment process or interferes with it. What the therapist expects to gain in time may be lost in diminished data and rapport.

The use of audio or videotaping requires permission of the patient and needs to be done before starting the interview. When requesting permission from a patient to use these techniques, the therapist needs to realize the imbalance of power patients experience. They may believe no real choice exists. Even if the patient has given permission for the taping, it is the responsibility of the therapist to protect the patient from the embarrassment of sharing intimate information on tape.

Complete documentation of the interview needs to be done immediately after the interview, when the therapist's recall of information is most reliable. When scheduling time for the interview, the therapist may include the time needed for recording the information afterward. If the therapist has written down a sequence of desired topics in preparation for the interview, it may serve as an outline for organizing the documentation.

TECHNIQUES FOR SPECIFIC INTERVIEWING SITUATIONS

People Who Are Hostile or Aggressive

When interviewing a person who is overtly hostile or aggressive the therapist may need to adapt techniques to facilitate the task. Often anger arises from a person's sense of losing control or a lack of being respected, a fear of the unknown, or as a symptom of the illness.[4] In response to these possibilities, the therapist needs to meet briefly with the patient to initiate the first step of an interview, the introduction, explaining the need for an interview and the amount of time needed, and to set a time for the interview. This preliminary technique gives the patient time to collect his or her thoughts, to think about the interview, and to feel a sense of control. When conducting the interview, the therapist needs to focus on the patient's affect immediately after briefly repeating the introduction and statement of purpose.[5] The therapist's attention to the patient's anger and listening to expressed needs before focusing on the planned content implies respect and concern. An intentional avoidance of the patient's expressions of anger will diminish the accuracy and amount of data that will be shared and will increase the anger.[5] The therapist's own feelings need to be monitored and controlled so that the patient's anger is not personalized and the therapist can provide a response that is helpful to the patient, rather than one that is based on the therapist's lack of comfort.[5] This requires that the therapist not react out of fear when a patient uses a loud voice or strong language. If the therapist uses communication techniques to accept a person's anger and to empathize, the feelings often will be defused, permitting discussion of the reasons for the anger.[5]

A therapist needs to be alert if a patient begins to act out the anger and become violent. Therapists have the right to safeguard their own physical and mental safety.[6] Agencies have procedures for responding to violence. The therapist needs to know how to begin the procedures before beginning an interview. If the therapist is afraid and needs reassurance, a second opinion or supervision needs to be requested.[6] Preferably, the request would be made before initiating the interview; however, if during an interview a therapist becomes frightened, the interview can be stopped early. If, before the interview, the therapist is concerned about the patient becoming violent, the therapist can plan to hold the interview where assistance will be readily available. Throughout the interview, the therapist sits at least an arm's length from the patient, at or below eye level, does not make any abrupt movements, and does not make provocative comments. Also, the therapist's hands need to be visible to the patient, and an exit door should be available for the patient and the therapist.[6]

People Who Are Frightened or Suspicious

Fear arises from a person's concern about psychological or physical harm, powerlessness, or the unknown. Anger may be used to mask the patient's fear.[4] Some patients who have fear as a primary affect need the therapist to be sensitive to nonverbal behavior and to recognize that they may not state their concerns in words. By attending to the patient's affect, rather than words, and behaving in a consistent, predicable, low key, tactfully firm manner, the therapist will encourage trust. The therapist should avoid being reassuring or providing rational explanations that contradict the patient's experience.[5] The therapist needs to have his or her name and identity badges where they can easily be read. By clearly stating his or her name, role, and purpose of the meeting before any questions are asked of the patient, the therapist provides structure and control for the patient. By encouraging discussion of any concerns the patient may have about the therapist or the meeting, the therapist allows the patient to attend to any suspicions or concerns. The therapist should sit at the patient's eye level or lower in a room that is familiar to the patient, if possible, and arranged so the patient can sit with his or her back to the wall and can watch the door, windows, and the interviewer. The room needs to be large enough so the patient does not feel penned in or that he or she is receiving the "third degree." Throughout the interview, the therapist should help the patient feel some control over the process. For the patient labeled paranoid or with paranoid tendencies, the therapist needs to know that many such patients believe they are in danger and may fear for their lives. When patients are viewed from this defensive perspective, rather than as aggressive toward others, an empathetic therapist can react in a way that calms the patients.

People Who Are Silent

Due to illness or fear, some patients are unable or unwilling to talk with a therapist. As stated earlier, an interview is by definition an oral interaction. The therapist then may have to choose another method of assessment. The skill of observation is critical when patients are silent. Careful observation of the patients' behavior allows the therapist to communicate and accept the silence by validating feelings. "I can appreciate this is a traumatic time for you." The focus is on communicating the therapist's acceptance of the silence. If patients are willing to perform tasks that do not demand an oral response, the therapist needs to use other occupational therapy assessment tools. A strength of occupational therapy is that patients can communicate through their performance, even when they cannot voice their concerns.

Patients who are withdrawn may respond to a special technique. A set of short but frequent visits by the therapist may help the person start to talk. Five minutes in the morning and afternoon at scheduled times connotes a concern and acceptance of a person, although one is not talking or doing. During visits, it is important that the therapist not ask any questions or make demands of the patient. The therapist's name and function are stated along with concern for the patient. This is accomplished using a statement, so the patient feels no pressure to respond. The therapist then sits in a nearby chair, is quiet, and remains so for the allotted time. It is critical that the therapist not do paperwork, talk to other staff or patients, or family members, or read magazines. The idea is to send the message, using non-verbal behavior, that the therapist is available without conditions. At the end of the stated time, the therapist may make a statement reflecting the patient's implied experience or affect. "It can be frightening to come into an unfamiliar setting." If an implication seems too intrusive, the therapist thanks the patient for the time and states a time for a return visit. The critical thing is to make no demands and to non-verbally communicate caring. After three or four short visits, most patients will ask why the therapist is doing this. The therapist briefly responds about concerns for the patient's well-being. This begins the relationship and sets the stage for an interview.

Often people who lack speech are severely depressed. They can probably respond with one or two words, but cannot provide details or lengthy responses. Some patients report that they cannot keep a thought longer than a few seconds, so they forget what they started to say and have forgotten the question. Others state that their heads are so full of thoughts that the question gets muddled in their heads, and they cannot sort out an answer. The therapist needs to select a few critical questions that are short, clear, and concrete. Using questions that require one or two answers may be easier for patients. The pace needs to be adjusted to their level of concentration. The interview should be kept short, as these patients tend to become overwhelmed or exhausted.

People Who Have Incoherent Speech

A person whose words and ideas do not follow the rules of secondary process are exhibiting cognitive limitations.[8] This information by itself is vital to functional assessment. Cognition assumes a significant role in fulfilling the task and interpersonal demands of daily life. If the patient cannot use information in thinking, planning, or problem solving, the therapist can infer severe disruptions in life roles and relationships.[24] The therapist who knows symbolism and listens carefully may identify some themes in the communication. The message may come from words that suggest the patient is frightened, feels trapped or wounded, or wants a sense of power. "I can't sit in the chair! Only humans sit in chairs!" The speech reflects a feeling or need. The therapist reflects on the core message, "You are feeling unworthy. You feel you don't deserve to sit in a chair." Often the person can verify the response or continue to clarify it. An example of a woman speaking in more disguised language is, "I'm bleeding to death. My throat is cut, and I'm bleeding." The therapist responded, "You feel hurt by what happened? You feel out of control?" The patient said, "Yes, I didn't mean to do it." Often, the more the therapist can respond with reflections or interpretations of the comments, the more the patient can communicate.

Besides listening for themes in the language the therapist listens to the non-verbal messages. People who have specific brain disorders, such as Alzheimer's, may maintain the inflection appropriate to their message, even though the words do not fit. If it sounds like a typical "Good morning," yet the words are incoherent, the therapist should respond to the non-verbal cues. "Good morning. It's nice to see you." If that was the intended message, the patient will usually continue. If that was not the intended message, the patient will speak again in incoherent words, but the non-verbal cues will again help the therapist identify the intended meaning.

During an assessment interview, the therapist needs to listen to the patient's incoherent speech, without questioning or emphasizing the inconsistency. To do so may provide information and connote to the patient that the therapist cares and is willing to listen. This accepting behavior from the therapist helps the patient share his or her thoughts and feelings. With the reduction of stress, the patient's thinking and therefore communication may become more coherent.

The therapist needs to acknowledge that part of the message is not being understood. To pretend to understand patients' incoherent speech is not helpful and is often disrespectful. Arguing with patients regarding their delusions, hallucinations, or other statements is not helpful and may alienate patients. Some optional responses that therapists may use are: "I don't know about that. Let's talk about something that we both know." "It seems that it's important to you. That's not how I experience it, but I'd like to understand how you experience it." In an assessment, the focus is on understanding how the incoherent speech and thinking relate to performance, rather than on convincing or confronting the patient.

People With Rapid Tangential Speech

The patient may speak quickly, with poor associations or tangential thoughts, making it difficult for the therapist to understand the message. If the patient can tolerate interruptions, the therapist may ask for a slower pace. The patient may be able to slow the speech for a short time before reverting to the rapid speech. Some patients can tolerate the therapist's providing periodic requests for slowing down, while it will frustrate others. The therapist needs to be alert to the patient's reactions and stop asking, if it appears to engender anger. When the therapist chooses to not request slowed speech, or the patient does not voluntarily speak slowly, other techniques may be helpful. The therapist may identify what seems to be a key word and highlight it, which may help the patient focus and increase the associations of their thought processes. As the patient's thinking again becomes tangential, the therapist highlights another key word or phrase. If a core message is identified, the therapist can reflect it, which may help the patient focus on a given topic. It is important the therapist include an affect or a feeling, when reflecting the message so that the patient will focus on reactions. If the therapist reflects only the content of the message, the patient may be encouraged to provide more explanations or rationalizations.

With patients who speak rapidly, but with meaningful associations in their thinking, the interviewer might ask them to speak slowly or to take a deep breath to relax. This is an important clinical decision as it suggests that the patient is the problem and must meet the needs of the therapist. To initiate the request with a brief comment that the therapist wants to understand the patient's situation will keep the focus on the patient's welfare.

SUMMARY

The interview is a valuable assessment tool that focuses on how patients perceive their occupational performance and on establishing a patient-therapist relationship. To effectively interview, the therapist needs knowledge and a set of attitudes and skills. The knowledge of psychiatric conditions and their effect on occupational performance areas helps the therapist set the topics and structure needed for an interview. A theoretical frame of reference gives the therapist guidelines to determine function and dysfunction, and serves as a base for interpreting the data. The attitudes of acceptance, openness, respect, self-awareness, and cultural sensitivity enable the therapist to be non-judgmental and genuine in the interaction and to support the well being of the patient. The communication skills provide the techniques necessary for patients to talk about difficult personal topics and permit the therapist to send a caring, knowledgeable response.

REFERENCES

1.   Reilly M. Research potentiality of occupational therapy. *Am J Occup Ther*. 1960;14(4)207.
2.   Smith HD. Assessment and evaluation: an overview. In Hopkins H, Smith H. *Willard and Spackman's Occupational Therapy*, 8th ed. Philadelphia, Pa: JB Lippincott Co; 1993:170-172.
3.   Downs CW. Effective interviewing. In *Effective Interviewing: The Virtual Interviewing Assistant*. http://www.ukans.edu/cwis/units/coms2/via/index.html. University of Kansas: Department of Communication Studies; 1996.
4.   Shipley KG. *Interviewing and Counseling in Communicative Disorders: Principles and Procedures*. New York, NY: Merrill, Macmillan Publishing Co; 1992:7,243.
5.   Morrison J. *The First Interview: A Guide for Clinicians*. New York, NY: The Guilford Press; 1993:1-2,30.
6.   Lukas S. *Where to Start and What to Ask: An Assessment Handbook*. New York, NY: WW Norton & Co; 1993:1,7.
7.   Purtillo R, Haddad A. *Health Professional and Patient Interaction*, 5th ed. Philadelphia, Pa: WB Saunders Co; 1996.
8.   Mosey AC *Psychosocial Components of Occupational Therapy*. New York, NY: Raven; 1986.
9.   American Occupational Therapy Association. Revision: Standards of practice for occupational therapy. In Hopkins H, Smith H. *Willard and Spackman's Occupational Therapy*, 8th ed. Philadelphia, Pa: JB Lippincott Co; 1993: Appendix B,883.
10.   Allen C. *Occupational Therapy for Psychiatric diseases: Measurement and Management of Cognitive Disabilities*. Boston, Mass: Little, Brown and Co; 1985:115-120.
11.   Fidler, G. The challenge of change to occupational therapy practice. In Cotrell R. *Psychosocial Occupational Therapy*. Rockville, Md: American Occupational Therapy Association; 1993:15-19.
12.   King M, Novik L, Citrenbaum C. *Irresistible Communication: Creative Skills for the Health Professional*. Philadelphia, Pa: WB Saunders Co; 1982:9.
13.   American Occupational Therapy Association. Occupational therapy code of ethics. *Am J Occup Ther*. 1994;48(11):1037-1038.
14.   Falk-Kessler J, Momich C, Perel S. Therapeutic factors in occupational therapy groups. *Am J Occup Ther*. 1991;45(1):59-66.
15.   Schwartzberg S. Therapeutic use of self. In Hopkins H, Smith H. *Willard and Spackman's Occupational Therapy*, 8th ed. Philadelphia, Pa: JB Lippincott Co; 1993:269.

16. Bernstein L, Bernstein R. *Interviewing: A Guide for Health Professionals*, 4th ed. Norwalk, Conn: Appleton-Century-Crofts; 1985.

17. Pedersen PB, Ivey A. *Culture-Centered Counseling and Interviewing Skills: A Practical Guide*. Westport, Conn: Praeger Publishing; 1993.

18. Egan G. *You and Me: The Skills of Communication and Relating to Others*. Monterey, Calif: Brooks/Cole Publishing Co; 1977:87-88.

19. Rogers, C. Speaking personally. In: Kirschenbaum H, Henderson V. *The Carl Rogers Reader*. Boston, Mass: Houghton Mifflin; 1989.

20. Koslow D, Salett, E. *Crossing Cultures in Mental Health*. Washington, DC: SIETAR International; 1989:18-20.

21. Satir V. *Peoplemaking*. Palo Alto, Calif: Science and Behavior Books, Inc; 1972.

22. DeGangi G, Geenspan S. Affect/interaction skills. In Royeen, C. *Neuroscience Foundations of Human Performance*. Rockville, Md: AOTA Press; 1980.

23. Turner IM. The healing power of respect—a personal journey. *OTMH*. 1989;9(1):17-22.

24. Fine S. Looking ahead: Opportunities for occupational therapy in the next decade. *OTMH*. 1987;7(4):3-12.

BIBLIOGRAPHY

Baker KA. Workshop model for exploring one's own cultural identity. In Koslow D, Salett E. *Crossing Cultures in Mental Health*. Vol 1. Washington, DC: SIETAR International; 1989.

Fleming M. Aspects of clinical reasoning in occupational therapy. In Hopkins H, Smith H. *Willard and Spackman's Occupational Therapy*, 8th ed. Philadelphia, Pa: JB Lippincott Co; 1993:871-873.

Peloquin SM. The patient-therapist relationship: beliefs that shape care. *Am J Occup Ther*. 1993;47(10):935-941.

3

Client-Centered Assessment: The Canadian Occupational Performance Measure

Susan Baptiste, MHSc, OT(C)
Sarah Rochon, MSc(T), OT(C)

Client-centered practice has been a construct within literature and the clinical domain for the past 60 years. Introduced by Carl Rogers just prior to World War II, this innovation in individual counseling and therapy gained popularity throughout the following two decades,[1] being of particular interest and appeal to the social work profession. Over the past 20 years in Canada, occupational therapy and occupational therapists have been seeking a clear framework to guide the unique contribution provided to the health care system by this professional group.[2] During this fascinating process of evolution, client-centeredness has become a constant and seminal construct, adopted as an organizing paradigm for the practice of occupational therapy across Canada, with growing interest and commitment within the United States.[3,4] The Department of National Health and Welfare (DNHW) and the Canadian Association of Occupational Therapists (CAOT) worked together, beginning in 1980 through a joint Task Force, to develop guidelines for client-centered practice.[5] The Task Force recommended that further work should be undertaken that would allow for the development of an outcome measure of occupational performance. This project was funded in 1988 and resulted in the Canadian Occupational Performance Measure (COPM),[5,6] which was built upon the constructs of occupational performance and client-centeredness.

In the spirit of this exciting basis for discussion, this chapter will address the concept of client-centeredness in detail, in the context of its application to mental health occupational therapy practice, and with recognition of the wider scope of application as a more universal practice approach. Client-centeredness, both as an overriding conceptual base of practice and as a methodology for intervention, is presented. The discussion is organized into three parts. The first addresses client-centeredness in relation to the following five categories: the foundational philosophical base, link to client intentionality and goal attainment, support for client autonomy, and enhancement of client/therapist collaboration and partnership.

Part two presents the COPM, an outcome measure, designed upon client-centered principles and used to establish intervention goals, review progress, and measure outcomes of occupational therapy.[3] The measure is outlined, along with research findings pertaining to its application. The COPM is illustrated in two brief case studies.

The COPM is only one tool that illustrates the use of a client-centered approach. Client-centered principles have long been applied in the practice of occupational therapy and are well-acknowledged in the theory and practice of occupational therapy.[2] However, the operationalizing of principles into practice can be difficult when therapists face demands to simply practice in a technical mode or face pressures from a health care team that adopts a symptom-reduction mandate associated with a medical model approach.[7-11] The application of the COPM, whose beauty lies in its simplicity of application, is its congruence with the client-centered essence of occupational therapy and power in the integration of a client partnership in goal setting, which can mitigate the subtle social press toward a medical model approach.

Part three reviews issues and implications of client-centered practice of the occupational therapist and the team. Emerging research, which suggests the "fit" between therapists' self-conceptions and the foundational constructs of client-centeredness needed for successful enactment in practice, is explained in relation to historical, theoretical, and educational factors. This section closes by proposing broader use of the COPM outside of occupational therapy, namely as an outcome measure for the work of entire rehabilitation teams. Current and proposed research questions related to the COPM and client-centered practice are proposed.

PART 1

Client-Centeredness: The Foundational Philosophical Base

The most important element of a client-centered approach to practice is that it is flexible and dynamic. This method allows for the development of functional and relevant knowledge of the client, obtained by creating a facilitative climate for shared exchange. Clients retain an active, key role in determining problems which are defined from their perspective. Inquiry and learning are purposeful, meaningful, and related to the client's own needs, goals, and values. These learning experiences encourage and enhance the client's involvement, stimulating individual desires to discover and understand, making each treatment plan unique and unpredictable. Client-centeredness is, by definition, individualized, leading, therefore, to creative thinking and applications of interventions that are useful to the client. Problem-solving abilities are developed and enriched, and the individual is encouraged to develop a responsible approach to learning and concomitant growth. The true theoretical basis of client-centered interactions have evolved from learning theory, the construct of self, and the dynamics of interpersonal relationships.[1]

In mental health, where the identified client can be a person who is in an acute psychosis or afflicted with chronic dementia, client-centeredness can be difficult to reconcile.[9] In such situations, two issues must be considered: first, whether the treatment wishes or long-term goals of the client are being gathered in a fashion that can be determined genuinely and applied to guide therapy; and second, a more salient issue, involving the identity of the "real" client.[9] In the case of the person suffering in an acutely psychotic state, at an existential level, perhaps the real client is a society that cannot tolerate the person's psychotic behavior; or, rather, the individual's goal, evident in either advance directives or pattern of past health care choices, is to get the psychosis under medical control and relieve symptoms. The goals for rehabilitation, would then be kept on hold until medical stability is regained.

Similarly, the person with steady-state or deteriorating dementia is not likely the client. The caregivers, be they family or institution, are more likely the true client, seeking help from occupational therapy for such intervention as determining behavior-management strategies and advising regarding optimal seating and safety strategies. In either of these situations, a therapist can function in a client-centered fashion by defining and responding to this client.

Six principles contribute to the philosophical basis of client-centered practice. These include a belief that the client is capable of choice, a valuing of flexibility and an individualized approach to intervention, a conviction that the therapist should act as an enabler, a certainty that success is measured by the client's own attainment of goals, the need for contextual congruence in intervention, and, finally, an understanding of client readiness to use a therapist's expertise.

The Client as Capable of Choice

Central to client-centeredness is the fundamental belief that all clients are capable of choice. Weiner has proposed that such a view is aligned with attributional theories of human motivation.[12] These theories suggest that the behavior of a human is not solely the result of instincts, drives, or needs, as one might derive from the tenets of Freud or Maslow. Nor is one's behavior simply the result of shaping by one's learning and environment. Attributional theories are founded on a premise that people are capable of choice and that choices predict and guide behavior.[13,14]

Such a view elevates individuals beyond the mechanistic view that they and their behavior are the result of innate predispositions or environmental pressure. The therapist is more than a "tinker," adjusting an imprinted individual. Instead it requires, as a basis for therapy, the engagement of clients' imagination, vision of their future, and choice, as actors in rich and varied lives.

Flexibility and an Individualized Approach

The environment within which a truly client-centered service can best operate is one that is low in bureaucratic expectations and in which therapy is a dynamic process. There will be situations in which different levels of client-centeredness will be utilized by therapists. However, when one reflects on the traditional hierarchical, therapist-centered environment, it becomes clear that a more client-centered environment will provide more options and perspectives from which to approach the whole treatment endeavor. As a practitioner, one must be guided by client directions and not limited by established program protocols. The client-centered treatment environment challenges therapeutic creativity and returns to the roots of occupational therapy as a dynamic process. Each assessment and intervention process must be totally individualized, providing the environment for the client to evolve a plan and process, rather than having the expectation that clients will fit into programs, processes, and plans that are created either for a diseased population or a group with common problems.

This emphasis on individualization can put occupational therapy at a disadvantage in a culture, such as health care, that values standardized responses, and in which science and truth are judged solely by results of strictly controlled trials, involving multiple subjects. Schon has referred to the thinking that supports such a view of science as "technical rationality."[7,15] He argues the need to avoid such limitations in support of a true understanding of and connection with one's clients. Mattingly and Fleming illustrated that within the "underground" practice of occupational therapy there is a devaluing of the large scale, standardized approach and a recognition that an individualized strategy is more compatible with the true tenets of occupational therapy.[10] A client-centered approach demands that a therapist take a truly individualized and flexible approach within a health care context that may, at the very least, shun and even punish such an endeavor.[9]

The Therapist's Role as an Enabler

A client-centered intervention is based on the client's vision and values. It is steered by a sense of mutual respect that builds on the clients' strengths and ability to know what is best for them. It is critical, however, that therapists become skilled in recognizing their values and biases, and how these may limit the therapeutic partnership.

Within a client-centered context, there is a redefinition of power.[12] The clients are, in essence, empowered and enabled to be the central figures in the determination of their present and future. Clients will define the occupational performance priorities and direct the intervention process through actively engaging with the therapist in assessment and developing treatment/intervention goals and outcome indicators. The truly client-centered relationship is a participatory and interdependent partnership.[16]

The process of care in a client-centered sense is important in and of itself. Skills of listening and understanding and the use of language are critical and essential. One cannot become an effective client-centered therapist if one focuses on one's own beliefs and values and assumes the content of an assessment or interview, based on previous clinical experiences or population health data. The client-centered process is reflective, inquisitorial, and based on trial, re-evaluation and sometimes experimentation.

The therapist's role is to use accurate and active listening to determine, with the client, specific goals for intervention. The therapist must be open to obtain and use client feedback to revise strategies, as client goals are met or changed. The successful client-centered therapist exhibits an openness and honesty within the clinical relationship. The therapist will recognize the client's own drive and need for growth and development and will be open to sharing knowledge and providing relevant information, without assuming an "expert" stance.

Enabling involves taking the lead from the client and shaping the treatment environment based upon the client's own goals. It implies an openness and non-presumptive stance. The goals for therapy must be those conveyed and ratified by the client. They cannot be goals presumed to be the client's, based upon expert opinion of the therapist or treatment team. One clinician, in struggling with enacting client-centeredness, has stated:

> On one of the task forces that I'm on to look at program management, I've noticed that I often will say—it's really important that whatever we do, that we set up with the person's goals in mind. What I'm realizing is that my definition of goals is quite different from the treatment team's. For example, I'd say, I'd like to see team meetings run based on the client's goals and just have those goals focused on within the meeting, and, I'd like to see charting set up with the goals in mind. But nursing seem to have their own system and it's their own opinion of what's going on vs. having the person state what they feel is their problem ...They'll (referring to the health care team members) have their own view and will say—these are the client's goals, but it's their goals as opposed to the client's own goals.[9]

Instead of being the consultant, expert, or oracle, the therapist now engages *with* the client in a mutual partnership where knowledge is shared and pooled to come to a logical treatment plan, based on expressed goals and objectives. The client brings knowledge of personal situations and experiences in which the therapist brings a pool of specialty knowledge and unique clinical skills on which the client draws to learn, adapt, and move forward. The therapist becomes a facilitator, mentor, and coach.

Success Is Measured by the Client's Attainment of Goals

The client's goals, clearly stated, ratified, and documented at the outset of therapy guide the collaborative work between therapist and client. They direct the course of treatment and become beacons by which progress between client and therapist is measured. Attaining client goals becomes the reason for intervention. The effectiveness of therapy in attaining these goals is the prime indicator of success. Clear bench marking, using visual analogue scaling within the COPM, keeps both parties honest in reviewing progress objectively.

The Need for Contextual Congruence

One of the most critical factors in client-centered practice is the importance of the client's roles, interests, environments, and culture to the overall therapy process. If the therapeutic experience does not make sense to the client, then the chance of engaging that client in a positive process is slim. Similarly, if the offer of help and intervention comes at a time when the client is not ready or does not see the sense in or purpose of such efforts, involvement in therapy and with the therapist will reap minimal rewards, if any. It is from such incongruence of time and purpose that labels of non-compliance and being a "difficult client" emerge. However, when the therapist takes the time to explore with the client what is most meaningful and valued for that client at that time, there are no limits to the success that can be experienced.

Client Readiness to Use Therapist's Expertise

Client readiness is significant within this model of practice. It accounts for the model's inability to justify occupational therapy imposed in a prescription to "rehabilitate" clients against their will and without their engagement. This concept may appear self-evident and, therefore, ludicrous. Consider, however, how many therapists have received and accepted referrals to "motivate" or "activate" a depressed client. In reality, the intervention, if successful, involves engaging the client's own inner hopes and dreams, rather than the therapist's manipulating or adjusting the individual from the outside.

The Intentions of Both Parties Related to Goals for Therapy Are Made Evident

The process of care in a client-centered sense is important in and of itself. Skills of listening and understanding the client's choice of language are critical. The therapist cannot make an assumption that what the client wishes to focus on and what the client's goals turn out to be are necessarily what is best for that client at that time. An intricate balance must be attained between a) advising, providing information, and assisting in planning and implementing; and b) informing of unethical, immoral, or illegal ramifications of choices and actions. Being client-centered does not mean allowing the client to determine every direction and detail. The importance of a true partnership becomes clearly obvious in this component of the discussion. The therapist can assert professional reservations and in extreme circumstances inform the client that he will be unable to treat, based solely on client goals. When client goals are judged as detrimental to well being, the therapist has a professional responsibility to identify this situation. A dialogue is opened up between the two parties, and each can "draw the line" specific to negotiation. Choices are made by both parties without coercion or manipulation. Goals derived in this open dialogue remain viable and motivating targets for both the client and therapist.[17]

Support of Client Autonomy

All clients are unique and have the right to make decisions for themselves. Each client also has the right to be in an environment and a therapeutic relationship that will nurture and facilitate dignity and integrity. The client should have access to information that will enable decision making. Therapists have been trained to function in the health care service and to be proud of the level of skill, knowledge, and expertise that has been achieved through academic preparation and, later, through clinical experiences. From these bases can stem an exceptional liaison, enriched and nurtured through shared knowledge and collaboration. Relinquishing this position of credibility and potential respect is a hard lesson to learn. Most dramatically, it is very difficult for a caring clinician to allow a client room to take what may seem to be risks and to either succeed or fail, based on personal choices, rather than on listening to expert advice and avoiding the possibility of further harm or, at least, a challenge to safety and security. There may come a point where the client goes beyond what the therapist believes to be right or wise. It is then the responsibility of that therapist to openly and honestly discuss the situation with the client and, finally, disengage from the therapeutic partnership if the conflict of views, values, and beliefs is too great. Assurance of alternative support and assistance should be identified in the event that the client wishes to move forward with another facilitator and guide.

Enhancement of Client/Therapist Collaboration and Partnership

In a client-centered context, there is redistribution of power. Clients are, in essence, empowered and enabled to be the central figures in determining their own present and future. Underlying values of a client-centered client/therapist partnership are those of openness, honesty, and the creation of a climate that supports mutual respect. For this to work, the therapist must shed the professional's mantle of power and become intimate with knowledge concerning the client's culture, values, and beliefs. The therapist must engage the client from a position of wanting to know and understand the client's unique qualities and contributions to his or her world and environment. The therapist must become a role model in the creation of a partnership.

PART II

The COPM

At the beginning of the 1980s, the DNHW in Canada, together with the CAOT, called for the formation of a task force to develop guidelines for quality assurance, relative to Canadian occupational therapy practice. This plan was completed, with the Task Force continuing along a more conceptual path, developing the model of occupational performance, definitions for common occupational therapy terminology, and process guidelines. Three independent publications resulted from the work of this Task Force[18-20] and are published in one volume.[5] Most recently the CAOT supported a national project to develop another iteration of how Canadian occupational therapists view their profession, with a view toward the new millennium against the backdrop of massive changes in health care delivery systems and organizational models.[21]

Intervention Guidelines for the Client-Centered Practice of Occupational Therapy suggested strongly that "a tool or set of tools...be developed...specifically for occupational therapy."[19] Consequently, in 1988, the Canadian Occupational Therapy Foundation (COTF) and the National Health Research Development Program (NHRDP) jointly funded a project to develop an outcome measure of occupational performance.

Development of the COPM

Since the publication of *Toward Outcome Measures in Occupational Therapy*,[22] there were clear criteria which were expected to be met in the newly developed outcome measures. The measures should:

1. Be based on the model of occupational performance
2. Focus on performance in self-care, productivity, and leisure as primary outcomes
3. Consider performance components (physical, mental/emotional, sociocultural, and spiritual) as secondary outcomes, measured only for their contribution to occupational performance
4. Consider the client's environment, developmental stage, life roles, and motivation
5. Be sensitive to clinical change relevant to occupational therapy goals, including development, restoration, and maintenance of function, and prevention of disability
6. Not be diagnosis-specific
7. Be modular for use in whole or in part
8. Incorporate measurement properties of reliability, responsiveness, and validity
9. Be usable in terms of format, administration, time, ease of scoring, and client acceptability
10. Be able to be scored numerically.

The authors consulted with colleagues in both clinical and academic settings, and explored the literature to identify existing outcome measures that could meet some, if not all, of the defined criteria. In total 136 measures were identified, with 54 surviving the first review phase, which addressed the first two criteria and went on to examination against the remaining eight criteria. Fifteen more measures were removed from the potential list at that time.[23]

The researchers were determined not to reinvent and had planned to adopt or adapt existing measures whenever possible. However, despite this intention, it appeared from the detailed literature review that no compatible measure existed. Therefore, work began on the development of an outcome measure that would address the 10 stated criteria and that would be based on the construct of "occupational performance," the end point of which was the COPM.

Features of the COPM

The Canadian Occupational Performance Measure (COPM):

- is based on an explicit model of occupational therapy
- encompasses the occupational performance areas of self-care, productivity, and leisure as primary outcomes
- recognizes the performance components as essential to the process of occupational performance
- incorporates the roles and role expectations of the client
- considers the importance of performance areas to the client
- measures client-identified problems
- incorporates reassessment of identified problem areas
- focuses on the client's own environment, thereby ensuring the relevance of the problems to the client
- considers the client's satisfaction with present performance
- engages the client from the beginning of the occupational therapy experience, and increases the client's involvement with the therapeutic process
- can be used across all developmental levels
- can be used with all disability groups
- supports the notion that clients are responsible for their health and their therapeutic process
- permits the client and the therapist to identify and deal with life span issues
- permits the evolution of the use of purposeful tasks and activities
- allows for input from members of the client's social environment if the client is unable to answer on his or her own behalf.[23]

Administration of the COPM

This measure is administered as a semistructured interview by an occupational therapist with the client or with someone responding for the client, as necessary, identifying and weighting problems. The whole process incorporates five steps: problem definition, problem weighting, scoring, reassessment, and follow-up. The reader should refer to the COPM handbook for details of these steps in the total process.[6]

Testing of the COPM

The development and testing of the COPM was a three-phase process. The first phase encompassed initial testing by the authors within their local communities. This phase addressed the format, directions, and wording of the measure. In the second phase further testing, focused on identifying clinical measurement issues that arose from clinicians administering the tool, was completed within the local communities and across Canada. During the third phase more detailed information was collected concerning the style and outline of the manual, administration guidelines, demographics of the clients with whom the measure was used, and the associated scores. Comments and questions from therapists have been valuable in the ongoing development of the COPM. One key question addresses whether the COPM is a standardized instrument. It is standardized in the manner in which the instructions and guidelines for administering and scoring are provided. However, since the clients compare themselves over time in relation to goals they have identified, the administration of the test is individualized.[6]

Research on the COPM

Occupational therapy clinicians chose to be involved in the further evolution of the COPM by exploring its use. Several research studies were undertaken with this goal in mind. A group of therapists working in a community-care environment completed a qualitative study examining the measure's clinical utility. Positive attributes of the tool were the semistructured interview design; the support of client-centered assessment, helping clients focus on their own issues; and its applicability to the community setting.[24]

A user survey also was undertaken that was added to the results of the pilot testing to help develop the second edition in which specific changes were made to ease the tool's use in the clinical setting.

Since the COPM was first published in 1992, many studies have been conducted by members of the research team and others to evaluate, in particular, the instrument's reliability and validity:

- In a study of 27 seniors attending an outpatient day program, the COPM was administered initially and on a second occasion within 2 weeks of the first assessment. Under ordinary circumstances, measurable changes are not expected in this population of varied impairments, including stroke, Parkinson's Disease, hip fractures, and arthritis. The test-retest reliability for the performance and satisfaction scores of the COPM, calculated using interclass correlation coefficients were 0.63 for performance and 0.84 for satisfaction. Measurements between 0.60 to 0.80 are considered good, and over 0.80 is considered excellent.
- Pilot studies conducted by the COPM research group have collected reassessment data for 139 clients for performance scores and 138 for satisfaction scores. The mean change scores in performance and satisfaction (statistically significant: $p .0001$) indicate that the COPM is responsive to changes in perception of occupational performance by clients.
- The COPM in a mental health setting is known to be holistic, client-centered, and motivating. It also helps clients with mental health problems gain or enhance insight. However, the COPM can tend to be time-consuming and may be difficult initially for some clients to comprehend.

Other studies and results are reported in the *Canadian Journal of Occupational Therapy*[24] and referenced in the handbook of the second edition of the COPM (1994).

PART III

Case Studies: Drawing Key Issues of Occupational Performance from Clinical Experiences

Case Example A

The foci of this case are upon the following:
- Client's own goal setting and attainment
- Collaboration
- Overcoming therapist's biases
- Client readiness
- Client cues and adaptive incorporation of magical thinking.

This case describes a slow process of adaptation that, without a client-centered approach and the application of the COPM, could easily have been derailed early on in treatment. At the outset of therapy, the client was engaged as a partner. This distributed or collaborated sharing of power, whereby the client felt he or she was in control, diminished the potentially destructive influence that is derived from the therapist's own value-laden empathy.

The client was a 43-year-old male, diagnosed with an atypical schizophrenoform illness, with some paranoid-like delusional and magical thinking (DSM III-R) of approximately 3 years duration. The client, Jim Smith, was a physician who had practiced for the last 10 years as a primary care physician in a remote northern community in Manitoba. He had no partner and often was flown to emergency cases, necessitating that he be away from his practice for periods of time. Serious cases, emergencies, and those requiring complicated or long-term care were flown to a large urban center 400 miles away.

This single man had reportedly lived a quiet social life, stating he enjoyed fishing, reading, and weekly dart tournaments at a local pub. He kept in touch by phone and the Internet with his mother and sister, who lived in the same city as the medical center where he was receiving treatment. They were his main sources of support.

Dr. Smith was referred to a specialized outclient occupational therapy unit for assessment and vocational "adjustment." He had two brief inpatient admissions necessitated by his not taking care of himself, and his lethargy, appearing to respond to internal cues or hallucinations (although he never owned up to having them), and holding some vaguely formed delusions more akin to magical thinking.

This latest admission was voluntary but had been prompted by his mother and sister after they had received several nocturnal phone calls from him in which he appeared fearful. When asked the cause of his ill health, he said that something had snapped in his head on the last medical flight he had taken and that "nothing was working right" in his brain.

On admission he had appeared unkempt and had poor hygiene. Language was stilted and obtuse. He appeared to avoid direct questions, often answering with phrases such as "you know" or "what do you expect?" On the unit he was described as having an "obstinate streak," a reputation earned in his interactions with health professionals, by his insistence on being called "doctor," and his refusal to acknowledge that he was having hallucinations.

During both earlier admissions he had been referred for vocational assessment. His license was under suspension and his psychiatrist wanted guidance from vocational testing to help him determine Dr. Smith's competence to practice. On each occasion Dr. Smith had come for one brief session, touring the department and stating that the various standardized assembly tasks and job stations had nothing to offer him. He discharged himself from occupational therapy each time.

Upon arrival Dr. Smith greeted the therapist politely and wandered around her office. Seeing her diploma, he remarked that she had graduated from the same university as he had. He then proceeded to state that his troubles at this medical center were because all the doctors there had graduated from another, "less prestigious" medical school. The establishment of the common alma mater set a tone of openness. He then agreed to sit and talk.

After some standard history had been gathered, he was asked to describe any problems he was having related to his daily routine, work, or activities he did for fun. He said that he needed help getting his brain to "work straight" (problem 1). He wanted to work again (problem 2) and thought that "having a pretty girl to talk to" would be nice (problem 3). He also cited having to tolerate the angry staff on the unit, "who forget that I am a doctor;" feeling sure they were jealous because he went to a "far superior university than they did" (problem 4), and feeling bored with nothing to do but watch others watching television (problem 5). Using the COPM, he rated the importance (from 1-10: not important at all, to extremely important) of each problem as:

Problem 1—Getting brain to "work straight"—10
Problem 2—Wanting to work again—10
Problem 3—Talking to a "pretty girl"—3
Problem 4—No respect from hospital staff—7
Problem 5—Boredom—4

He then went on to give an estimation of how he thought he was performing (1-10: not at all well, to extremely well), giving the following scores:

Problem 1—4
Problem 2—10, commenting, "Just give me a lab coat..."
Problem 3—1, commenting, "I can't find anyone in this stupid city!"
Problem 4—2, commenting, "The staff are really against me."
Problem 5—10, commenting, "Anyone can watch the tube! It doesn't take any brains to do that!"

He then was asked to rate his satisfaction with how well he could do the activity now. His response was that this whole thing was getting so formal. Couldn't he please go back to the inclient unit. The first session ended at that point.

Treating a professional colleague could have led to some assumptions on the part of the therapist. Empathy could have been based on identification with Dr. Smith's loss of control, influence over clients, and opportunity to apply his hard-learned medical knowledge. The questions elicited in the COPM made Dr. Smith's reasoning apparent and quickly made his goals appear in a direct and open manner.

In the next interview, the therapist began by recapping Dr. Smith's goals and negotiating regarding the treatment team's concern about his readiness to practice medicine. Clearly he was willing to consider this question, provided his needs related to "getting his brain to work straight again" and "wanting to work again" were dealt with. An occupational therapy assessment was agreed to, with the therapist suggesting that he could expect the following considerations—he would be addressed as "Doctor" at all times and, in that role, he could be part of understanding and choosing the components of his assessment. He also could ask for an explanation of how each test or activity might help both him and the therapist understand how his brain "was working" at the time. As he wanted to get back to work, Dr. Smith's definition and expectations related to work were explored. As he spoke, it became evident that work meant occupation or activity to him, a way of fighting boredom. It also represented a source of prestige or esteem. The therapist, picking up on this, offered him a white lab coat to wear throughout his assessment and, eventually, in the extensive work-adjustment placements that followed. The working contract was forged and cemented by these simple, respectful insights and offerings contributed by both the client and the therapist. This collaborative starting point broke through Dr. Smith's previous refusal of therapy and supported his readiness to begin on a 4-year path of slow rehabilitation.

The direct and open COPM methodology allowed the therapist quick insight into this client's own wishes, and the extent and importance of his "magical" notions. These notions were manifestations of Dr. Smith's very real and natural fears of loss of status, competence, and control. The early dialogue around goals clearly set forth the rules for client/therapist relationship and allowed Dr. Smith to choose to risk and become involved. A less open approach would have further ignited his fears and likely diminished any chance of an early meaningful connection between the two partners in rehabilitation.

With the solid footing upon which the partnership commenced, Dr. Smith progressed through assessment, which revealed marked impairment, to carefully negotiated and staged work practice or adjustment placements around the hospital. Each placement chosen allowed him to wear his lab coat and well-earned salutation. Cues from Dr. Smith related to relinquishing these provisos were taken as indicators of his readiness to consider alternative work. Work placements at a private pharmaceutical firm led to gainful employment as a drug sales representative. Four years after his initial "break," through medical intervention and occupational therapy, Dr. Smith was gainfully employed, engaged to be married, and reporting that he was satisfied that things were as good as they could be, given the challenges of his illness.

The use of the COPM set the tone of partnership that helps to engage this man even at a time when his own ability to make judgments could be deemed to be impaired. Indeed, the therapist's willingness to respect the judgments he could still make made the essential connection.

Case Example B

The foci of this case are upon the following:
- Client's own goal setting and attainment
- Therapeutic partnership
- Team-client collaboration
- Relevance to client view of life priorities.

This case describes a situation in which a client, suffering with a chronic pain syndrome, was faced with additional problems, when coping with the aftermath of a stroke. From the beginning the client and the rehabilitation team seemed to be "at odds," despite good intentions on both sides.

Mrs. Z was a 63-year-old woman who had experienced an automobile accident 10 years previously. The accident had resulted in a chronic upper back and neck problem, as well as severe and frequent headaches. She had managed well with her home and personal tasks in the intervening time period but had decided to use drug therapy to assist her in keeping her feelings of depression and failure under some measure of control. Mrs. Z had engaged actively in a pain-management program, where she was a resident in a 5-day-a-week unit participating in cognitive-behavioral modalities and psychotherapy, with a strong focus on occupational therapy as a core discipline. Overall, Mrs. Z had accomplished a relatively high level of control over her pain problems and had returned home with minimal follow-up, when 6 months later, she experienced a stroke. This seemed to be the end of it all for her; she was responding in a very depressed manner and was virtually non-verbal with both staff and fellow clients. The rehabilitation team leader requested a consultation for future involvement from the occupational therapist who had been working with Mrs. Z in the pain program. And this next phase of their therapeutic relationship began with a re-evaluation of which problems were seen as paramount.

Mrs. Z, however, upon interview, was crying constantly and expressing statements of "wishing she were dead." The occupational therapist spent some time with her, providing support, but realized that she would need to attend a team meeting to get a sense of the broader scope of the current situation. When the team expressed their understanding of the problems, it became apparent that the team members were very frustrated that this woman would not engage with them in the rehabilitation program that they felt was best suited to her immediate needs. First, they felt she needed to accomplish stair climbing to become more functional, independent, and closer to being discharged. Mrs. Z was adamantly opposed to going anywhere near a set of stairs. The occupational therapist managed to secure the agreement of the team for her to complete a COPM-based interview with Mrs. Z to identify her priorities for immediate attention.

When Mrs. Z was a client within the pain management program, she used the COPM format on two previous occasions and, therefore, was comfortable with the process.

The second interview with the occupational therapist began smoothly with Mrs. Z identifying some key issues for her, albeit through some quiet tears. She started by declaring that she wished she could get up and about more easily (problem 1), and then collapsed into much deeper sobs and sighs. She stated that the team kept pushing her to participate in exercise classes and she hated doing exercises—she had never liked it—also, she did not care at all about stairs and rough walking outside, as she knew she would never be able to do her housework as she had done before this stroke. After all her hard work, following the car accident, it was all for nothing (problem 2). Her grief and sadness became even more profound when she started talking about her work with her friends in the congregation of her church. Mrs. Z was used to being a leader among the ladies at the Ukrainian Orthodox Church in the heart of the city. She spoke proudly of her accomplishments in organizing the annual bazaar and in designing a special cross-stitch Christmas tree ornament every year as the drawing card of the craft stall. Mrs. Z was devastated and believed that she would never be able to do embroidery again or even participate in church events (problems 3 & 4).

Using the COPM, Mrs. Z rated the importance of the identified problems to her:
Problem 1—Getting "up and about"—6
Problem 2—Managing her housework—8
Problem 3—Participating as a leader at church—10
Problem 4—Doing handwork and design—10
She went on to determine, in her view, how well she thought she was doing these activities now:
Problem 1—3, commenting, "I just don't have the interest."
Problem 2—2, commenting, "I'm not home so I can't say, but I think I'd be pretty hopeless."
Problem 3—0, commenting, "Oh, dear, dear ..." and crying.
Problem 4—0, commenting, "I fear I'll never do this again."

When Mrs. Z began to rate her satisfaction with being able to perform these activities at that time, she broke down, stating that she felt totally helpless and useless, and did not know which way to turn.

Using the COPM at this stage of Mrs. Z's recovery was critical in helping the team develop an intimate understanding of the true picture of her helplessness and apparent lack of focus. Following a lengthy team discussion, the occupational therapist was comfortable in the mandate from her colleagues that she should proceed with her treatment planning, involving Mrs. Z from the beginning and using the problems identified by the client in the first COPM interview.

Mrs. Z agreed to contact her best friends at church and to set up a time for them to visit her at the rehabilitation center, with the intention of reestablishing her connections and developing a plan involve her in planning the bazaar and in craft activities. Even though she found it very difficult, if not impossible, to sew at this time, she was able to design her tree ornament for the current year and work with her friends to begin planning in earnest. During the process of enhancing her creative skills and her social interactions, Mrs. Z found that she was able to get in and out of a car with greater comfort. She could manage to climb a couple of steps to and from the church and was able to get ready to attend meetings at the church. She also was able to visit her home on weekends and help prepare the Sunday meal.

Despite starting on the rehabilitative path at a different point from that the rehabilitation team would have chosen, Mrs. Z was able to reclaim a certain degree of control over her life and was able to at least return part of the way to the degree of mastery that she had achieved over her pain and mood problems in the past. By using the COPM, the rehabilitation team opened the door for a different approach to problem definition and, therefore, a fresh look at treatment planning and outcome measurement.

IMPLICATIONS OF CLIENT-CENTERED SERVICE FOR THE REHABILITATION TEAM IN CURRENT HEALTH CARE CONTEXTS

Historically, rehabilitation teams have functioned from a context of empowerment within a larger medical model.[25,26] Rehabilitation health professionals have prided themselves on their ability to frame their therapeutic input, based on client and family needs and prioritized problems; however, despite this positive background, the essence of client-centeredness remains somewhat blurred to the majority of rehabilitation teams. This is not intended as a revolutionary declaration of inadequacy, but rather as a call to those teams to awaken to the changing needs of clients and their support systems at a time in the history of health care delivery when the consumer movement and client self-advocacy are paramount. The client-centered philosophy of occupational therapists should be seen, and accepted, as a move into a truly client-oriented model of facilitation and care. While most of the investigation and research into this approach to client/therapist partnerships has stemmed from the occupational therapy literature over the past few years,[17,24,27,28] this should by no means be seen as a profession- or discipline-specific initiative. Much of what has been found through the exploration of occupational therapy assessment and treatment planning using a client-centered model, can easily be translated into a wider rehabilitation-based application.

Since the advent of the COPM, members of other health care disciplines have been intrigued by the use of this measure, and have approached the authors to ask about the feasibility of adopting the process to suit their discipline's mission and mandate. While the COPM is, by definition, an occupational therapy tool based on the model of occupational performance, the essence of the process can be applied to reinforce the tenets and desired outcomes of other professional groups, such as social work, physical therapy, and nursing.[24]

SUMMARY

A client-centered approach to occupational therapy practice provides practitioners with the opportunity to frame their investment in client/therapist partnerships in a manner that addresses the true essence of occupational therapy as a discipline. Given the framework of occupational performance, the focus on person, environment, and occupation, and the interfaces between these elements, a client-centered practice model allows the occupational therapy clinician to refine the unique contributions that can be offered to the clients and the health care system as a whole. This comes at a time when it is becoming imperative that resources be used in the most effective way possible and that occupational therapists do not remain seduced into believing that they are able to provide everything to everyone at any point in time. The key elements of a client-centered model of practice highlight the importance of approaching the therapeutic interface from the viewpoint of what is important to the client by identifying priority needs and focusing limited resources to facilitate positive change and growth, while respecting the individual attributes of each client, taking into consideration culture, beliefs, values, and roles, recognizing the importance of evolving a therapeutic partnership at the right time in the client's mission for empowerment and actualization, and approaching this partnership with the desire to enhance mutual skills, knowledge, and expertise.

> Therapists must use their skills to select the appropriate method for the particular client and adapt it to the situation. It is not easy. It requires flexibility, interpersonal skill, active listening, empathy, and patience. It may be much more comfortable to use a standardized measure to assess a performance component, than it is to open the discussion to whatever the client may want to deal with. But, it is essential to establishing a relationship with a client and will guide the rest of the therapeutic process.[29]

Since goal setting is a truly profound piece of the whole treatment endeavor, it is critical that the client/therapist partnership begin on the right foot. The COPM provides that opportunity, and, within this context, is an important tool.

> If the client is to become committed to the therapeutic process, both client and therapist must share a view about why engaging in any particular set of treatment activities makes sense. Coming to share such a view requires the therapist and client to see how these treatment activities are going to move the client toward some future she or he can care about. Such a view is not reducible to a general prognosis or even to a shared understanding of a treatment plan. Therapist and client must come to share a story about the therapeutic process, must come to see themselves as 'in the same story.' This kind of future story, a story of what has not yet happened or has only partly happened, as in a yet-unfinished story.[10]

Many questions remain to be addressed from clinical, educational, and research points of view:

- How does the occupational therapy practitioner engender understanding and acceptance of this approach to care?
- Can occupational therapy clinicians withstand the onslaught of respected colleagues when they attempt to change their roles, which have been long established?
- How can student occupational therapists be best prepared to approach their clinical roles given this emerging mandate and paradigm?
- How can occupational therapy practitioners work together with researchers to emphasize and prove the value and positive impact of a client-centered approach to practice?

Answers to such questions will not come easily; however, it behooves the occupational therapy profession to grasp this challenge with both hands, accepting it as a positive move into creating and reinforcing strong future roles. If this challenge is accepted in this proactive manner, the groundwork for a healthy, powerful, and meaningful role will be ensured for occupational therapy in the coming health care environment.

REFERENCES

1. Rogers C. *Client-centered Therapy*. Boston, Mass: Houghton Mifflin; 1951.
2. McColl MA, Law M, Stewart D. *Theoretical Basis of Occupational Therapy: An Annotated Bibliography of Theory in Professional Literature*. Thorofare, NJ: SLACK Incorporated; 1993.
3. Law M, Baptiste S, McColl M, Opzoomer A, Polatajko H, Pollock N. The Canadian Occupational Performance Measure: An outcome measurement protocol for occupational therapy. *Canadian Journal of Occupational Therapy*. 1990;7:82-87.
4. Townsend E, Brintell S, Staisey N. Developing Guidelines for Client-Centred Occupational Therapy Practice. *Canadian Journal of Occupational Therapy*. 1990;57(2):69-76.
5. Canadian Association of Occupational Therapists. *Occupational Therapy Guidelines for Client-Centred Practice*. Toronto, ON: CAOT Publications ACE; 1991.
6. Law M, Baptiste S, Carswell A, et al. *Canadian Occupational Performance Measure*, 2nd ed. Toronto, ON: CAOT Publications; 1994.
7. Schon, DA *The Reflective Practitioner: How Professionals Think in Action*. New York, NY: Basic Books; 1983.
8. Schon, DA. *The Reflective Turn: Case Studies in and on Educational Practice*. New York, NY: Teachers' College Press; 1991.
9. Rochon, S. *Theory from practice: A reflective curriculum for occupational therapist*. Unpublished master's thesis. Hamilton, ON: McMaster University; 1994:98.
10. Mattingly C, Fleming MH. *Clinical Reasoning: Forms of Inquiry in Therapeutic Practice*. Philadelphia, Pa: FA Davis Co; 1994:245-246.
11. Yerxa, EJ. Some implications of occupational therapy's history for its epistemology, values and relation to medicine. *Am J Occup Ther*. 1992;46(1):79-83.
12. Weiner B. *Human Motivation: Metaphor, Theories and Research*. Newbury Park, Calif: Sage Publications; 1992.
13. Kelly G. *The Psychology of Personal Constructs* (volume 1). New York, NY: WW Norton & Co; 1955.
14. Kelly G. *Theory of Personality: The Psychology of Personal Constructs*. New York, NY: WW Norton & Co; 1963.
15. Schon DA. *Educating the Reflective Practitioner: Toward a New Design for Teaching and Learning in the Professions*, 1st ed. San Francisco, Calif: Jossey-Bass; 1987.

16. Sumsion T. Client-centred practice: the true impact. *Canadian Journal of Occupational Therapy.* 1993;60(1):6-8.

17. Law M, Baptiste S, Mills J. Client-centred practice: what does it mean and does it make a difference? *Canadian Journal of Occupational Therapy.* 1995;62(5):250-257.

18. Department of National Health and Welfare, and Canadian Association of Occupational Therapists. *Guidelines for the Client-Centred Practice of Occupational Therapy.* Cat. H39-33/1983E. Ottawa: Author; 1983.

19. Department of National Health and Welfare, and Canadian Association of Occupational Therapists. *Intervention Guidelines for the Client-Centred Practice of Occupational Therapy.* Cat.H39-100/1986E. Ottawa: Author; 1986:21.

20. Department of National Health and Welfare, and Canadian Association of Occupational Therapists. *Toward Outcome Measures in Occupational Therapy.* Cat. H39-114/1987E. Ottawa: Author; 1987.

21. Canadian Association of Occupational Therapy. *Enabling Occupation: A Canadian Perspective.* Toronto, ON: CAOT Publications ACE; 1997.

22. Department of National Health and Welfare, and Canadian Association of Occupational Therapists. *Toward Outcome Measures in Occupational Therapy.* Cat. H29-114/1987E. Ottawa: Department of National Health and Welfare; 1987.

23. Law M, Baptiste S, Carswell-Opzoomer A, et al. *Canadian Performance Measure Manual.* Toronto, ON: CAOT Publications; 1991:9.

24. Toomey M, Nicholson D, Carswell A. The clinical utility of the Canadian Occupational Performance Measure. *Canadian Journal of Occupational Therapy.* 1995;62(5):242-249.

25. Brown JA, Kirlin BA, Watt S. *Rehabilitation Services and the Social Work Role: Challenge for Change.* Baltimore, Md: Williams and Wilkins; 1981.

26. Baptiste S. An ecological perspective on the social work role. In Brown J, ed. *Rehabilitation and the Social Work Role: Challenge for Change.* Baltimore, Md: Williams & Wilkins; 1982.

27. Brockett M. *An Ethic of Respect for Client-Centred Partnerships.* Unpublished thesis. Toronto, ON: Ontario Institute for Studies in Education, University of Toronto; 1993.

28. Healey H, Greenberg E. *A Pilot Study of the Use of the Canadian Occupational Performance Measure.* North York, ON: Discoverability: Career Education and Assessment for Ontario Young People With Physical Disabilities; 1993.

29. Pollock N, McColl MA. Assessment in client-centred occupational therapy process. In Law M, ed. *Client-Centered Occupational Therapy.* Thorofare, NJ: SLACK Incorporated; 1998:103.

4

The Occupational Performance History Interview

Alexis D. Henry, ScD, OTR/L, FAOTA
Trudy Mallinson, MS, OTR/L, NZROT

The Occupational Performance History Interview (OPHI-II) is a semistructured interview designed to gather information about an individual's work, play, and self-care performance history.[1] The OPHI-II represents a substantive revision to the original OPHI[2-4] that was first developed over 15 years ago. This chapter presents a brief history of interviewing in occupational therapy and discusses the development of the OPHI-II, based on empirical studies over the past 15 years. In addition, the interview content, rating scales, and narrative report format of the OPHI-II are described.

THE INTERVIEW PROCESS

Interviews involve an exchange between two people, organized around the asking and answering of questions, and range from being highly structured to unstructured.[5] While many interview formats fall somewhere in between, ideal structured and unstructured research interviews are characterized by two different methodological traditions. The quantitative tradition employs structured interviews as a survey data collection method, while the qualitative or ethnographic tradition employs the unstructured interview as part of field methods. The logic of both these approaches will be discussed here briefly.

Structured interviews, typically used in survey research, strive for consistency and neutrality on the part of the interviewer, so that differences in responses can be attributed to differences among the interviewees.[6] During a structured interview, the interviewer presents the same questions in the same wording to each interviewee, uses only non-directive, often predetermined probes to elicit additional information and records responses in a standardized manner. The interviewer attempts to minimize the personal aspects of the interaction by refraining from telling personal stories or expressing personal opinions related to the content of the interview so as not to influence the interviewee's responses.[6] According to Lincoln and Guba the structured interviewer "knows what he or she does not know" and frames questions to find it out.[7]

The unstructured interview is used most often in ethnographic or qualitative field studies as part of broader participant-observation methods. In unstructured interviews, the interviewer seeks, as the interview progresses, to achieve greater understanding of the unique viewpoint of the interviewee.[7] The emerging understanding on the part of the interviewer guides further questioning; the interviewer and interviewee jointly engage in interpretation of the data. In the unstructured interview, the interviewer "does not know what he or she doesn't know," and, thus, must rely on the interviewee to help him or her come to an understanding of the questions to be asked.[7] In contrast to the structured interview, in the unstructured interview the interviewer strives for genuineness and uses the personal aspects of the interaction to develop trust with the interviewee and to encourage the interviewee to be forthcoming to achieve as complete an understanding of the interviewee's viewpoint as possible. The unstructured interview is conversational in style; it is a form of discourse that is jointly constructed by the interviewer and the interviewee.[5]

Insights from both traditions are relevant to clinical interviews. Most often, the clinical interview takes the form of a semistructured interview that attempts to maximize the strengths of both the structured interview and the unstructured interview. Semistructured clinical interviews may be organized around a theoretical model that guides the nature of the questions asked and the interpretation of the data obtained.[8] In the clinical setting, the interview is often one of the first interactions between a therapist and a patient. The goals of the initial clinical interview include 1) determining the nature of the problem, 2) developing and maintaining a therapeutic relationship, and 3) communicating information and beginning the implementation of intervention.[9] A degree of structure is useful in clinical interviewing, eg, using specific, detailed questions, allowing the interviewer to gather specific information that will lead to a clearer formulation of the problem. On the other hand, a more open-ended, unstructured approach allows patients to fully tell their stories and aids the clinician in coming to an understanding of patients' unique perspectives on their situations and problems.

THE OCCUPATIONAL THERAPY INTERVIEW

Smith suggested that an occupational therapy interview is most often done as part of the initial evaluation of a patient.[10] It serves to collect information about the patient pursuant to treatment planning, to inform the patient about the purpose of occupational therapy, and to give the patient an opportunity to discuss his or her situation and goals for treatment. She pointed out the importance of therapists having a theoretical knowledge base from which to develop questions and interpret the data from the interview. Pedretti proposed an initial interview aimed at seeking information about family and friends, community and work roles, education history, leisure and social interests, the living situation to which the person will return, and how the person spends and manages time.[11] Trombly suggests that in addition to providing information about the patient's former and future roles, interests and goals, an interview can provide insight into the patient's cognitive abilities such as memory, sequencing, and orientation.[12] Other authors have emphasized the importance of taking a patient-centered approach to assessment and have advocated using an interview to evaluate occupational performance, satisfaction with occupational performance, and to identify priorities for intervention, all from the patient's perspective.[13,14]

LIFE HISTORY INTERVIEWING IN OCCUPATIONAL THERAPY

Although clinical interviews may take many forms, the interviews that have been developed in occupational therapy are generally historical in nature, focusing on how an individual's involvement in occupations, such as work, play, and daily living tasks, has changed over time.

As a natural outgrowth of the occupational behavior tradition, Reilly first proposed the importance of life history interviewing in occupational therapy practice in the early 1960s.[15] Moorhead, a student of Reilly, developed *The Occupational History*, generally acknowledged to be the first serious attempt at developing an interview that reflected occupational therapists' concerns.[16] The Occupational History, a lengthy, semistructured interview, based in the occupational behavior perspective, was designed to gather qualitative information about the individual's functioning in occupational roles. Although Moorhead's interview yielded extensive information, the procedure lacked any systematic method for analyzing and organizing the data that was obtained. More recent interviews represent a range of adaptations to and departures from the format first presented by Moorhead. These procedures include the Occupational Role History,[17] the Occupational Role History Interview,[18] the Occupational Case Analysis Interview and Rating Scale (OCAIRS),[19] the Assessment of Occupational Functioning (AOF),[20] the Role Activity Performance Scale (RAPS),[21] the Worker Role Interview (WRI),[22] the Work Environment Impact Scale (WEIS),[23] the Canadian Occupational Performance Measure (COPM),[14] and the Occupational Performance History Interview (OPHI).[3] While each interview has its own unique set of characteristics, all provide strategies for gathering information about the patient's occupational functioning. The remainder of this chapter will discuss the development of the Occupational Performance History Interview and the research that has been conducted with it thus far.

THE OCCUPATIONAL PERFORMANCE HISTORY INTERVIEW

Occupational therapy has recognized the need for the development of standardized instruments.[24] Well-developed data gathering procedures provide the basis for assessment and treatment of patients, and allow for the implementation of sound research studies to investigate the effectiveness of interventions. Consequently, the American Occupational Therapy Association (AOTA) determined to fund projects that would lead to standardized instruments for use by occupational therapists. With funding provided by the AOTA and the American Occupational Therapy Foundation (AOTF), the original version of the OPHI was designed to gather relevant historical information on occupational performance, to be used with a wide variety of patients, and be compatible with a variety of conceptual practice models.[3] Thus, the content of the OPHI needed to be broad enough to reflect the concerns of therapists working from different theoretical perspectives and with patients of varying ages and with varying disabilities or disorders.

Unlike some occupational therapy interviews, eg, AOF or OCAIRS, which have tended to be designed for specific populations, the original OPHI was intended for use with adolescent, adult, and geriatric patients with both physical and psychiatric diagnoses. Although the content of the OPHI is consistent with the occupational behavior perspective, the original OPHI was specifically designed to be compatible with more than a single conceptual practice model.[2] The interview consisted of a set of recommended questions, an accompanying rating scale, and a method for reporting narrative data gathered during the interview.

DEVELOPMENT OF THE OPHI AND OPHI-II

The psychometric properties of original OPHI have been extensively studied since it was developed more than 15 years ago.[2-4] This section will present a review of research on the OPHI and describe how the empirical evidence from these studies provided the foundations for the OPHI-II revisions. The original OPHI was designed to provide both quantitative and qualitative information about patients.[3] Like the OPHI-II, it included a semistructured interview, rating scale, and life history narrative.

The original OPHI scale consisted of two items in each of five areas: 1) organization of daily living routines; 2) life roles; 3) interests, values, and goals; 4) perception of abilities and assumption of responsibility; and 5) environmental influences. Following the interview, each of the items was scored, using a 5-point rating scale (ranging from 1-maladaptive to 5-adaptive) for both the patient's past and present occupational adaptation, resulting in 20 ratings. Environment items were rated on a separate 5-point rating scale.[3]

In the original OPHI, past and present were defined by a demarcation point, ie, a point at which the patient's occupational functioning changed, that the therapist and patient together identified at the beginning of the interview. The items were scored to represent functioning before and after the demarcation point to identify any changes between past and present occupational functioning that might follow such events as a traumatic life incident or onset of impairment.

RELIABILITY STUDIES

The OPHI scale was originally studied with a sample of 154 occupational therapy patients from psychiatric, physical disability, and gerontology practices in the United States and Canada.[2] The study asked whether pairs of therapists who listened to an audiotape of the interview would demonstrate interrater reliability and whether the scores would be stable across two different therapists who administered the interview to the same patient (test-retest reliability). Results of this investigation showed minimally acceptable test-retest and interrater reliability.[2] The original AOTA/AOTF requirement that the OPHI be compatible with multiple theories obligated the investigators to avoid basing the OPHI on a specific occupational therapy theory. However, the investigators in this first study found that pairs of therapists who shared the same conceptual practice model were more likely to agree on patient ratings than pairs of therapists who used different practice models. This finding suggested that designing an interview to be used with multiple theories was not compatible with achieving maximum reliability.

Consequently, a second study, also funded by AOTA/AOTF, sought to improve reliability by developing clearer guidelines for rating the items, following two theoretical approaches, an eclectic approach and the model of human occupation.[4] The original rating scale was retained, but the investigators developed guidelines for conducting the interview to arrive at the ratings from each theoretical approach. This second reliability study failed to demonstrate substantially improved psycho-metric properties.

The investigators for the second study[4] noted that better reliability had been achieved with two other interviews, the Occupational Case Analysis Interview and Rating Scale (OCAIRS)[19] and the Assessment of Occupational Functioning (AOF).[20] Since these rating scales contained items explicitly connected to concepts from the model of human occupation, it seemed reasonable to expect that the reliability of the OPHI could be improved if the items better corresponded with theoretical concepts. Consequently, the OPHI scale was revised (OPHI-R) to include 21 items specifically related to concepts from the model of human occupation. This study also failed to find acceptable reliability for the new scale.[25] Moreover, low item-to-total correla-tions in this study suggested that individual items were not working well with the total scale.

Development of the OPHI had followed a traditional psychometric approach by first assessing stability of the scale across time (test-retest reliability) and raters (interrater reliability). This approach followed the conventional wisdom that a scale could not have validity if it lacked reliability. More contemporary perspectives in measurement theory argue that development of a scale must begin with establish-ing the construct validity of the scale, ie, assessing how well items, collectively and individually, capture the construct that the scale seeks to measure.[26,27] One study, reporting on the construct validity of the OPHI, found significant correlations between OPHI scores and measures of depression and pain in patients following traumatic spinal cord injury.[28] However, psychometricians have criticized the approach of correlating an instrument with other constructs prior to establishing the internal validity of an instrument because there is no evidence that the instrument in fact captures the relevant, observable elements of the domain of interest.[26]

In a recent study, new methods of analysis were applied to examine the con-struct validity of the OPHI-R.[29] Rasch analysis has become increasingly popular in health services research in recent years. This method is based on the common-sense expectation that when the items of an assessment operate as a true measure, ie, like a ruler, some items will be harder for patients to do well on, and some patients will do better on more items. Of course, to compare patients on an assessment or between admission and discharge, we expect those items that are more difficult to always be more difficult, and those items that are easier for patients to always be easier. We also expect patients with better occupational adaptation to do better on the more difficult items than less-able patients. This set of expectations is referred to as the Rasch Measurement Model. Rasch analysis involves a comparison between these expectations (the measurement model) and the data actually obtained. If unex-pected patterns occur, eg, very adaptive patients do poorly on an easy item, we say that the item misfits the measurement model. In practical terms, this means that the item is not measuring the same thing as other items in the scale, since patients are responding differently on this item than on other items in the scale. In short, not all the scale items are working together to form a single construct.

Using Rasch analysis, Mallinson, Mahaffey and Kielhofner found that the 21 items of the OPHI-R did not measure a single trait (construct) of adaptation, but rather captured three separate factors.[29] One factor was related to how people saw themselves and saw opportunities for participating in occupations. A second factor was related to what persons believed they actually did. The third factor was related to supports and constraints in the environment. It is likely that Gutkowski found low item-to-total correlations, in part, because the items captured three separate constructs rather than a single construct of occupational adaptation.[25] This discovery pointed toward the need to develop three separate scales for each of these three constructs, rather than a single overarching scale of occupational adaptation.

VALIDITY STUDIES

While the previous studies all were helpful in developing the OPHI-II, other research supported the idea that the OPHI was a worthwhile assessment. Lynch and Bridle found that OPHI scores correlated with a measure of activity involvement among people with spinal cord injury (SCI), and that subjects showed decreased OPHI scores for the present, ie, post-SCI, in comparison with past scores.[28] Similarly, Mauras-Nelson and Oakley found lowered present OPHI scores among subjects undergoing bone marrow transplant, when the demarcation between past and present was set at the time the subject was first diagnosed with cancer.[30] Fossey examined therapists' perspectives on the use of the OPHI with people who had psychiatric disabilities.[31] Therapists in this study reported that the flexibility in the OPHI allowed the interview to be tailored to the individual needs of the patient and provided qualitative information that was important for problem identification. In a short-term follow-up study of adolescents and young adults hospitalized for a first episode of psychosis, Henry found present OPHI scores to be a significant predictor of community functioning 6 months after discharge from the hospital.[32]

NARRATIVE ANALYSIS OF DATA FROM THE OPHI

An important feature of the OPHI is its focus on eliciting a patient's life history narrative. That is to say, the OPHI encourages a patient to relate the events of his life and the motivations for and reasons why events unfolded as they did. As noted previously, the original OPHI included the idea that a qualitative narrative of the patient's life was important since the rating scale could not capture all the relevant information from a life history. Mattingly and Fleming have suggested that when therapists think about the meaning of disability in a patient's life and the role of therapy in treating that disability, they reason from a narrative perspective.[33] Narrative reasoning involves considering the specifics of the patient's life story, rather than just the generalities of symptoms or diagnosis. When taking a narrative perspective, a therapist attempts to understand how the patient's present circumstances fit into the larger life story that the patient is living. Thus, the therapist considers how the patient views his or her life circumstances, why the patient behaves in the way he or she does, whether the patient's current situation is congruent with his or her life view, etc. "Narratives make sense of reality by linking the outward world of actions and events to the inner world of human intention and motivation."[34]

This recognition of the importance of the life story to a patient's self-understanding, behavior and therapy experience led to a closer examination of the life history narratives elicited by the OPHI. Kielhofner and Mallinson examined the narrative features of OPHI-generated life histories by analyzing 20 videotaped interviews of inpatients with psychiatric disorders originally made for the second reliability study of the OPHI.[35] They found that the interviews often failed to elicit narrative accounts from respondents and that the structure of the OPHI interview was more conducive to obtaining descriptive lists or characterizations than narrative data. Kielhofner and Mallinson identified those interviewing strategies that were more successful in eliciting stories and suggested ways to incorporate these strategies to make interview situations more conducive to obtaining narrative accounts.[35]

Using the same set of interviews, Mallinson, Kielhofner, and Mattingly found that patients connected the events of their lives into a coherent story to which they ascribed meaning by using metaphorical images.[36] They argue that metaphors, eg, when a person describes his or her illness as "imprisoning" him or her, represent a "working version" of how the patient views his or her life story, and that "the OPHI implicitly, if not explicitly, is an interview which is about what is wrong and needs fixing in a person's life."[36] Metaphors give the patient a way of naming the problem and provide suggestions to the therapist for ways to intervene. Understanding metaphors gives therapists a way of building the collaborative relationship. Mallinson, et al argue that, for interventions to be effective, they should resonate with or "match" the patient's perspective.[36]

SUMMARY OF PAST RESEARCH ON THE OPHI

To date, the studies that have been conducted with the OPHI point to both the strengths and limitations of the interview. The reliability studies indicated that, while the total scores of the original OPHI (particularly past scores) demonstrated acceptable stability, some subscale scores were less stable than desirable. In addition, past and present ratings did not form separate constructs, but rather items cohered around the constructs of identity and competence. Clinically, it had been reported that dividing a patient's life into two distinct periods had proven problematic.[31] Consequently, the OPHI-II no longer employs a demarcation point nor separate past and present ratings. The interview continues to focus on capturing the whole life history, noting important changes and transitions, rather than a single demarcation, and discerning where the patient's life seems headed.

FORMAT OF THE OPHI-II INTERVIEW

The OPHI-II consists of three parts: the semistructured interview, rating scales, and life history narrative.[1] The first part of the OPHI-II is the semistructured interview, which is organized around five thematic areas: 1) Activity/Occupational Choices, 2) Critical Life Events, 3) Daily Routine, 4) Occupational Roles, and 5) Occupational Behavior Settings.

The thematic areas of the OPHI-II have been developed to more accurately reflect theoretical constructs within the model of human occupation[37] and are designed to elicit information more directly related to the content of the rating scale items. Interview questions, with alternatives, are provided within each of the thematic areas. Therapists can conduct the interview by covering these thematic areas in any sequence, or move back and forth between thematic areas. Because of the flexible nature of the interview, it is more easily adaptable to both the style and experience of the clinician.

The second part of the OPHI-II is composed of the three rating scales. They are: 1) the Occupational Identity Scale, 2) the Occupational Competence Scale, and 3) the Occupational Behavior Settings Scale. The three scales provide a means of converting the information gathered in the interview into three measures. *Occupational Identity* measures the degree to which a person has internalized a positive occupational identity, eg, having values, interests, confidence, seeing oneself in various occupational roles, and having an image of the kind of life one wants. *Occupational Competence* measures the degree to which a person is able to sustain a pattern of occupational behavior that is productive and satisfying. *Occupational Behavior Settings* measure the impact of the environment on the patient's occupational life.

The final part of the OPHI-II is the Life History Form. Completing this form involves constructing a time line as a brief graphical representation of the patient's life and writing a brief narrative of the person's life history.

ADMINISTRATION OF THE OPHI-II

Determining Whether the OPHI-II Is Appropriate

The first stage of administering any evaluation is to determine whether a particular evaluation is appropriate to use. In determining the appropriateness of the OPHI-II for a particular patient, consideration should be given to the ability of the patient to participate meaningfully in the interview process and the use of the instrument within the demands of a particular treatment setting. The OPHI-II is designed for use with an occupational therapy patient who is capable of responding meaningfully to a life history interview. Factors that are important to consider when deciding if a particular patient is appropriate for the interview include age, emotional and psychological state, and cognitive/linguistic ability.

The OPHI-II is a valuable tool for establishing the therapeutic relationship; providing detailed, intimate information regarding a person's past life and future goals; and setting a framework for therapeutic intervention. Given the amount of time required to administer and score the OPHI-II (45-60 minutes) and given the detailed information elicited through the interview, the OPHI-II is most appropriate in settings in which the therapist expects to have an ongoing relationship with the patient. A briefer version of the OPHI-II (approximately 20-30 minutes) is currently under development. It is anticipated that this more brief version will be more appropriate for use in those settings in which therapists have only a short time with the patient, such as in acute care, but which require the contextual and environmental information that the OPHI-II elicits to assist them in making, for example, placement or discharge decisions.

Conducting the Interview

The interview involves conducting a conversation or a series of conversations with the patient to learn about his occupational life history. Before doing the interview, the therapist should gather any relevant information about the patient that will enhance the interview. In some cases, the therapist may wish to administer other assessments before doing the interview. These may include performance assessments or they may include paper and pencil assessments, such as the Role Checklist,[38] Interest Checklist,[39] the Occupational Self Assessment,[40] or other self-reports that provide preliminary information about the patient. As narratives are specific, rather than general, such data gathering before the interview helps the therapist tailor the interview to the patient's circumstances. For example, after asking a patient to complete the Role Checklist,[38] a therapist may begin the OPHI-II interview by asking the patient about his or her notation that he or she no longer considers himself or herself a worker and how that perception has changed in the last year.

Using the Rating Scale

As noted previously, there are three scales that correspond to the content of the interview. The three scales are a) the Occupational Identity Scale, composed of 11 items; b) Occupational Competence, composed of nine items; and c) Occupational Behavior Settings, also composed of nine items. The OPHI-II uses a 4-point rating scale to reflect a patient's level of adaptation for a given item. Assigning a rating requires the therapist to use the information gathered in the interview to make a judgment about the item that is being rated. This judgment requires that the therapist clearly understand the item being rated, the scoring system, and the information gathered in the interview. Ratings of 4 and 3 reflect two levels of satisfactory occupational functioning. Ratings of 2 and 1 reflect two levels of unsatisfactory occupational functioning. The 4-point rating system is as follows: 4, exceptionally competent occupational functioning; 3, good, appropriate, satisfactory occupational functioning; 2, some occupational dysfunction; and 1, extremely occupationally dysfunctional.

Although the meanings of ratings 1, 2, 3, and 4 are constant across all items, the actual definitions of satisfactory or unsatisfactory occupational functioning vary from item to item. Consequently, criteria that the therapist should consider in assigning ratings are written next to each item on the rating form. Typically in occupational therapy assessments, these criteria are provided in the manual, not on the rating form. This results in therapists' having to frequently return to the manual to refer to the meanings of ratings for individual items.

The OPHI-II requires that a therapist make judgments about what constitutes adaptive occupational functioning within the culture and other relevant contexts to which the individual belongs. Rating accuracy is enhanced when the therapist and the patient share an appreciation of health and well-being maintenance or enhancement in the person's culture, the meaning of illness and disability in his or her culture, and the satisfying of reasonable expectations or norms of his or her occupational behavior settings.

Writing the Narrative Report

Completing the life history narrative involves developing a time line of the life history, as told by the patient; validation of the life history with the patient; completing written documentation of the life history narrative; and establishing a framework for undertaking the therapeutic process. These tasks are not necessarily completed in sequence, and the therapist may work back and forth between them. The time line graphically presents the occupational choices and events that the patient considers to be most significant in shaping his or her life story and whether those events had a positive or negative impact on the direction in which his or her life was heading. The direction of the line between events is the narrative slope. The narrative slope indicates where a person's life has been and where it is headed. The therapist can have the patient construct a time line prior to beginning the interview, then use it to facilitate the telling of the life story. Alternatively, the therapist or patient may create the time line after the interview is completed. In either case, the events are placed horizontally on the time line in chronological sequence and displaced vertically—up to represent events that had a positive impact on the patient's life, down to represent negative-impact events.

The narrative is intended to briefly summarize the meaning and implications of the story, and should include any descriptive phrases, metaphors, or other characterizations of the impact that an event had on the patient's life.

RESEARCH ON THE OPHI-II

Findings from a recent international study suggest that the reliability and construct validity of each of the three rating scales of the OPHI-II are much improved over its predecessors.[40] Sixty-four occupational therapists from four countries (Australia, Belgium, Finland, and United States) participated in the study. Data was collected on 44 physically or psychiatrically disabled patients from four countries. To ensure that the OPHI-II evaluated people effectively across a broad range of occupational functioning, 38 people with no medical diagnosis also were assessed. In addition, all the therapists viewed and rated a common videotaped interview to ensure that they were using the three scales consistently. The three rating scales were analyzed, using Rasch analysis. The construct validity of each of the scales was supported, since all items fit for each scale. Reliability for each scale was high (.90 - .96). Additionally, rater consistency was high, despite the interviews having been conducted and rated in three different languages.[41] The OPHI-II is currently distributed by the AOTA and has been translated into eight languages, including Chinese, Finnish, Flemish-Dutch, Dutch, Japanese, Portuguese, Spanish, and Swedish.

SUMMARY

Interviews are a rich source of information and a valuable tool in the occupational therapy evaluation process. Interviews not only provide data regarding a patient's occupational functioning over time, but also insight into the patient's perspective, or life story, and an opportunity to develop rapport and a collaborative relationship with the patient. These functions of interviews have important implications for intervention.

Data that describe how patients are functioning now and how they have functioned in the past allow clinicians to make predictions about how the patients will function in the future. Among patients with psychiatric disorders, past functioning has been shown to be a consistent predictor of future functioning.[42] Knowing which factors are most likely to place an individual at risk for dysfunction in the future allows clinicians to better target interventions to those factors. Moreover, having insight into the patient's perspective allows clinicians to design more personally relevant and meaningful interventions. A collaborative relationship, one in which the patient is an active partner in the treatment planning process, can facilitate the attainment of those treatment goals.[43,44]

REFERENCES

1. Kielhofner G, Mallinson T, Crawford C, et al. *A User's Manual for the Occupational Performance History Interview*, Version 2. Chicago, Ill: Model of Human Occupation Clearinghouse, University of Illinois at Chicago; 1998.

2. Kielhofner G, Henry AD. Development and investigation of the occupational performance history interview. *Am J Occup Ther*. 1988;42:489-498.

3. Kielhofner G, Henry AD, Walens D. *A User's Guide to the Occupational Performance History Interview*. Rockville, Md: American Occupational Therapy Association; 1989.

4. Kielhofner G, Henry AD, Walens D, Rogers ES. A generalizability study of the occupational performance history interview. *Occupational Therapy Journal of Research*. 1991;11:292-306.

5. Mishler EG. *Research Interviewing: Context and Narrative*. Cambridge, Mass: Harvard University Press; 1986.

6. Fowler FJ. *Survey Research Methods*. Beverly Hills, Calif: Sage Publications; 1984.

7. Lincoln YS, Guba EG. *Naturalistic Inquiry*. Newbury Park, Calif: Sage Publications; 1985:269.

8. Kielhofner G, Mallinson T. Gathering and reasoning with data during intervention. In Kielhofner G. *A Model of Human Occupation. Theory and Application*, 2nd ed. Baltimore, Md: Williams & Wilkins; 1995:189-203.

9. Lazare A, Bird J, Lipkin M, Putnam S. Three functions of the medical interview: An integrative conceptual framework. In Lipkin M, Putnam S, Lazare A, eds. *The Medical Interview*. New York, NY: Springer; 1989:103.

10. Smith HD. Assessment and evaluation: an overview. In Hopkins HL, Smith HD. *Willard and Spackman's Occupational Therapy*, 8th ed. Philadelphia, Pa: JB Lippincott Co; 1993:169-191.

11. Pedretti LW. *Occupational Therapy: Practice Skills for Physical Dysfunction*, 4th ed. St. Louis, Mo: CV Mosby; 1996.

12. Trombly CA. *Occupational Therapy for Physical Dysfunction*, 4th ed. Baltimore, Md: Williams &Wilkins; 1995.

13. Pollock N. Client-centered assessment. *Am J Occup Ther*. 1993;47:298-301.

14. Law M, Baptiste S, Carswell A, McColl MA, Polatajko H, Pollock N. *Canadian Occupational Performance Measure*, 2nd ed. Toronto, ON: Canadian Association of Occupational Therapists; 1994.

15. Reilly, M. Occupational therapy can be one of the great ideas of 20th century medicine. *Am J Occup Ther*. 1962; 16:1-9.

16. Moorhead LC. The occupational history. *Am J Occup Ther*. 1969; 23:329-334.

17. Florey LL, Michelman SM. Occupational role history: A screening tool for psychiatric occupational therapy. *Am J Occup Ther*. 1982;36:301-308.

18. Kielhofner G, Harlan B, Bauer D, Mauer P. The reliability of a historical interview with physically disabled respondents. *Am J Occup Ther*. 1986;40:551-556.

19. Kaplan K, Kielhofner G. *Occupational Case Analysis Interview and Rating Scale*. Thorofare, NJ: SLACK Incorporated; 1989.

20. Watts JH, Brollier C, Bauer D, Schmidt W. The assessment of occupational functioning: The second revision. *OTMH*. 1989;8:4:7-27.

21. Good-Ellis MA, Fine SB, Spencer JH, DiVittis A. Developing a role activity performance scale. *Am J Occup Ther*. 1987;41:232-241.

22. Velozo C, Kielhofner G, Fisher G. *A User's Guide to the Worker Role Interview*, research version. Chicago, Ill: Department of Occupational Therapy, University of Illinois at Chicago;1990.

23. Moore-Corner R, Kielhofner G, Olson L. *The Work Environment Impact Scale*. Chicago, Ill: Model of Human Occupation Clearinghouse, University of Illinois at Chicago; 1998.

24. Bonder B. Issues in assessment of psychosocial components of function. *Am J Occup Ther*. 1993; 47:211-216.

25. Gutkowski M. *A Generalizability Study of the Revised Occupational Performance History Interview*. Chicago, Ill: University of Illinois at Chicago. Unpublished master's thesis; 1992.

26. Nunnelly J, Bernstein I. *Psychometric Theory*. New York, NY: McGraw-Hill; 1995.

27. Wright B, Stone M. *Best Test Design*. Chicago, Ill: MESA Press; 1979.

28. Lynch KB, Bridle MJ. Construct validity of the occupational performance history interview. *Occupational Therapy Journal of Research*. 1993;13:231-240.

29. Mallinson T, Mahaffey M, Kielhofner G. The Occupational Performance History Interview: Evidence for three underlying constructs of occupational adaptation. *Canadian Journal of Occupational Therapy*. 1998,65:219-228.

30. Mauras-Nelson E, Oakley F. *Bone marrow transplantation: Implications on function*. Poster presentation at the AOTA annual conference. Chicago, Ill; April 1996.

31. Fossey E. Using the occupational performance history interview (OPHI): therapists' reflections. *British Journal of Occupational Therapy*. 1996;59:223-228.

32. Henry AD. *Predicting psychosocial functioning and symptomatic recovery of adolescents and young adults with a first psychotic episode: A six-month follow-up study*. Unpublished doctoral dissertation. Boston University;1994.

33. Mattingly C, Fleming MH. *Clinical Reasoning. Forms of Inquiry in a Therapeutic Practice*. Philadelphia, Pa: FA Davis Co; 1994.

34. Mattingly C. The narrative nature of clinical reasoning. *Am J Occup Ther*. 1991;45:998-1005.

35. Kielhofner G, Mallinson T. Gathering narrative data through interviews: Empirical observations and suggested guidelines. *Scandinavian Journal of Occupational Therapy*. 1995;2:63-68.

36. Mallinson T, Kielhofner G, Mattingly C. Metaphor and meaning in a clinical interview. *Am J Occup Ther*. 1996;50:338-346.

37. Kielhofner G. *A Model of Human Occupation Theory and Application*. Baltimore, Md: Williams & Wilkins; 1995.

38. Barris R, Oakley F, Kielhofner G. The Role Checklist. In Hemphill B. *Mental Health Assessment in Occupational Therapy*. Thorofare, NJ: SLACK Incorporated; 1988.

39. Rogers J. The NPI Interest Checklist. In Hemphill B. *Mental Health Assessment in Occupational Therapy*. Thorofare, NJ: SLACK Incorporated; 1988.

40. Baron K, Kielhofner G, Goldhammer V, Wokenski J. *A User's Manual for the Occupational Self Assessment*. Chicago, Ill: Model of Human Occupation Clearinghouse, University of Illinois at Chicago; 1999. (Distributed by American Occupational Therapy Association.)

41. Kielhofner G, Mallinson T, Lai J-S. Reliability and validity of the Occupational Performance History II (OPHI-II): An International Study. Manuscript in preparation. University of Illinois at Chicago.

42. Henry AD, Coster WJ. Predictors of functional outcome among adolescents and young adults with psychotic disorders. *Am J Occup Ther*. 1996;50:171-181.

43. Neistadt ME. An occupational therapy program for adults with developmental disabilities. *Am J Occup Ther*. 1987;41:433-438.

44. Neistadt ME. Methods of assessing clients' priorities: A survey of adult physical dysfunction settings. *Am J Occup Ther*. 1995;49:428-436.

5

Role Change Assessment: An Interview Tool for Older Adults

Joan C. Rogers, PhD, OTR/L, FAOTA
Margo B. Holm, PhD, OTR/L, FAOTA, ABDA

The Role Change Assessment by Jackoway, Rogers, and Snow[1] was developed to describe the perceived role participation of older adults. It included an examination of past and current role participation, changes in role participation, and the value or importance of roles. The Role Change Assessment was recently revised by Rogers and Holm[2] to simplify the role items and definitions, structure the measurement of role change, and improve the format for use by clinicians and researchers.

This chapter begins with an overview of the significance of the concept of role to occupational therapy and specifically to practice with older adults. A description of the instrument and its development, including the revision, follows. Clinical and research applications of the instrument are then detailed.

THEORETICAL BASE

Role participation is of particular interest in older adults because late life is generally characterized by multiple role changes. In fact, social gerontologists[3-4] view aging as a succession of changes in the number and content of social roles. These changes vary in the extent to which they are scheduled, voluntary, and have positive or negative connotations. For example, for most older workers retirement is voluntary and having the freedom to do the things they have not had the time to do previously is viewed as pleasurable.[5] For some older workers, however, retirement is precipitated by illness rather than personal choice. Further, having or not having the financial resources to realize retirement goals is a critical determination of satisfaction in late life.[6] Similarly, relocation from Northern Michigan to a retirement community in Southern Arizona reflects a planned choice to adopt a different lifestyle. However, relocation to a nursing home to accommodate increased disability is likely to be perceived as a less desirable move. The stress of widowhood is due in part to its unscheduled nature, although the extent of stress itself is moderated by the overall quality of the spousal relationship, the abruptness of the spouse's death, and the degree to which social relationships are disrupted.

Retirement, relocation, institutionalization, and widowhood are examples of late life-role transitions. Common to these role changes, whether they are scheduled or unscheduled, voluntary or involuntary, perceived as positive or negative, is the adaptation required to adjust to change. Change disrupts the present dynamic, and adaptive processes are needed to restore equilibrium. Resources in terms of time, energy, or space need to be re-evaluated and reallocated.

While role change is characteristic of late life, this change is more often of role loss and decrease than gain and increase.[7] This is especially the case when frailty develops due to the accumulation of disease-associated and age-related impairments, and task performance becomes difficult or impossible. Of particular concern is the loss of the most valued roles, for example, those of worker, spouse, and home maintainer. In part, self-identify is formed while participating in social roles. Role participation reaffirms that one can fulfill the expectations inherent to holding a particular status. To the extent that self-identity is attached to a role that is lost, role loss will threaten a person's sense of identity and self-sameness. Thus, role loss has the potential for exerting wide-ranging effects on well being. Role loss implies the loss of rewards associated with a position, including social status and social contacts as well as any financial considerations. In addition, intrinsic loss of activity may lead to changes in life satisfaction.

Role in Occupational Therapy With Older Adults
The domain of occupational therapy encompasses function and dysfunction in three hierarchically organized areas of behavior—the components of occupational performance, occupational performance, and occupational role performance. Occupational performance refers to the performance of tasks in three fundamental activity areas, namely, self-care, work and productivity, and play or leisure. The components of occupational performance are the physical, cognitive, and affective substrates of behavior that underlie skilled task performance. For example, to write a letter, a person must have, among other things, the motoric ability to hold and move a pen, the cognitive abilities to compose a text, and the motivation to initiate and complete the letter. Impairments in these abilities will likely result in occupational performance dysfunction or disability. While the components of occupational performance reflect a breakdown of tasks into their basic abilities, occupational role performance represents the organization of multiple tasks according to function. For example, to be a caregiver, a person must be able to do the myriad tasks involved in performing personal self-care and home management tasks for the care recipient.

Tasks are pivotal in occupational therapy practice, with their segmentation the focus of the components of occupational performance and their aggregation the focus of occupational role performance. Because tasks are organized functionally into roles, the assessment of role performance provides critical information about clients' task priorities. If the homemaker role is essential to a person's self-worth, and critical tasks, such as cooking and food shopping, are threatened by depression, dementia, or other pathologies, these tasks must be addressed in occupational therapy.

Development, Description, and Revision of the Role Change Assessment
The Role Change Assessment (RCA) is a semistructured interview tool designed specifically to assess the role function of older adults. Several principles were used to guide the development of the RCA. These principles were:
1. The instrument was to include a comprehensive list of older adult roles. This was to be achieved in part by defining roles in terms of several functionally related or functionally similar activities, rather than a single activity. Thus, sports-participant was listed as a role in preference to hunter or golfer.

2. Inquiry was to focus on perceived stability and change in role participation. Role change included the addition and loss of roles, as well as increases or decreases in the time or intensity of participation. The birth of the first grandchild is an example of the addition of a role, while the death of a spouse reflects a role loss. Moving from full-time to part-time employment represents a decrease in worker-role participation, while doubling the time of one's volunteer commitment represents an increase in the volunteer role.

3. Questioning about role participation was to be structured. However, the interviewer was to have the freedom to clarify the respondent's answers and to pose additional, exploratory questions, as suggested by the respondent's answers, to facilitate a better understanding of role change.

4. Administration time was to take less than 1 hour.

Reliability

Reliability refers to the stability of measurement. Test-retest reliability is the degree to which the same results will be obtained if the same test is re-administered to the same subject under the same conditions. To appraise the stability of the RCA[1] over time, test-retest reliability with a 3- to 4-week retest interval, was calculated on five subjects. Results from the test and retest administrations were compared by computing percent agreement scores. Percent agreement was defined as the percentage of scores in the "Present," "Past," and "Change" columns that were identical in both administrations, divided by the number of items in those columns in which there was an answer on either administration of the tool. Average percent agreement for roles held in the present and 1 year ago was 95%, while for perceived change in level of role participation it was only 66%. Thus, there was greater stability in regard to perceptions of static parameters of role participation than to change in role participation.

Test-retest reliability of the RCA (version 2.0)[2] is based on a convenience sample of 11 retirees, five males and six females, with a mean age of 67 years. Subjects were retested 1 day after testing, and "Past" was designated as 1 year ago. Percent agreement for Past, Present, Value (Time), and Value (Meaning) ranged from 84% to 97% (Table 5-1), with an average of 91%. Subjects were most stable in their responses to Value (Time) (mean = 93%), followed by Value (Meaning) (mean = 91%), Present (mean = 89%), and Past (mean = 90%).

Therefore, the sample was more consistent when responding to items that had a value connotation than with items that pertained to level of participation in a role, ie, Present, Past. The Change Value item, for which subjects were asked to identify whether changes from Past to Present are Positive, Neutral, or Negative yielded an overall percent agreement of 86%. Percent agreement for changes considered Positive was 97%; followed by Neutral, 95%; and Negative, 65%. Subjects had no difficulty with consistent responses if they initially deemed a change to be positive or neutral, but if they deemed a change to be negative, responses at retest were consistent with initial testing only 65% of the time, with retest being 35% more positive. Except for the Negative Change item, the test-retest stability of the 2.0 version of the RCA is substantial.

Table 5-1
Test-Retest Reliability of the Role Change Assessment (Version 2.0)*

Role Categories	Past	Present	Value Time	Value Meaning
Relationships	84	88	95	95
Self-care/ Home Maintenance	87	91	90	90
Productivity	94	88	94	91
Leisure	86	87	94	86
Organizational	90	88	92	91
Health/Wellness	97	97	94	94

*Percent agreement

Content Validity

Content validity refers to the extent to which the items on a test adequately sample the desired behavioral domain. In reference to the RCA, the behavioral domains of concern were role categories and roles. A review of the literature on late life roles and of role instruments led to the identification of six role categories and a master list of specific roles.[7-16] The master list of roles was condensed by consolidating role descriptions that were functionally-related or functionally similar into one broader role. Specific roles were then assigned to one of the six role categories. The role categories, along with the specific roles assigned to them, were submitted to four experts in geriatrics (a physician, a nurse, and two occupational therapists) for logical analysis. They were instructed to critique the comprehensiveness of the role categories, the assignment of roles to the categories, the role definitions, and the sequencing of role categories and roles within each category. During pilot testing of the RCA, subjects were asked to identify roles they currently held that they felt were not adequately covered on the instrument. In response to the feedback of the pilot subjects, contact with other relatives was added to the family and social category, musician was added to the leisure category, trustee/director was added to the work category, and professional and special interest organizations were added to the organizational category. Thus, content validity of the RCA was based on a review of the relevant literature, logical analysis of clinical experts, and feedback from pilot subjects.

DESCRIPTION OF THE ROLE CHANGE ASSESSMENT (VERSION 2.0)

The RCA[1] was revised by Rogers and Holm[2] to simplify the role items and definitions, structure the measurement of role change, and improve the format for clinical and research use. To accomplish these objectives, adaptations were made in the role categories and specific items, the response format, and the administration method; interpretation of the data yielded by RCA (version 2.0) remains essentially the same. The format of the RCA was updated to reflect these changes.

Role Categories and Items

The RCA (version 2.0) is organized around six role categories—relationships, self-care/home maintainer, productivity, leisure, organizational, and health and wellness. Thus, in the revision, the title of the family and social category was changed to relationship, the self-care category to self-care/home maintainer, the vocational category to productive, and the health care category to health and wellness. Use of the instrument with psychiatrically disabled populations favored a reordering of the categories. The revised placement of the categories on the instrument is as follows: relationship, self-care/home maintainer, productive, leisure, organizational, and health and wellness.

Relationship roles are defined as spouse, parent, grandparent, son/daughter, sibling, other relatives, friend, neighbor, and pet owner. Visitor was deleted from the specific roles because it overlapped with other relationships or organizational roles. The question about preferences for interacting with people of specific ages was also eliminated. Self-care/home maintainer roles are defined as self-carer, cook, housekeeper (light), housekeeper (heavy), launderer, shopper, driver, gardener, and repairer. When these items are compared to the original items, the title of personal-carer was changed to self-carer, and the house cleaner role was divided into housekeeper—light and heavy. Productive roles are described as worker for pay, caregiver, and student. Reduction of this category from 10 to three specific roles reflects the deletion of the various formats of work for pay, eg, part-time, full-time, consultant, relief, self-employed part-time, self-employed full-time, and of the volunteer and trustee/director roles that overlapped with organizational roles. Leisure roles are identified as hobbyist/craftsperson, musician/artist, sports participant, dancer, collector, aerobics participant, game player, traveler/tourist, observer/reflector, reader, and event attender. Reader was added to the original list of roles, and walking was broadened to aerobics participant and observer to observer/reflector. The classification of leisure roles, taking place primarily at home or away from home, and alone or with others, was deleted.

Organizational roles are classified according to the type of organization—religious, civic, political, senior citizens, social, support/self-help, educational, and professional. The revision reflects the addition of the educational group. When rating participation in organizational roles, role assignment is based on the function that the organization serves for the individual. For example, membership in the National Audubon Society could serve the purpose of a social group, a political organization (conservation and environmental action), or a social organization (contact with people with interest in birds). Information about participation as a leader or member was transferred to the response format (see following page). The health and wellness category represents a reconceptualization of the health care category. The roles of chronic, acute, and episodic are replaced with those of recipient of health care, recipient of therapy care or therapy/wellness participant. Thus, the revision consists of 43 specific roles in six categories: nine under relationships, nine under self-care/home maintainer; three under productive, 11 under leisure, eight under organizational, and three under health and wellness. Role definitions were simplified, and the definitions were added to the interview schedule.

Response Format

Each role is rated by the respondent in terms of present participation, past participation, and the connotation of perceived change. Present participation in a role implies that one is currently active in that role. Past participation in a role implies that one held the role in the past. Present participation is compared with past participation to determine whether participation has remained the same or changed. Any change in role participation is further identified as a gain or a loss of a role, or an increase or a decrease in participation. Present and past participation are rated by the respondent on a 5-point scale indicating the frequency of personal or telephone contact in the identified role, with 0 indicating low frequency of contact and 4 indicating greater frequency of contact. Role gain is indicated if there was no participation in a role in the past, but there is in the present. Role loss is indicated if there is no participation in a role in the present, but there was in the past. Role participation in the past as well as the present may still be marked by role change, characterized as a change in the intensity of role participation. Role increase occurs when the time devoted to a role has increased. Conversely, role decrease occurs when the time devoted to a role has decreased. Present ratings are subtracted from past ratings to obtain an index of increased or decreased participation in a role. Perceived role changes are rated on a 3-point scale, indicating a positive, neutral/no change, or negative connotation. The primary adaptation in the response format of RCA (version 2.0) from the original instrument lies in the introduction of the 5-point scale for rating past and present role participation and its potential to quantify role changes. The response option of role replacement has been deleted in the revised version because it overlaps with role gain.

When the Role Change Assessment was originally presented, the past was interpreted as the previous 12 months. Use of the instrument has suggested that various time frames may be appropriate to use, depending on the purpose of the assessment and the medical and disability status of the population. For example, with an inpatient, depressed geriatric population, we have found it useful to define the past as the premorbid or predepression period. Conversely, with a well, young-old population, little change in role functioning emerged over 12 months and we found it useful to expand the retrospective interval to 5 years. Within each role category, respondents also rank three roles that serve as the major organizers for the respondent's time and the three roles that are most valued. These ratings replace the open-ended questions that were included at the end of the original interview.

Data Interpretation

An overall profile of role performance is created in the Summary Table at the end of the instrument. This summarizes role gain, loss, increases, and decreases in each of the six role categories. As such, it facilitates an overall judgment of role behavior in terms of change and stability. This summary remains essentially the same as in the original instrument, but incorporates the revised response format.

Method of Administration

The Role Change Assessment is designed to be a semistructured interview. Guiding questions for each role are given in the Role Change Assessment Manual.[1-2] Within the parameters of the intent of the interview, the interviewer can reword the questions to enhance their clarity for a particular client. Further, additional questions can be added to facilitate an accurate picture of the respondent's role participation and pattern.

Role participation is to be examined in the order in which roles are presented on the semistructured interview protocol. Initially, present status is explored in each role category. After a general discussion of participation in each role within a category, the frequency of contact scale is presented on a 5 x 8 index card and respondents rate their participation. The examiner then proceeds to explore the next role until all roles within a category have been considered, eg, spouse, grandparent, son/daughter.

The past is then defined for the respondent, as it is to be interpreted during the interview. The past is then examined for the first role, eg, spouse, in the category just completed for present status. The examiner then identifies any role changes, ie, gains, losses, increases, or decreases, inherent to a comparison of past and present role participation. The respondent confirms these changes and rates their change value. The examiner then proceeds to explore the next role until all roles within a category have been discussed. Before moving to the next category, the respondent rank orders the three roles within that category that a) take the most time and, therefore, serve as major time organizers, and b) are most valued or most important. The interview then progresses to the next category until the semi-structured interview is completed. Before concluding the interview, the interviewer completes the Summary Table to verify impressions with the respondent.

Research Using the Role Change Assessment

Research studies are based on the original RCA, and all three studies involved community-dwelling older adults. Jackoway[17] administered the RCA to 25 healthy, community-dwelling older adults, with a mean age of 77 (range 70 to 85). There were 15 women and 10 men; eight of the men and six of the women were married. The subjects were volunteers from senior centers and apartments. The mean number of roles held at the time of the interview was 24.5, with a range of 15-33. The mean number of roles held 1 year prior to the interview was 25.3, with a range of 18-32. Overall, there was a mean decrease of 2% in the number of roles held. Eleven roles—parent, grandparent, friend, member of a religious organization, personal-carer, cook, shopper, house cleaner, traveler, observer, and walker—were held by at least 80% (n = 20+) of the sample. No one participated as a consultant, was self-employed full time, or belonged to a support or self-help group. In general, subjects were not equally involved in the social and family, organizational, and leisure categories. Rather, they tended to concentrate their participation in one or two of these categories.

In the open-ended question, the roles named most often as being most influential for organizing time were home maintainer, church member, and volunteer. The roles cited as most important were church member, being a reader, and participation in social activities. Thus, the roles mentioned as most influential for time use differed from those given as most important. Six of the 25 subjects stated that nothing prevented them from being more active, as they were already as active as they could or desired to be. Lack of time was mentioned by five subjects as a limiting factor, closely followed by lack of energy and problems with eyesight. Health was overwhelmingly perceived as the primary determinant for maintaining current activity levels.

Role gain was experienced by 36% of the subjects and role loss by 56%. Increases in role participation were perceived by 88% and decreases by 96%. Thus, there is a tendency toward a decline in both the number of roles and in the time spent in roles. The organizational role category evidenced the most change, followed by health care, leisure, self-care, family, and vocational. The specific roles lost most often were acutely ill, neighbor, visitor, part-time worker, student, hobbyist, and episodically ill.

The relationship between role participation and life satisfaction was also examined in this study. Cantril ladders[18] were used to assess life satisfaction at present and 1 year ago. A 10-rung ladder was presented and respondents were asked to use the ladder to rate their satisfaction in relation to the best (10) and worst (1) they could imagine. In general, they expressed considerable life satisfaction, with a mean life satisfaction of 8.2 for the present and 8.0 for the past. Change in life satisfaction from past to present was found to be correlated with the number of roles lost ($r = .43$, $P < .05$), with loss of roles contributing to increases in life satisfaction. This finding supports the selective optimization concept of Baltes and colleagues[19] by which older adults reduce their participation in some roles so that they can function more effectively in others.

Bonder and Fisher[20] used the Role Change Assessment to examine the activity balance of adults 64 years of age and older. Of the 88 subjects, two-thirds were women; 80 percent were white and the remainder were black. The sample was one of convenience. It consisted of essentially well, community-dwelling older adults, as those with obvious disabilities, such as hemiplegia and dementia, were excluded. Subjects were interviewed only in reference to their present role participation. Hence, change in role participation over time was not examined. Also, questions were not asked about health care roles. Almost 80 percent of the subjects (70 of 88) enumerated roles in at least four of the five role categories. The range in number of roles was 3 to 11, with a mean of 6.4. Roles in the organizational and vocational categories were mentioned least. Of the 45 roles included in the interview, 35 were mentioned at least once, suggesting that older adults fill a wide range of roles.

In a third study of the community-dwelling elderly,[21] 10 older adults—nine women and one man—from a senior citizens' center lunch program were recruited. All participants were over age 75, and the mean age was 85. A retrospective interval of 5 years was selected for comparison with the present. In the family and social category, the subjects participated in seven of the nine roles. Given the age of the sample, it was not surprising to find that the participants were no longer in the spousal or son/daughter roles. Role decline was seen in reference to the roles of friend, sibling, visitor, and pet owner. All participants were active in religious and senior citizen organizations; and 60 percent (n = 6) were active in social groups. The high participation in senior citizen organizations is an artifact of the subject selection mechanism. Decreased participation was observed in all roles, except senior citizen, political, and support/self-help groups; participation in the latter two organizations was low. Participation in the vocational category was currently restricted to the volunteer role, with losses over the past 5 years taking place in part-time and full-time work and in caregiving. In regard to leisure, subjects were active in eight of the nine possible roles, with no engagement seen in sports-participation. Declines were seen in the roles of hobbyist, collector, traveler, event attender, game player, and walker, but not in observer. In the self-care category, the subjects were active in seven of eight possible roles, with repair person being the role excluded. Even though these individuals were living in the community, declines were perceived in roles associated with cooking, shopping, doing the laundry, driving, and gardening. House cleaning and performing personal care were stable. In the organizational category, subjects were active in six of eight possible roles, with no activity detected in professional or special-interest groups. In the health care category, an increase was seen in regard to chronic care, a slight decrease in acute care, and stability in episodic conditions. In general, role changes were perceived as positive or neutral. This seemed to be due, in part, to the fact that changes occurred in roles that were not as highly valued as other roles or that were not perceived as desirable in late life. Thus, reductions in worker, leisure, and self-care roles were viewed as positive.

SUMMARY

The Role Change Assessment is a tool that enables therapists and older adult patients to examine role changes that have occurred and whether those role changes have been positive or negative. It helps therapists to target tasks that are related to role loss for further assessment and intervention. Overall role loss can also be an indicator of decrements in health, as well as the need for support services. Further research is needed on the revised RCA and will help to identify the relationships among role change, disability, and impairment, as well as outcomes following occupational therapy intervention.

REFERENCES

1. Jackoway IS, Rogers JC, Snow T. The Role Change Assessment: An interview tool for evaluating older adults. *Occupational Therapy in Mental Health.* 1987;7:17-37.
2. Rogers JC, Holm MB. *The Role Change Assessment (version 2.0): An Interview Tool for Evaluating Older Adults.* Pittsburgh, Pa: Unpublished role assessment tool; 1995.
3. Reilly MW, Foner A, Hess B, Toby ML. Socialization for the middle and later years. In Goslin DA. *Handbook of Socialization Theory and Research.* Chicago, Ill: Rand McNally College Publishing Co; 1969.
4. George LK. *Role Transitions in Later Life.* Monterey, Calif: Brooks/Cole Publishing Company; 1980.
5. Goudy R. Changing work expectations: Findings from the Retirement History Study. *Gerontologist.* 1981;21:644-649.
6. Streib GF, Schneider CJ. *Retirement in American Society: Impact and Process.* Ithaca, NY: Cornell University Press; 1971.
7. Blau ZS. *Aging in a Changing Society.* New York, NY: Franklin Watts; 1981.
8. Albrecht R. The social roles of old people. *J Gerontol.* 1951;6:138-145.
9. Bengston VL. Differences between subsamples in level of present role activity. In Havighurst RJ, Munnichs MA, Neugarten BL, Thomas H. *Adjustment to Retirement: A Cross-National Study.* New York, NY: Humanities Press; 1969.
10. Cavan RS, Burgess EW, Havighurst RJ, Goldhammer H. *Personal Adjustment in Old Age.* Chicago, Ill: Science Research Associates; 1949.
11. Clark M, Anderson B. *Culture and Aging: An Anthropological Study of Older Americans.* New York, NY: Arno Press; 1980.
12. Cumming E, Henry W. *Growing Old: The Process of Disengagement.* New York, NY: Basic Books; 1961.
13. Havighurst RJ, Albrecht R. *Older People.* New York, NY: Longmans, Green and Co; 1953.
14. Morgan LA. Social roles in later life: Some recent research trends. In Eisdorfer C. *Annu Rev Gerontol Geriatr.* 1982;3:55-79.

15. Oakley F. *The Model of Human Occupation in Psychiatry.* Unpublished master's project. Richmond, Va: Department of Occupational Therapy, Virginia Commonwealth University; 1982.

16. Williams RH, Wirths CG. *Lives Through the Years.* New York, NY: Atherton; 1965.

17. Jackoway IS. *Role Change in Older Adults.* Unpublished master's thesis. Chapel Hill, NC: Division of Occupational Therapy, University of North Carolina; 1985.

18. Cantril H. *The Pattern of Human Concerns.* New Brunswick, NJ: Rutgers University Press; 1965.

19. Baltes PB, Baltes MM. Psychological perspectives on successful aging: The model of selective optimization with compensation. In Baltes PB, Baltes MM. *Successful Aging: Perspectives From the Behavioral Sciences.* Cambridge, England: Cambridge University Press; 1990.

20. Bonder BR, Fisher AG. Roles and activities of the elderly. *Gerontologist.* 1990; 30:139A.

21. Mitcham MD, Cartin AE, Krause CA, Mannix CV, Mayhugh ME, Melton PS. *The Effects of Role Changes on the Life Satisfaction of Independent Elderly Adults.* Presented at the Great Southern Occupational Therapy Conference, Lexington, Ky: October 27, 1994.

PART III:
FUNCTIONAL ASSESSMENTS

6

The Bay Area Functional Performance Evaluation

James P. Klyczek, PhD, OTR

The purpose of this chapter is to describe the historical development of the original and revised Bay Area Functional Performance Evaluation (BaFPE), the administration and scoring of the two BaFPE components, the Task Oriented Assessment (TOA) and the Social Interaction Scale (SIS); and standardization of the BaFPE, including numerous studies examining the validity and reliability of the TOA and SIS. Samples on which current norms have been developed for the TOA are described, as well as research testing the influence of various factors, such as age, education, gender, and culture, on the development of norms. Clinical application of the BaFPE to psychiatric inpatients, patients with eating disorders, and skilled nursing residents is reviewed, and a description of how the TOA and SIS have been used to evaluate patient progress in research studies is provided. Finally, suggestions for further research on the BaFPE are provided with an invitation to therapists to take part in the continued development of perhaps the most widely used and researched standardized occupational therapy functional performance evaluation.

THEORETICAL BASIS

While the theoretical foundation of the BaFPE shares some features characteristic of psychoanalytic, developmental, and biopsychosocial models, Bloomer and Williams[1] based the BaFPE primarily on the acquisitional,[2] occupational behavior, adaptational, and functional restoration frames of reference. The underlying principles of the BaFPE, "like those of the acquisitional frame of reference, imply that functional performance can be measured...(and that patients) may be helped to become more functional through exposure to situations in which more adaptive behavior can essentially be practiced."[1]

The necessity of maintaining a balance among the daily life tasks of work, play, rest, and sleep is emphasized in the occupational behavior frame of reference, as is the focus on occupational role and acquisition of skills and habits necessary to facilitate the development and performance of occupational behavior.[3,4] Dysfunction is viewed by Bloomer and Williams as "the lack or loss of skill acquisition... (and that) functional behavior be considered a prerequisite to the acquisition of occupational behavior."[1]

King described adaptation as "an active response evoked by specific environmental demands."[5] Bloomer and Williams viewed adaptation as critical to an individual's overall functional performance and was an important consideration in developing the BaFPE.[1]

The underlying principles of the BaFPE are also thought to be consistent with the theory and application of occupational therapy as described by Spencer, in that a basic premise of occupational therapy "is the use of performance as feedback to the patient to assist him or her in becoming involved in self-initiated, purposeful activity."[6]

The BaFPE is also viewed as consistent with the model of human occupation developed by Kielhofner and others.[7-11] The model is used to describe how occupational behavior is motivated, organized, and performed. Underlying the ability to perform occupational behavior are communication/interaction skills, process skills, such as planning and problem solving, and perceptual-motor skills. The BaFPE is used to evaluate the "functional parameters that underlie these component skills."[12]

Bloomer and Williams stated that there are two skills necessary for general function in the environment—the ability to engage in goal-directed and task-oriented activities with objects in the environment, and the ability to interact with other people in the environment in a socially acceptable way.[13] Their goal was to develop a valid and reliable tool that would appropriately assess general components of functioning needed to perform activities of daily living.[14]

HISTORICAL DEVELOPMENT

The BaFPE was developed by Judith Bloomer and Susan Williams in 1977 and 1978 at Langley Porter Psychiatric Institute at the University of California Medical Center in San Francisco to meet the need for a standardized assessment of functional performance.[15] Williams and Bloomer defined functioning as "employing useful activity to achieve an active mode of adaptation to the environment. This process or activity would include the ability to satisfy physiological and psychological needs through interaction with both people and objects in the environment. The term *functional* "...pertains to this definition of functioning, and is a descriptive adjective connoting purposeful activity and active adaptation to the environment."[14]

Williams and Bloomer also stated that activity can be classified into the functional areas of self-care, work, and leisure, and that functional skill is the foundation of everyday performance that integrates the motoric, social, cognitive, psychological, and sensory-integrative performance components. They use the term functional to pertain to "an individual who is able *to perform*, synthesizing these components."[14]

The present BaFPE is composed of the TOA and SIS. The TOA assesses one's ability to act on the environment in goal-directed ways and contains five tasks used to provide information about the patient's cognitive, performance, and affective areas of functioning. The SIS assesses social behaviors observed in five different settings. Originally conceptualized as a single evaluation, with the TOA and SIS as two subtests from which an overall BaFPE score was derived, the BaFPE was later revised with the TOA and SIS used together or separately, but with no overall BaFPE score. The authors cautioned that information from either the TOA or SIS alone is not a measure of functional performance. Functional performance, as defined by the test authors, requires evaluation of the patient's ability to interact with both objects and people in the environment.

The BaFPE was revised based on feedback from clinicians and the results of data analysis, and was published in a second edition in 1987.[14] The purposes of revision were to reduce ambiguity of some of the functional parameters, clarify administration instructions, and to provide additional guidance in score interpretation and reporting. According to Williams and Bloomer,[14] the main revisions were as follows:

1. Separate use and scoring of the TOA and SIS.
2. The TOA Bank Deposit Slip task was changed to the Money and Marketing task, because the former task may have been biased against patients without checking accounts. The revised task is more common and retains the processes of the former task.
3. The TOA House Floor Plan task was changed to the Home Drawing task, because it was difficult to score and may have been subject to local house design. A more common list of room names and more carefully defined residence are provided in the revised task.
4. One of the original 10 TOA parameters was dropped (decision-making), three were revised (paraphrase, thought disorder, task completion), and three new parameters were defined (errors, efficiency, general affective impression), resulting in 12 functional parameters.
5. The functional parameters were newly organized into cognitive, performance, and affective components to facilitate scoring and interpretation of results.
6. Timing was formalized as part of the performance component.
7. The Qualitative Signs and Referral indicators section was added to the TOA rating sheets to screen for organicity.
8. Rather than using one single overall rating for the SIS, five settings are now specified for evaluating social behavior.
9. A Self-Report of Social Interaction, similar to the SIS, was developed for patients as a means to assessing clients' perceptions and insights related to their own social functioning.
10. The TOA and SIS rating sheet formats were revised and summary score sheets were developed to facilitate reporting results.

Since publication of the second edition of the BaFPE, numerous studies have been conducted, examining the validity and reliability of the TOA, and norms on psychiatric inpatients and patients with eating disorders have been developed. Research to develop a third edition of the BaFPE is underway. Similar to revisions of the first and second editions, the test authors plan to incorporate feedback from clinicians and data from the numerous studies conducted thus far. The feasibility of developing a shortened version of the TOA also is being examined for the third edition.

ADMINISTRATION AND SCORING

TOA

Description

The TOA is designed to gather information about an individual's functioning in a one-to-one setting through five task-oriented activities. The TOA was originally developed for use in inpatient or outpatient psychiatric settings, but, as discussed later, has been used with other populations and is appropriate in any situation in which information about an individual's task-oriented functioning is desired.

TOA Tasks

The TOA is composed of five tasks that include a range of difficulty and structure:

1. Sorting Shells: 10 categories of shells are sorted by size, shape, and color.
2. Money and Marketing: The amount of money needed to purchase specific items is calculated; the ability to purchase the items with available money and a mock check is determined; and the amount of change from the transaction is calculated.
3. Home Drawing: A floor plan for a home is drawn, following specific instructions about what should be included.
4. Block Design: A block design is duplicated from memory or with the use of a cue card if needed.
5. Kinetic Person Drawing: A person doing something is drawn.

The TOA begins with a pre-assessment interview to elicit information about the patient's current or past functioning and to develop rapport, and explain what the patient will be doing during the assessment. The patient is tested at a table or desk in a room with as few distractions as possible. Testing materials for the five tasks are prepared by the examiner prior to the test.

Scoring the Functional Parameters

The individual is rated on 12 functional parameters during each task. Ratings range from (1) markedly dysfunctional or inappropriate to (4) almost always functional or appropriate. Behavioral guidelines are provided on rating sheets for evaluating the 12 parameters for each task. The parameters are organized into three components:

Cognitive Component
1. Memory for written and oral instructions
2. Organization of time and materials
3. Attention span
4. Evidence of thought disorder
5. Ability to abstract
Performance Component
6. Task completion
7. Errors
8. Efficiency
Affective Component
9. Motivation and compliance
10. Frustration tolerance
11. Self-confidence
12. General affective and behavioral impression

At the beginning of each task, the therapist reads instructions to the patient, which the patient is asked to restate. If the patient cannot restate the general idea of the task after one repetition of instructions, the task is not completed. The patient's performance is scored during the task, using the rating sheet provided for each task. A stopwatch is used to time each task, and the patient is asked to stop if the maximum allowable time has been used. Some areas on the task rating sheets may be scored after the task has been completed, but, with experience, the therapist should be able to complete all ratings during testing.

Qualitative Signs and Referral Indicators

Following completion of each task, the therapist completes the Qualitative Signs and Referral Indicators (QSRI) section of the rating forms by checking off any of the observations noted during testing. The QSRI contains general and task specific observations that indicate possible organic factors, suggesting the need for referral for further evaluation.

Summary Score Sheet

Scores on the five task rating sheets are then transferred to the TOA Summary Score Sheet, and the scores are then summed up to derive parameter, component, task, and total TOA scores. Check marks recorded on the QSRI section of the task rating sheets are summed up and transferred to the TOA Summary Score Sheet. Although the QSRI scoring is not included in the formal TOA score, if more than 20 of the 141 symptoms are checked, or if any starred QSRI items are checked, consultation or further testing is considered.

Interpretation

TOA scores may be interpreted in three ways. They may be interpreted first by examination of parameter and component scores, which provides information about the client's strengths and needs in various area of functioning. For example, a patient may score well in the performance areas, but low in the affective areas. The second way is by examination of task scores. Because the tasks range in difficulty and structure, performance trends may become evident, for example, when the patient performs better in more structured tasks. The third way of interpreting TOA scores is by comparison to norms, which allows the therapist to compare the patient's performance to an appropriate reference group. This avenue of interpretation will become more useful when more extensive norms are developed for the TOA.

Social Interaction Scale

Description

The SIS is used to assess seven categories of verbal and non-verbal social interaction behaviors considered important to overall functioning. It is intended to be completed within 24 hours of the TOA to obtain a valid assessment of the two types of functioning. Behavior is assessed in five social setting situations:

1. One-to-One Interview—during an interview or administration of the TOA.
2. Mealtime—a group setting in which group interaction must be possible, such as several individuals eating together at the same table.
3. Unstructured Group Situation—a group setting in which there is no expectation regarding the patient's performance, such as a common-living or group-gathering area. There should be no stimuli, such as a TV being played, that preclude the opportunity for social interaction.

4. Structured Activity Group—a planned group activity or recreational game setting in which social interaction is expected. The difference between the unstructured and structured group settings is the presence of a leader who expects the patient to participate.

5. Structured Oral Group—any group that fosters discussion among members, ranging from oral group therapy to any type of discussion group, such as a community meeting or current events group. The difference between structured activity and structured oral groups is a focus on doing or actively participating in a group activity or task in the former, and a focus on oral interaction in the latter.

Williams and Bloomer cite research indicating that multiple observations across situations is necessary for accurate assessment of social skills.[16-20] They suggest that the SIS is best completed with frequent observations by the therapist, supplemented by observations of other staff working with the patient, and in multiple situations.[14]

Scoring the Functional Parameters

An individual is rated on a 5-point scale on seven functional parameters across five social situations. Behavioral guidelines for the ratings are provided on the rating forms. Ratings range from 1 to 5, with 1 indicating that assessment was not possible due to the degree of dysfunction. The ratings of 2 through 5 are used to reflect a continuum of performance from (2) markedly dysfunctional or inappropriate to (5) almost always functional or appropriate.

The seven parameters of social interaction rated on the SIS scoring form include:

1. Verbal Communication—quantity and quality of verbal interaction.
2. Psychomotor Behavior—motor effect of psychological processes, reflected in hypo- or hyperactivity.
3. Socially Appropriate Behavior—quality of behavior in relation to cultural and social expectations.
4. Response to Authority Figures—quality of interaction with and response to people who influence power or control over the individual.
5. Independence/Dependence—appropriateness of self-reliance and self-direction.
6. Ability to Work With Others—quantity and quality of peer interactions in work or task-oriented settings.
7. Participation in Groups or Program Activities—ability to take part in activities that require social interaction.

Not all seven parameters are scored in each situation. The SIS is completed through direct observation by the examiner, although corroboration by other team members is desirable. A minimum of 10 minutes of observation in each social setting is recommended, with the SIS completed within a 1 to 2 day period.

SIS Scoring Sheet

Parameter scores are derived by summing up the ratings for each situation and dividing this number by the number of rated observations. For example, scores of 4, 2, 2, 3, and 2 for the verbal communication parameter across the five situations yield a parameter score of 13/5 or 2.6. The situation scores are derived by summing up all parameter scores for that situation. The total SIS score is derived by totaling the five situation scores. For interpretation of situation scores, the sum of the parameter scores for a situation is divided by the number of parameters scored.

Interpretation

Methods for interpreting SIS scores are similar to that of the TOA. Parameter and situation scores may be examined to identify a patient's strengths and needs in relation to the seven categories of verbal and non-verbal interaction, and in relation to structured versus unstructured and group versus one-to-one situations. SIS normative data on two reference groups are provided in the BaFPE manual,[14] but the small number of subjects (n = 20, n = 35) makes comparison of patient scores difficult. As with the TOA, this avenue of interpretation will become more useful when more extensive norms are developed.

STANDARDIZATION

Test standardization is a long and complex process that involves developing a consistent protocol for administration and scoring, testing of the tools' validity and reliability, and definition of norms. The administration and scoring of the BaFPE (summarized earlier) are clearly described in the manual provided with the test kit. The focus of this section is to describe a number of studies that have been conducted to examine the validity and reliability of the original and revised BaFPE. First, a brief overview defining the various types of validity and reliability testing conducted on the TOA and SIS is provided.

Validity and Reliability

Validity of a tool, in a general sense, refers to whether the tool is measuring what it was intended to measure. *Concurrent validity* refers to the correlation between scores on the tool under study and scores for the same individual on another tool, with established or accepted validity measuring the same construct concurrently. The correlation should be high enough to indicate that the new tool is valid, but not so high as to suggest that the new tool is identical to the existing tool. New tools may be developed because they are less expensive, easier or quicker to administer and score, and are more reliable than existing tools.[21] *Discriminant validity* is a measure of the ability of a tool to differentiate between various groups. For example, can a functional assessment distinguish differences in ability between functionally disabled individuals and non-impaired individuals? Is the tool useful for determining which individuals are in need of intervention? *Predictive validity* is the extent to which the scores on one measure successfully predict a particular outcome. For example, how well do lower scores on a discharge ADL evaluation relate to the need for increased caregiver support post-discharge? *Construct validity* is a measure of whether a tool tests the construct for which it was intended, such as functional performance in the case of the BaFPE.

The reliability of a tool refers to whether the measurements obtained are consistent and predictable. *Interrater reliability* or *interrater agreement* refers to the consistency of measurements obtained by different raters.[22] *Intrarater reliability* or *test-retest reliability* refers to the consistency of measurements by the same rater.[21] Refer to Chapter 22 for a thorough review of validity and reliability.

TOA

Validity on the Original Version

Concurrent

Bloomer and Williams[1] conducted a concurrent validity study on the original TOA with the Functional Life Scale (FLS)[23] and the Global Assessment Scale (GAS).[24] Correlations between the TOA and the FLS and GAS were .43 and .45, respectively. Correlations between the composite BaFPE (TOA and SIS) and the FLS and GAS were .52 and .57 at $P < .001$, respectively. Bortone also found a positive, but not statistically significant, correlation between the BaFPE and GAS scores of 23 schizophrenic and borderline patients.[25]

Cheeseman[26] tested 20 patients diagnosed with brain vascular disease with the TOA, FLS, and Jebsen Hand Function Test.[27] The correlation between the composite BaFPE and the FLS was .62, which was consistent with Bloomer and Williams' original field study results ($r=.52$).[1] Cheeseman reported a statistically significant correlation ($P < .0005$) between BaFPE scores and the Jebsen for the non-affected hand that suggested that "adequate motor skills are necessary to successfully perform tasks on the TOA."[12]

Kaufman[28] studied the concurrent validity of the TOA by comparing TOA scores of 16 psychiatric inpatients with their scores on the Kohlman Evaluation of Living Skills (KELS)[29] and reported that the composite BaFPE and TOA correlations to both were .84 at $P < .001$. The highest correlation between the KELS and TOA tasks was with the House Floor Plan task with $r=.82$.

Discriminant

Several studies lend support to the discriminant validity of the original TOA. In initial field testing, it was found that patients exhibiting higher degrees of psychotic behavior scored lower on the BaFPE.[1] Bortone found that patients diagnosed with borderline personality disorder scored higher on the BaFPE than patients with schizophrenic disorders.[25] Also, patients with borderline personality disorder scored lower on the TOA than the SIS, but the reverse was true for patients with schizophrenia.

Wener-Altman, Wolfe, and Staley examined the use of the BaFPE with adolescents.[30] They tested 19 male and 29 female psychiatric inpatients ranging in age from 13 to 17 years with a mean of 15.45 years. Primary diagnoses of subjects were conduct disorders (48%), adjustment disorders (21%), schizophrenia or affective disorders (18%), and character disorders (13%). They found a significant correlation between diagnosis and TOA, but those with more severe impairments, such as schizophrenia, scored less well.

Other researchers report different findings. Olson and Jamal completed the most extensive published study on the original BaFPE with 211 inpatients.[31] They found no statistically significant differences in TOA or composite BaFPE scores by diagnosis among patients diagnosed with schizophrenia, depression, or manic depression.

Brockett examined the discriminant validity of the BaFPE and reported significant differences in scores of 50 patients tested at a Canadian general hospital from scores of patients tested in San Francisco.[32] They suggested that the differences might have been due to cultural differences and, therefore, questioned the validity of the BaFPE.

Predictive

The relationship between the TOA, the Nurse's Observation Scale for Inpatient Evaluation (NOSIE-30),[33] and an adaptation of the Comprehensive Evaluation of Basic Living Skills (CEBLS)[34] was studied by Accardi.[35] His sample of seven males and 12 females, primarily white, ranged in age from 21 to 72, with a mean age of 40.5 years. Correlations between the TOA and NOSIE-30 were .66 ($P<.001$); and .63 ($P<.005$) between the TOA and the adapted CEBLS. Houston, et al. stated that "Accardi's findings support the use of the BaFPE as a predictor of functional performance, as determined by two other functional assessments given concurrently."[12]

In addition to their research on the BaFPE discriminant validity, Olson and Jamal reported that TOA scores correlated significantly with aftercare residential placement.[31] Also, BaFPE-based recommendations regarding legal conservatorship correlated significantly with actual treatment-team decisions regarding conservatorship.

Construct

Bloomer and Williams established the initial construct validity of the BaFPE via their findings that patients' BaFPE discharge scores were significantly higher than admission scores. They also found high correlations between the TOA tasks and parameters with most in the .70 to .89 range.[1] Wener-Altman, et al. reported positive correlations between the TOA parameters and total TOA score ranging from .25 to .88.[30] Olson and Jamal also found high internal correlations for the TOA, SIS, and composite BaFPE.[31] Finally, Mason found that most of the TOA parameters did not correlate significantly with the SIS parameters, suggesting that the TOA and SIS are measuring different aspects of functional performance.[36]

Francis and Cermak's study with 20 patients with schizophrenia and 20 non-diagnosed subjects supported the validity of the sorting shells and house floor plan tasks on the original TOA.[37] They randomly divided subjects into original and modified task groups, each composed of 10 diagnosed and 10 non-diagnosed subjects. Subjects in the original group performed the original tasks, while subjects in the modified task group used buttons instead of shells for the sorting task and were given a simplified five-room square house instead of the 10-room L-shaped house as in the original TOA. It was hypothesized that subjects would perform better on the modified tasks because they were more relevant and familiar than the existing tasks. Diagnosed subjects performed more poorly than non-diagnosed subjects on both tasks as expected, but "he use of a different medium did not differentially affect the performance of the patients with schizophrenia,"[37] thus lending support to the validity of the existing tasks.

Validity on the Revised Version

Concurrent

The concurrent validity of the TOA has been tested with the revised Allen Cognitive Level Test (ACL), the Global Assessment Scale (GAS), three subtests of the Wechsler Adult Intelligence Scale (WAIS), Part 1 of the American Association on Mental Deficiency Adaptive Behavior Scale (AAMD-ABS), and the Scorable Self-Care Evaluation (SSCE).

Newman[38] studied the relationship between TOA scores and cognitive level, as assessed with the revised ACL Test[39] with 21 inpatients. All TOA tasks, except sorting shells, correlated significantly with the ACL at $P <.05$. Newman also reported that the TOA and ACL correlated significantly with the GAS.

Testing the hypothesis that intelligence influences functional performance, Thibeault and Blackmer[40] examined the relationship between scores on the TOA and three subtests of the WAIS[41] with 26 male and 34 female subjects, ranging in age from 21 to 75 years. Subjects were diagnosed with either schizophrenia (n = 31) or depression (n = 29). Correlations between the total TOA score and the digit symbol, block design, and picture completion subtests were .60, .67, and .58 ($P <.05$), respectively. The authors stated that these positive correlations are evidence of the TOA validity, "but the correlations are not so high as to suggest that the two tests assess the same dimensions of human functioning."[40]

Klyczek and Mann[42] tested the concurrent validity of the TOA with Part I of the AAMD-ABS.[43,44] The sample included 67 psychiatric inpatients with a mean age of 30.8 years, 73% of whom were male. The correlation between the TOA and the total ABS Part I score was .32 at $P <.05$. Correlations ranged from -.19 between the eating subdomain of the ABS and the Kinetic Person Drawing task of the TOA, to .58 between the socialization domain of the ABS and the Sorting Shells task of the TOA. The authors suggested that the ABS' fair reliability may have resulted in the low correlation between the two tests.

Mercer, Castilla, and Klyczek[45] examined the relationship between parameter, component, and total task scores on the Kinetic Person Drawing (KPD) task of the TOA and the personal care, housekeeping chores, work and leisure, and financial management subscales of the SSCE[46] to determine the extent to which scores on a projective drawing task (TOA-KPD) correlate with measures of functional performance (SSCE). Correlations between the tests ranged from .10 to -.42 (inverse scoring) and were not statistically significant. The correlation between the total TOA and total SSCE scores was -.28 and was not statistically significant. The authors concluded that the KPD is not a valid measure of functional performance when used alone.

Discriminant

The discriminant validity of the TOA has been tested with a number of samples, including psychiatric inpatients versus outpatients, patients with eating disorders versus non-diagnosed, adult psychiatric patients versus non-diagnosed adults, and elderly psychiatric patients versus non-diagnosed elderly.

Curtin and Klyczek published the first study examining differences in TOA scores for inpatient and outpatient samples.[47] Subjects included 31 psychiatric outpatients in an adult day-training program and 29 psychiatric inpatients matched by age and years of education. Outpatient subjects had an average age of 58.6 years and 9.5 years of education. Inpatient subjects had an average age of 53.6 years and 10.8 years of education. The majority of subjects were white females in both groups. The inpatient group scored significantly higher on the Sorting Shells task and on all cognitive and performance parameters, except attention span and evidence of thought disorder. The inpatient group scored significantly lower on all affective component parameters except self-confidence. The total TOA score was 6.8 points higher for the inpatient group, but this difference was not statistically significant.

The authors noted that the inpatient group had almost twice as many subjects with a diagnosis of mood disorder than with schizophrenia, while the outpatient group had almost four times as many subjects with a diagnosis of schizophrenia than mood disorder. Longer psychiatric histories were also noted for subjects in the outpatient sample. The authors concluded that differences between inpatient and outpatient TOA scores do exist, but suggest that these differences may be due to diagnosis and chronicity.

Konieczny reported very good discriminant validity of the TOA with 63 patients diagnosed with eating disorders and a sample of 64 non-diagnosed subjects.[48] The samples were matched on age, race, gender, occupation, education in years, educational degree, and marital status. The age range of subjects was 14 to 58 years in the diagnosed group, and 14 to 54 years in the non-diagnosed group. The mean age was 24.4 years in both groups. There were no significant differences between groups on any of the matching variables. Diagnosed subjects scored significantly lower on the total TOA score, all five task scores, all three component scores, and all parameter scores, except evidence of thought disorder. The largest differences were observed in the affective component and parameters, and the smallest differences were observed in the performance component and parameters.

Lissner examined the discriminant validity of the TOA with 60 individuals with a diagnosis of mental illness and 60 non-diagnosed subjects.[49] The samples were matched on gender, age, ethnicity, education level, years of education, and marital status. Each sample included 18 male and 42 female subjects. Subjects' ages ranged from 19 to 59 (M = 27.7) in the diagnosed sample and from 19 to 66 (M = 27.4) in the non-diagnosed sample.

Based on discriminant analysis, Lissner concluded that 18 of the 21 ratings analyzed (12 parameter, three component, five task, total) have sufficient discriminant validity. Three parameters, including memory for written/oral instructions, evidence of thought disorder, and motivation and compliance, do not possess discriminant validity.

Stoffel matched 20 non-diagnosed subjects over 60 years old with 20 subjects with a DSM-III-R diagnosis receiving treatment in an adult psychiatric day treatment program.[50] Subjects in the diagnosed sample had diagnoses of schizophrenia (55%), mood disorder (30%), or psychoactive substance-use disorder, organic mental disorder, or other psychotic disorders (15%). Subjects' ages ranged from 61 to 85 with a mean of 71.65 years in the diagnosed sample and 72.75 years in the non-diagnosed sample. There were no significant differences between samples on age, gender, ethnicity, or years of education. The results showed that the diagnosed subjects scored lower on all TOA ratings, except the motivation/compliance parameter. Differences between the groups were statistically significant for the total TOA score and cognitive and performance component scores, and for six of the 12 parameter scores. Stoffel stated that her findings indicate that discriminant validity does exist on the TOA for the cognitive component, performance component, and total TOA scores, but that further research, with a larger sample, is necessary to validate the lack of difference between the samples on the affective component score.

The TOA as the Standard

Interestingly and indicative of growing support for the validity of the TOA, two studies have been conducted testing the concurrent validity of other tools with the TOA.

Tardif[51] examined the concurrent validity of the Functional Needs Assessment (FNA)[52] with the TOA with 10 male and 17 female patients, ranging in age from 33 to 85 years with a mean age of 58.9 years. Subjects were diagnosed with schizo-phrenia (63%), organic mental disorders (22%), or mood disorders (15%). She found that the sorting shells and home drawing tasks significantly correlated with four of the six clinical program scores on the FNA. The TOA cognitive component scores significantly correlated with all six FNA clinical program scores and that the total TOA and total FNA scores correlated with $r = .54$ at $P < .01$.

As a *show-me* assessment, the FNA is used to evaluate actual functional per-formance. The premise that the TOA is useful for evaluating the functional parame-ters underlying component skills was supported by the largest correlation ($r = .59$, $P < .001$), which was found between the total TOA score and the preplacement clin-ical program of the FNA, composed of the following skills: care of living quarters, laundry skills, social etiquette, planning and decision making, and leisure skills.

Rogers[53] failed to establish the concurrent validity of the Milwaukee Evaluation of Daily Living Skills (MEDLS)[54] with the TOA with seven male and eight female psychiatric outpatients. Ages of subjects ranged from 17 to 66, with a mean age of 40. The majority of correlations were low and nonsignificant. Scores on only four of the 20 MEDLS subtests correlated significantly with the total TOA. These included use of transportation ($r = .80$), medication management ($r = .70$), use of money ($r = .61$), and brushing teeth ($r = .50$), all at $P < .05$. Rogers stated that her findings are limited by a small non-randomly selected sample.

Reliability

Original Version

Bloomer and Williams tested the interrater reliability of the TOA with 62 diag-nosed and 20 non-diagnosed subjects.[1] Correlations for the TOA total and BaFPE total were .99. A field study conducted in 1981 with 51 diagnosed and 50 non-diag-nosed subjects showed correlations ranging from .86 to .99 for the total TOA score, and .82 to .97 for the BaFPE total.

Revised Version

Williams and Bloomer reported that the interrater reliability of the revised TOA is higher than the original.[14] They evaluated interrater reliability with four pairs of OTRs. Each team evaluated 25 patients with a DSM III diagnosis. Complete data on 91 subjects were evaluated with Pearson's Product-Moment Correlation Coefficients. Approximately 80% of the correlations equalled or exceeded .80. The average correlations for the total TOA and the cognitive, performance, and affective components were .96, .93, .96, and .85, respectively. According to Williams and Bloomer, "correlation coefficients for 10 of the original 16 scales on the TOA improved...three were lower, and three remained about the same. The items added to the revised instrument showed high correlations."[14]

Evaluation of the internal consistency of the revised TOA showed the overall range of correlations to be .29 to .84, with an average of .60. The intercorrelations for the parameters and component areas were higher than for the tasks, but not "high enough to suggest that any item or task should be eliminated from the TOA format."[14]

Conducting further analysis on the TOA data collected on 266 psychiatric patients from which the 1991 standard scores for the TOA were developed,[55] Mann and Huselid reported that the internal reliability of the TOA "is excellent (alpha coef-ficient = .93),"[56] which indicates high intercorrelation among the items on the test.

Social Interaction Scale

It should be noted that little research has been conducted with the SIS in comparison to the numerous studies that have examined the TOA. As will be discussed later in the Further Research section of this chapter, few therapists have reported using the SIS.[57]

Validity on the Original Version

Concurrent

Bloomer and Williams examined the concurrent validity of the SIS with the FLS and GAS, and reported correlations of .46 and .53 respectively.[1] The correlation between the SIS and the socialization component of the FLS was .42 at P <.001. Accardi found that correlations between SIS scores and NOSIE-30 and adapted CEBLS scores ranged from .46 to .69 at P <.05.[35] Kaufman reported a correlation of .74 between the SIS and the KELS.[28]

Predictive

Olson and Jamal found positive correlations between TOA scores and aftercare placement; however, SIS scores did not correlate with those placements.[31] Wener-Altman, et al found a significant negative correlation ($r = -.39$, P <.01) between length of stay and total SIS score in a study with 48 adolescent psychiatric inpatients.[30]

Reliability

Original Version

The mean interrater reliability correlations on the original SIS ranged from .54 to .72 for the seven parameters and was .86 for the total SIS score.[1] Bortone reported moderate to perfect agreement among raters on all SIS parameters in an "interrater agreement analysis" of SIS scores for 30 schizophrenic and borderline patients.[25]

Revised Version

According to Williams and Bloomer, the interrater reliability for the revised SIS improved substantially from the original version, although the SIS correlations were lower than those for the TOA.[14] The interrater reliability on the original SIS ranged from .54 to .72, while the correlations ranged from .56 to .94 (P <.001) on the revised SIS. Interrater reliability on the five observation situations ranged from .74 to .94 (P <.001). Internal reliability of the SIS was also examined. The overall range of correlations was .35 to .87 (P <.001).

NORMS

While tests of validity are used to establish that an instrument actually measures what it was intended to measure, and tests of reliability are used to determine the consistency or predictability of scores, norms enable the therapist to compare a particular patient's score with the scores of a larger group of individuals similar to the patient tested. Normed scores are often presented in the form of standard scores. According to Mann, Klyczek, and Fiedler, "results of testing are more easily understood when presented in some form of standard deviation units and, thus, are more appropriate for clinical documentation."[58]

General Psychiatry

Mann, et al. published the first norms on the revised TOA, using data on 144 psychiatric inpatients.[58] These norms were later expanded to include data on 266 psychiatric patients.[55] The sample was composed of 118 male and 148 female subjects ranging in age from 14 to 70 years old, with a mean age of 30.7 years and a mean of 11.5 years of education. Standard scores were presented for each of the component task summary scores, component summary scores, parameter total scores, total task summary scores, and the total TOA score.

Eating Disorders

Stanton, Mann, and Klyczek presented percentile scores for anorexic (n = 37) and bulimic (n = 28) patient samples for TOA component total scores, and total TOA scores as well as mean scores and standard deviations for the three components and their respective parameters.[59] The anorexic sample was composed of one male and 36 females, ranging in age from 14 to 49 years with a mean of 22.8 years. The bulimic sample was composed of 28 females ranging in age from 16 to 58 years, with a mean of 27.4 years. The authors provide examples for reporting test results. They stated that their findings are limited in generalization, due to a small sample composed of patients from only one private psychiatric hospital, but further state that the TOA can be used to identify patient problems in cognitive processing and with actual performance.

Factors Affecting Norms

General

Thibeault and Blackmer's study with 60 psychiatric patients showed no significant differences in TOA scores that were based on type or dosage of medication.[40] However, in evaluating the effect of electroconvulsive therapy (ECT), they found that non-ECT patients (n = 41) scored significantly higher than ECT patients (n = 19) on the memory, organization, and attention span parameters; the cognitive component total; the Block Design Tasktotal; and the total TOA. They also found differences in TOA scores by education, with more highly educated patients scoring significantly higher than less-educated patients.

Age

Thibeault and Blackmer found that younger adult patients scored significantly higher on the TOA than older patients.[40] In contrast, Wener-Altman, et al. found that older adolescent patients scored significantly higher on the TOA and SIS than younger adolescent patients.[30] In a study with 30 adolescents receiving psychiatric services at a residential placement center, Peterson found that older adolescents scored higher on the TOA than younger adolescents but the differences were not statistically significant.[60]

Length of Stay

Thibeault and Blackmer reported no difference in TOA scores based on number of hospital admissions or total time in a hospital for adult psychiatric patients.[40] However, Wener-Altman, et al found a significant negative correlation: (r = -.39, P <.01) between length of stay and total SIS scores for adolescent psychiatric inpatients.[30]

Gender

Most studies have not identified differences in TOA scores by gender. Crouch tested gender differences on the TOA with 33 male and 33 female psychiatric patients matched on diagnosis, age, years of education, highest educational degree achieved, ethnicity, and marital status.[61] Both male and female groups were composed of 28 white and five African-American subjects. Males ranged in age from 15 to 68 years, with a mean age of 37.15 years and a mean of 9.88 years of education. Females ranged in age from 15 to 69 years, with a mean age of 37.61 years and a mean of 10.58 years of education. There were no significant differences between the male and female groups on any of the matching variables. Crouch reported no significant differences on any of the TOA parameter, component, task or total scores between groups. These findings are similar to those found with adult psychiatric patients,[40] and with adolescent psychiatric inpatients in which no gender differences were found on the revised TOA, original TOA or SIS, respectively.[30]

Tornabene used a non-diagnosed sample of 25 male and 25 female subjects to test gender differences on the TOA.[62] The two groups were matched on age, race, years of education, and marital status. There were no significant differences between groups on the matching variables. In contrast to previous research,[30,40,61] Tornabene found significant differences on four parameter and two component scores on the TOA, with females scoring significantly higher than males on the memory for written/oral instructions parameter and the cognitive component total, and males scoring significantly higher than females on the task completion, errors, efficiency parameters, and performance component total. There were no significant differences between groups on the total TOA score. Peterson also found that females scored significantly higher than males ($P =.01$) on the cognitive parameters in a study with adolescents at a residential placement center.[60]

Culture

Cultural factors were cited as a possible reason scores on the original BaFPE for 50 patients tested in a Canadian general hospital differed significantly from patients tested in San Francisco.[32] No further research into cultural differences was located in a recent search of the literature.

CLINICAL APPLICATION

Based on results of face-to-face, in-depth interviews with 30 occupational therapists from four cities who use the BaFPE, Managh and Cook identified seven primary reasons occupational therapists use the BaFPE.[57] These reasons include: 1) implicit departmental policy requires use of the BaFPE; 2) the BaFPE can be administered and scored more quickly than alternate assessments; 3) the BaFPE is used as a screening, either to determine if occupational therapy intervention is necessary for a patient or to place a patient in a particular occupational therapy group; 4) the BaFPE is used in response to the preference of multidisciplinary treatment teams for standardized rather than non-standardized assessments; 5) the BaFPE supports clinical observations and complements other life skills assessments; 6) the BaFPE is a therapeutic medium by which patient self-esteem and self-confidence can be enhanced; and 7) the BaFPE emphasizes the performance of action, rather than patient self-report.

Other researchers have reported that the TOA or SIS are useful in evaluating patients with eating disorders, some skilled nursing home residents, and patient progress in research studies.

Eating Disorders

In their research to develop TOA norms for the eating disorder population, Stanton, et al state that the TOA "results can be useful in confronting defense mechanisms, particularly patient denial that eating patterns have had any significant negative effects (and that) the House Floor Plan and Kinetic Person Drawing may be used by the skillful clinician as projectives, although this is not part of the standardized scoring system."[59]

Wozniak hypothesized that the sense of ineffectiveness experienced by patients with eating disorders, as measured by the ineffectiveness subscale of the Eating Disorders Inventory (EDI),[63] would be reflected in their scores on the self-confidence and general affective impression parameters of the TOA.[64] BaFPE-TOA and EDI scores for 63 patients diagnosed with eating disorders were analyzed. Low and non-significant correlations resulted in rejection of the hypothesis. However, these results are consistent with Stanton, et al., who stated that "feelings of ineffectiveness, often verbalized by anorexic patients are not always related to poor performance."[59] Interestingly, Wozniak reported a low to moderate but non-significant correlation between the total TOA score and the EDI perfectionism subscale score. Konieczny later found that the smallest difference in TOA scores between subjects with an eating disorder and non-diagnosed subjects were on the performance component total and the task completion, errors, and efficiency parameters.[48]

Skilled Nursing Residents

Applicability of the TOA with skilled nursing residents was studied by Mann and Small Russ.[65] They analyzed TOA data on 13 male and 29 female residents aged 47 to 93 years old (M = 75.4). Approximately 25% (range = 17 to 29%) of the residents were rated at the lowest possible score on the five TOA tasks suggesting that the "TOA is appropriate for nursing home patients at the middle and higher end of cognitive and physical abilities, but for some patients...it is not practical."[64] The authors offer a number of examples to illustrate how lack of stimulation in the nursing home environment influences resident behavior, which is reflected in poor performance on the TOA and interpretation of drawings completed in the Kinetic Person Drawing task.

The authors suggest various opportunities that should be afforded nursing home residents to improve quality of care. Although they suggest that the TOA may not be appropriate for up to 25% of this population, the use of such tools as the TOA possibly could help therapists develop appropriate treatment programs for residents.

Evaluation of Patient Progress in Research Studies

The TOA was reported useful for evaluating patient progress to compare the effectiveness of a cognitive rehabilitation treatment modality to a traditional one-to-one task-oriented approach for attention disorder in 29 patients with chronic schizophrenia. Although study results indicated no significant difference between the two treatment methods, patients showed significant improvement on scores in the

TOA Sorting Shells task and on the self-confidence and motivation parameters across four of the five tasks and on the efficiency parameter across all five TOA tasks.[66]

The SIS was used by Staron to evaluate changes in patients' interpersonal communication skills in a study in which the effectiveness of verbally oriented versus activities-oriented group treatment approaches in a psychiatric day treatment program were compared.[67] The SIS was administered prior to and at the completion of a 12-week treatment protocol. Eighteen patients received the oral therapy approach in 45-minute/once-per-week treatment groups, while 17 patients received the same amount of an activities-oriented approach. All patients continued to receive the same treatment services regularly provided in the program. Results indicated that there were no significant differences between the two treatment methods, but patients in both groups showed significant improvement in SIS scores.

FURTHER RESEARCH

Variations in BaFPE Administration

Results of the survey conducted by Managh and Cook described earlier, showed variations in occupational therapists' use of the BaFPE. Common variations included not using the QSRI, not using the SIS, modifying the administration and scoring of the TOA, and infrequent reference to the available normative data.[57]

Approximately 20% of therapists reported they never used the QSRI. Almost 50% of therapists who did use the QSRI only used it if the patient previously exhibited organic signs. Some therapists indicated they could identify signs of organic involvement in other situations without the QSRI. Lack of use of the SIS was attributed to lack of time to rate the SIS and because social interaction was already routinely assessed in therapy groups.

Common modifications to the TOA protocol involved altering task timing by allowing patients to finish tasks, even if allowable time had expired; altering the TOA verbatim instructions because they were viewed by some therapists as demeaning or because they wanted to ensure patient success on the task; and not following the scoring protocol due to lack of time. Few therapists used the TOA norms because of concern about the small sample size or lack of comparative reference for patients they were evaluating.

When variations such as these are made to test protocol, therapists are no longer administering a standardized test. Although lack of use of the SIS is apparently common, as demonstrated by Managh and Cook's survey results and the lack of published studies on the SIS (compared to the TOA), therapists are only assessing task-oriented behavior and not functional performance as intended by the test authors. Further research in this area is presently being conducted in preparation for development of the third edition of the BaFPE.

Development of a Shorter TOA

Development of a shortened version of the TOA, containing only 24 rather than 60 ratings, has been explored.[56] Using multiple regression and factor analyses on data originally used to formulate the 1991 TOA standard scores,[55] four parameter ratings were eliminated (attention span, evidence of thought disorder, efficiency, and motivation/compliance), as well as two tasks (home drawing and block design). The correlation of total TOA scores between the full and shortened versions of the TOA was high ($r = .94$). Further research on a shortened version of the TOA that takes into account patient diagnosis, age, gender, and education is being conducted.[68]

SUMMARY

Research on the use of the BaFPE continues. Therapists are invited and encouraged by the test authors to participate in the ongoing testing and refinement of the BaFPE, and in the development of national norms for the TOA and SIS. Therapists who do not see themselves as *researchers* or who cannot find the time to conduct research in their own clinics may become involved in BaFPE research by developing relationships with academics or other researchers currently working on the BaFPE. The therapist can serve an important role in the research process by securing approval from the clinic or hospital administration to collect research data in the therapist's department. It is important to note that graduate occupational therapy students have made useful contributions to the current research on the BaFPE. Developing relationships with graduate occupational therapy students, who may be studying the BaFPE, is another possible avenue for therapists to become involved in clinical research.

REFERENCES

1. Bloomer J, Williams S. *The Bay Area Functional Performance Evaluation*, research ed. Palo Alto, Calif: Consulting Psychologists Press; 1979:12,15.
2. Mosey A. *Three Frames of Reference for Mental Health*. Thorofare, NJ: SLACK Incorporated; 1970.
3. Reilly M. A psychiatric OT program as a teaching model. *Am J Occup Ther*. 1966;20:61-67.
4. Reilly M. The educational process. *Am J Occup Ther*. 1969;23:299-307.
5. King L. Toward a science of adaptive responses—1978 Eleanor Clarke Slagle Lecture. *Am J Occup Ther*. 1978;32:429-437.
6. Spencer E. Functional restoration. In Hopkins H, Smith H. *Willard and Spackman's Occupational Therapy*, 5th ed. Philadelphia, Pa: Lippincott; 1978:336.
7. Kielhofner G. A model of human occupation, part 2. Ontogenesis from the perspective of temporal adaptation. *Am J Occup Ther*. 1980;34:657-663.
8. Kielhofner G. A model of human occupation, part 3. Benign and vicious cycles. *Am J Occup Ther*. 1980;34:731-737.
9. Kielhofner G. The model of human occupation. In Kielhofner G. *Conceptual Foundations of Occupational Therapy*. Philadelphia, Pa: FA Davis; 1992:154-169.
10. Kielhofner G, Burke J. A model of human occupation, part 1. Conceptual framework and content. *Am J Occup Ther*. 1980;34:572-581.
11. Kielhofner G, Burke J, Igi C. A model of human occupation, part 4. Assessment and intervention. *Am J Occup Ther*. 1980;34:777-788.
12. Houston D, Williams S, Bloomer J, Mann W. The Bay Area Functional Performance Evaluation: Development and standardization. *Am J Occup Ther*. 1989;43:170-183.
13. Bloomer J, Williams S. The Bay Area Functional Performance Evaluation. In Hemphill B. *The Evaluative Process in Psychiatric Occupational Therapy*. Thorofare, NJ: SLACK Incorporated; 1982:255-308.
14. Williams S, Bloomer J. *Bay Area Functional Performance Evaluation*, 2nd ed. Palo Alto, Calif: Consulting Psychologists Press; 1987:1-2,11.

15. Bloomer J, Williams S, Houston D. In progress—short reports on psychosocial assessment, The Bay Area Functional Performance Evaluation. *OTMH*. 1980;1(2):41-42.

16. Bellack A. Recurrent problems in the behavioral assessment of social skills. *Behavior Research and Therapy*. 1983;21(1):29-41.

17. Carlsmith J, Ellsworth P, Aronson E. *Methods of Research in Social Psychology*. Reading, Mass: Addison-Wesley; 1976.

18. Kazdin A. *Behavior Modification in Applied Settings*. Homewood, Ill: The Dorsey Press; 1975:67-82.

19. Murphy K, Martin C, Garcia M. Do behavior observation scales measure observation? *Journal of Applied Psychology*. 1982;67(5):562-567.

20. Paul G, Lentz R. *Psychosocial Treatment of Chronic Mental Patients: Milieu Versus Social Learning Program*. Cambridge, Mass: Harvard University Press; 1977:111-126.

21. Stein F. Research analysis of occupational therapy assessments used in mental health. In Hemphill B. *Mental Health Assessment in Occupational Therapy, An Integrative Approach To the Evaluative Process*. Thorofare, NJ: SLACK Incorporated; 1988:223-247.

22. Ottenbacher K. *Evaluating Clinical Change*. Baltimore, Md: Williams & Wilkins; 1986:84-87.

23. Sarno J, Sarno M, Levita E. The Functional Life Scale. *Archives of Physical Medicine and Rehabilitation*. 1973;54:214-220.

24. Endicott J, Spitzer R, Fleiss J, Cohen J. The Global Assessment Scale. *Archives of General Psychiatry*. 1976;33:766-771.

25. Bortone J. *Functional Component Skills Associated With DSM-III Diagnoses of Schizophrenia and Borderline Personality Disorders* Thesis. New York, NY: New York University; 1984:51.

26. Cheeseman J. *An Investigation of the Concurrent Validity of the Bay Area Functional Performance Evaluation for Patients With Brain Vascular Disease*. Richmond, Va: Virginia Commonwealth University; 1980. Thesis.

27. Jebsen R, Taylor N, Trieschmann R, Trotter M, Howard L. An objective and standardized test of hand function. *Archives of Physical Medicine and Rehabilitation*. 1969;50:311-319.

28. Kaufman L. *A Comparison of Performance on the Bay Area Functional Performance Evaluation and the Kohlman Evaluation of Living Skills by Adult Psychiatric Patients*. Boston, Mass: Sargent College of Allied Health Professions, Boston University; 1982. Thesis.

29. McGourty L. *Kohlman Evaluation of Living Skills*. Seattle, Wash: KELS Research, Box 33201; 1979.

30. Wener-Altman P, Wolfe A, Staley D. Utilization of the Bay Area Functional Performance Evaluation with an adolescent psychiatric population. *Canadian Journal of Occupational Therapy*. 1991;58:129-136.

31. Olson B, Jamal J. *The BaFPE: Standardization and Clinical Application in Acute Adult Psychiatry*. Irvine, Calif: University of California Irvine Medical Center; 1987.

32. Brockett M. Cultural variations in Bay Area Functional Performance Evaluation scores—considerations for occupational therapy. *Canadian Journal of Occupational Therapy*. 1987;54:195-199.

33. Honigfeld G, Gillis R, Klett, C. NOSIE-30: A treatment sensitive ward behavior scale. *Psychological Reports*. 1966;19:180-182.

34. Casanova J, Ferber J. Comprehensive Evaluation of Basic Living Skills. *Am J Occup Ther*. 1976;30:101-105.

35. Accardi M. *The Bay Area Functional Performance Evaluation: A Validity Study*. Boston, Mass: Boston School of Occupational Therapy, Tufts University; 1985. Thesis.

36. Mason J. *Observer Ratings Versus Self-report of Social Interaction As Assessed by the Bay Area Functional Performance Evaluation*. Halifax, Nova Scotia: Dalhousie University; 1985.

37. Francis E, Cermak S. Comparison of two subtests of the Bay Area Functional Performance Evaluation. *OTMH*. 1987;7:99-114.

38. Newman M. *Cognitive Disability and Functional Performance in Individuals With Chronic Schizophrenic Disorders*. Los Angeles, Calif: University of Southern California; 1987. Thesis.

39. Allen, C. *Occupational Therapy for Psychiatric Diseases: Measurement and Management of Cognitive Disabilities*. Boston, Mass: Little, Brown; 1985.

40. Thibeault R, Blackmer E. Validating a test of functional performance with psychiatric patients. *Am J Occup Ther.* 1987;41:515-521.

41. Wechsler D. *WAIS Manual: Wechsler Adult Intelligence Scale.* New York, NY: The Psychological Corporation; 1955.

42. Klyczek J, Mann W. Concurrent validity of the Task-Oriented Assessment component of the Bay Area Functional Performance Evaluation with the American Association on Mental Deficiency Adaptive Behavior Scale. *Am J Occup Ther.* 1990;44:907-912.

43. Nihira K, Foster R, Shellhaas M, Leland H. *AAMD Adaptive Behavior Scale.* Washington, DC: American Association on Mental Deficiency; 1969.

44. Nihira K, Foster R, Shellhaas M, Leland H. *AAMD Adaptive Behavior Scale,* 1974 Revision. Washington, DC: American Association on Mental Deficiency; 1974.

45. Mercer Castilla L, Klyczek J. Comparison of the Kinetic Person Drawing Task of the Bay Area Functional Performance Evaluation with measures of functional performance. *OTMH.* 1993;12(2):27-38.

46. Clark EN, Peters M. *The Scorable Self-Care Evaluation.* Thorofare, NJ: SLACK Incorporated; 1984.

47. Curtin M, Klyczek J. Comparison of BaFPE-TOA scores for inpatients and outpatients. *OTMH.* 1992;12(1):61-75.

48. Konieczny T. *Discriminant Validity of the BaFPE TOA As An Evaluation Tool for Patients With Eating Disorders.* Buffalo, NY: D'Youville College; 1996. Thesis.

49. Lissner J. *Discriminant Validity of the Bay Area Functional Performance Evaluation Task Oriented Assessment.* Buffalo, NY: D'Youville College; 1996. Thesis.

50. Stoffel E. *Discriminant Validity of the Revised Bay Area Functional Performance Evaluation—Task Oriented Assessment for An Elderly Population.* Buffalo, NY: D'Youville College; 1994. Thesis.

51. Tardif M. *Concurrent Validity of the Functional Needs Assessment With the Task Oriented Assessment Component of the Bay Area Functional Performance Evaluation.* Buffalo, NY: D'Youville College; 1993. Thesis.

52. Dombrowski L. *Functional Needs Assessment Program for Chronic Psychiatric Patients.* Tucson, Ariz: Therapy Skill Builders; 1990.

53. Rogers E. *A Study of the Concurrent Validity of the Milwaukee Evaluation of Daily Living Skills With the Bay Area Functional Performance Evaluation.* Buffalo, NY: D'Youville College; 1992. Thesis.

54. Leonardelli C. *The Milwaukee Evaluation of Daily Living Skills: Evaluation in Long-Term Psychiatric Care.* Thorofare, NJ: SLACK Incorporated; 1988.

55. Mann W, Klyczek J. Standard scores for the Bay Area Functional Performance Evaluation Task Oriented Assessment. *OTMH.* 1991;11(1):13-24.

56. Mann W, Huselid R. An abbreviated Task Oriented Assessment (Bay Area Functional Performance Evaluation). *Am J Occup Ther.* 1993;47:111-118.

57. Managh M, Cook J. The use of standardized assessment in occupational therapy: The BaFPE-R as an example. *Am J Occup Ther.* 1993;47:877-884.

58. Mann W, Klyczek J, Fiedler R. Bay Area Functional Performance Evaluation (BaFPE): Standard scores. *OTMH.* 1989;9:1-7.

59. Stanton E, Mann W, Klyczek J. Use of the Bay Area Functional Performance Evaluation with eating disordered patients. *OTJR.* 1991;11(4):227-237,234-235.

60. Peterson B. *A Preliminary Examination of BaFPE-TOA Scores for Adolescents With Psychiatric Disorders.* Buffalo, NY: D'Youville College; 1996. Thesis.

61. Crouch A. *Gender Bias in the Bay Area Functional Performance Evaluation—Task Oriented Assessment.* Buffalo, NY: D'Youville College; 1994. Thesis.

62. Tornabene P. *Gender Differences of a Nonpatient Population on the Bay Area Functional Performance Evaluation.* Buffalo, NY: D'Youville College; 1995. Thesis.

63. Garner D, Olmsted M, Polivy J. Development and validation of a multidimensional eating disorder inventory for anorexia nervosa and bulimia. *International Journal of Eating Disorders.* 1983;2:15-35.

64. Wozniak L. *The BaFPE-TOA and the EDI In Relation To Individuals With a Diagnosis of Eating Disorders* Thesis. Buffalo, NY: D'Youville College; 1991:128.

65. Mann W, Small Russ L. Measuring the functional performance of nursing home patients with the Bay Area Functional Performance Evaluation. *Physical and Occupational Therapy in Geriatrics*. 1991;9(3):113-129.

66. Brown C, Harwood K, Hays C, Heckman J, Short J. Effectiveness of cognitive rehabilitation for improving attention inpatients with schizophrenia. *OTJR*. 1993;13(2):71-86.

67. Staron R. *The Effectiveness of Activity Versus Verbal Therapy in Improving Interpersonal Communication Skills*. Buffalo, NY: D'Youville College; 1992. Thesis.

68. Klyczek J, Bloomer J, Fiedler, R. *Analysis of a Shortened BaFPE Task Oriented Assessment*. Buffalo, NY; D'Youville College; 1999.

7

The Prevocational Assessment Process in Mental Health Occupational Therapy

Margaret L. Hunter, MS, OTR, MA, LLP

For individuals with mental disabilities, seeking employment is often critical to recovery. Self-esteem, social support, community involvement, and finding meaning in life are enhanced by obtaining work. Occupational therapy is based on the notion that work is an essential part of one's psychosocial well-being.[1]

Programs are being developed for patients accessing mental health services as a means of providing vocational training, employment skills training, employment acquisition, and support while on the job.[2] Such programs are based on the psychosocial rehabilitation model, which emphasizes patients advocating for their own needs in a caring, supportive, non-hierarchical setting. Training programs may stress that patients initiate their personal goals/objectives, as opposed to having mental health professionals determine patient needs. Patients are becoming role models for each other.[2] Employment opportunities are broadening, due to the passage of the American Disabilities Act (1990), which mandates equal access to employment for all disabled Americans. Traditional day programs, in which groups are led by mental health professionals in isolated, non-community-based settings, are quickly becoming outdated. Managed care providers as well as patient advocacy groups are insisting that therapists work with patients to develop "real world" employment opportunities with tangible outcomes. The traditional state mental institutions, whose tendency to allow for lengthened stays, are downsizing and integrating individuals into community settings.

Occupational therapy has responded to the changes in deinstitutionalization, managed care demands, and patient advocacy group needs, while recognizing occupational therapy history and theory are based on this paradigm shift. The basic human drive toward meaningful occupation is primary when providing occupational therapy for individuals with mental illness. The purpose of this chapter is to provide a guideline for occupational therapy assessment of prevocational skills of patients seeking mental health treatment.

The assessment process, ideally used when determining the needs and capabilities of individuals with mental illness, must reflect psychosocial sensitivity, functional outcomes, and patient preference. The occupational therapist can no longer decide independently which assessments are best to use without including the patient. Prior to establishing the assessment process, the occupational therapist has a thorough understanding of the diagnosis, medications, patient history, and interests.

ASSESSMENT PROCESS

Diagnoses/Background Information

Mental health patients have broad and often idiosyncratic illnesses. Needs are unique and require a sensitive approach when inquiring about the nature of the symptoms and how these affect an individual's ability to perform work activities. Occupational therapists who can use the *Diagnostic and Statistical Manual of Mental Disorders*, 4th edition, (DSM-IV)[3] will be able to follow the diagnoses provided by psychiatrists and psychologists. These tools are limited, however, and validity and reliability are minimal for both measurement tools. In addition, diagnostic categories are poor predictors of vocational success (12 in 13). Occupational therapists can turn to Claudia Allen's[4] levels of cognitive functioning to establish an understanding of a patient's status when chronic mental illness is present. Vocational assessment is based on a clear understanding of how symptoms interfere with functional skills over time. Adults experiencing psychotic symptoms will have different support needs than do individuals with chronic depression, anxiety disorders, or developmental delays. Occupational therapists can use behavioral observation, patient interview, patient records, and family interviews to obtain background information useful for vocational assessment.[5] Medications and their side effects; precautions, such as limited exposure to sunlight; and medical procedures related to certain diagnoses are beneficial to determine. All physical problems such as a history of back pain, chronic fatigue syndrome, old bone fractures, abnormal muscle tone, migraine headaches, and asthma should be identified as a means of establishing the vocational assessment.

Occupational Therapy Prevocational Assessment Process

The occupational therapy prevocational assessment package is designed to correlate with desired and available employment opportunities.[6] Performing standardized prevocational assessments that are unrelated to available employment will most likely not be reimbursed and will result in ineffective job placement.

The assessment process varies significantly when evaluating patients with chronic mental illness who have lost skills and self-image as an employed member of society, versus evaluating patients experiencing acute, episodic mental illness. A severe, yet brief depression can be a temporary period of unemployment in which skills are preserved. Individuals with acute and chronic illness need to be closely involved in determining appropriate assessments. An effective first step is to find a comfortable setting, preferably a non-clinical environment, if the patient is stabilized on medication, and determine a work history and current interests in employment, as well as the emotional impact of either returning to work, seeking training, or applying for a new job.

Occupational therapists practicing in mental health use the Interest Inventory to determine prevocational interests more than any other evaluation.[7] The Interest Inventory can be filled out after discussing its content in a friendly and open conversation.[8] Interest inventories can also include media, such as a slide presentation of various occupations,[9] or computer programs outlining occupational options and related skills. The method of gathering patient preferences needs to be determined by patients and therapists, working as a team, or by having successfully employed patients interviewing and educating less experienced patients.[2] Vocational interest inventories can be found in journals or created for specific programs, taking job market concerns into consideration. The focus of this process needs to be on skills, opportunities, and options versus deficits and failures. A narrative of the patient's work history can accompany an interest inventory.

Support/Needs/Accommodations

A significant indicator of the mental health patient's employment success is the level and type of support available.[10] When a patient has family, friends, and/or a community providing encouragement to work or receive training, the outcome is higher.[10]

Supported employment programs are available with some mental health programs in which either the employer or therapeutic staff assists the patient in training and provides support to stay on the job. The assessment should include discerning the kind of support needed to either enter or re-enter the workplace or to keep the job if acute phases of the illness occur. In addition, the occupational therapy assessment includes identifying support people in the patient's life who can provide encouragement to obtain a job.

This information can be obtained by asking the patient questions, such as:

1. Is there anyone close to you who would like you to work/get training?
2. When previous employment did not work out, would more support have helped you stay? What would that support have included?
3. What motivates you to stay employed?
4. Describe why you left your previous jobs.

Patients experiencing reactive depression; acute anxiety, with or without a phobic response; acute manic-depressive episodes; post-traumatic stress disorder resulting in anxiety or depression; or acute compulsive disorders need to be evaluated for job-related stressors that induce mental illness. Reasonable accommodations can then possibly be identified. Individuals experiencing somatic complaints, such as undiagnosed chronic pain, in which mental or emotional illness has either resulted from the pain or created the pain, need to be provided with questions similar to those for patients with diagnosed mental illness.

For patients of a mental health program who have lost skills or work-related behaviors, or who want to seek new training or a new type of job, the assessment includes evaluation of existing skills related to desired and available employment. Managed care providers are often unwilling to reimburse training costs if skills are sufficiently intact to permit the return to previous employment. Reasonable accommodations are often less costly than training.

The content of many vocational assessments often is not applicable to patients who are attempting to return to their original jobs.[1] The work force is moving away from unskilled factory jobs and toward the service industry.[11] This change is an example of the need for new psychiatric occupational therapy vocational assessments that mimic current job market trends and include the social and emotional aspects of new working environments.

Evaluating Skills

Deciding to evaluate prevocational skills as they correlate with specific job tasks or essential job functions is done when individuals have not retained skills to return to previously held jobs, or when time and reimbursement allow for seeking new employment. If the assessment reveals that more training is needed or that reasonable accommodations are appropriate, the patient, the potential employer, and the third-party payee can be provided with assessment results to determine reimbursement options.

Despite the theoretical emphasis on work in occupational therapy, few standardized work evaluations specific to the profession are available in the area of mental health practice.[1] Vocational evaluators have developed testing in the following areas: motor skills in tests, such as the Valpar; interest inventories such as the Strong-Campbell Vocational Interest Inventory;[12] aptitude and achievement tests; and work samples.[1] Occupational therapists use tests from the vocational rehabilitation profession, as well as from psychology, behavioral medicine, and sports medicine.[1]

With the emphasis on psychosocial rehabilitation, occupational therapy in community- and hospital-based programs can use the following assessments to determine prevocational skills:

1. Situational Assessment—observing a patient perform job tasks in a sheltered employment setting, either in a work-therapy unit or workshop where actual conditions of a job outside the unit are simulated.[5] A checklist of skills and behaviors can be used to identify strengths and needs.[13]
2. Functional Capacity Evaluation—observing and recording a patient's functional tolerances of lifting, motor coordination, finger and hand dexterity. Normative data are available.[14]
3. Work Tolerance Screening (WTS)—a physical and functional assessment of the injured worker. The emphasis is on tasks specific to a desired type of work. WTS evaluates the patient's physical and psychological abilities to perform work.
4. Job Try-Out—a final step of evaluation wherein the patient works for a brief period, at no charge to the employer, performing on the actual job. The occupational therapist evaluates performance, how motivated the patient is to proceed with getting the job, and the need for reasonable accommodations.
5. Work Samples—tasks, materials, and tools used in jobs, and range from simple to complex.[15] The Pennsylvania Bi-Manual Worksample[16] measures finger dexterity of both hands, gross movements of both arms, eye-hand and bimanual coordination, and the ability to use both hands in cooperation.[17]
6. The Bay Area Functional Performance Evaluation (BaFPE)—an assessment that uses tasks to determine a patient's ability to participate in goal-directed activity and his or her ability to demonstrate appropriate behaviors.[18]
7. The Baltimore Therapeutic Equipment Work Simulator (BTE)—objectively evaluates the functional capacity, using an instrument to determine strength, movement, force exerted, work done, and power output for specific tasks. Objective data is provided via a computer printout.[19]
8. The Valpar Component Work—work samples that eliminate reading and language skills. Several individual components are available to permit vocational exploration.[9]

Several assessments are available to determine motor coordination, including the Purdue Pegboard, Crawford Small Parts Dexterity Test, and the Bennett Hand-Tool Dexterity Test.[20]

Table 7-1

Psychiatric Occupational Therapy Prevocational Assessment Process

Gather Background Information
a. Work history, education, and training background
b. Current medications and their side effects
c. History of mental and physical illnesses
d. Factors/stressors influencing symptomatology

Determine Consumer Work Interests and Support Systems
a. Available emotional support persons
b. Cultural/familial influences affecting employment
c. Skills needed for most recent employment
    1. Is that job still available?
    2. Will employer rehire?
    3. Are skills still in place?
    4. Does patient want to return to the job?

Return to Most Recent Employment
a. Identify job stressors
b. Identify accommodations needed to stay employed
c. Identify strategies needed to be practiced to return to work (eg, relaxation techniques, medication management, cognitive therapy, etc)
d. If c. is not an option, which employment opportunities are considered desired by consumer?
    1. Which skills are needed for identified employment?
    2. What training is needed?
    3. Is a job analysis needed?

Assess Skill Level for Employment Opportunity
a. Determine assessments directly relating to employment tasks
    1. Work tolerance screening
    2. Functional capacity evaluation
    3. Simulated job try-out
    4. Work samples
    5. Standardized assessments for specific job tasks
b. Consider a work behavior assessment
c. Determine job interview skills

Assess for Reasonable Accommodations

Work behaviors are significant indicators of the ability to hold a job.[21] Vocational behaviors evolve as an individual develops (7 to 9 years of age). The cultural influences and childhood development of worker traits (attitude, punctuality, appearance, acceptance of supervision, attitude toward peers, productivity, and the degree to which work is valued within early family relationships) significantly affect vocational choice.[10] Several occupational therapy programs have developed evaluations of prevocational behaviors, such as the Prevocational Evaluation of Rehabilitation Potential, developed at Northville State Hospital in Michigan. The 20 items rate such behaviors as socialization, hostility, peer adjustment, and ability to work with others.[22] Behavioral tests can be completed with patients rating themselves and with sensitive feedback from the therapist.

All prevocational assessments can be used to assist the occupational therapist and the patient in identifying support needs and accommodations, as opposed to focusing on how the patient needs to change or become better able to work.

SUMMARY

Occupational therapy has a long and rich history of providing vocational evaluation and treatment, yet few standardized occupational therapy vocational assessments are available to use with mental health patients.[1] Mental health occupational therapy is moving into community-based centers, where psychosocial rehabilitation is the foundation for treatment. Patients of mental health and occupational therapists now need to work as mutual members of the therapeutic team. Providing vocational assessments requires a match between patient interests, motivation, skill level, and job market opportunities.

The assessment process moves from a casual interview and obtaining background information, to an actual job try-out. Employers, community members, and therapeutic staff can all be part of the process of determining suitable employment for mental health patients. For an overview of the assessment process, see Table 7-1.

REFERENCES

1.   Velozo CA. Work evaluations: Critique of the state of the art of functional assessment of work. *Am J Occup Ther.* 1993;47:203-209.
2.   Tappen BE. New opportunities for mental health OTs. *OT Week.* 1996;10(9):16-17.
3.   American Psychiatric Association. *Diagnostic and Statistical Manual of Mental Disorders,* 4th ed. Washington, DC: Author; 1994.
4.   Allen CK. Activity: Occupational therapy's treatment method. *Am J Occup Ther.* 1987;41:565-575.
5.   Lloyd C, Fiqir N. Vocational evaluation: The use of work samples. *Australian Occupational Therapy Journal.* 1990;37:185-189.
6.   Oxley C. Devising an assessment package for an employment rehabilitation service. *British Journal of Occupational Therapy.* 1992;55:448-452.
7.   Anderson AP. Work potential evaluation in mental health. *Am J Occup Ther.* 1985;39:659-663.
8.   Smith PC, Bohmfalk JS. Vocational evaluation in the private sector: An occupational therapy approach. *Occupational Therapy in Health Care.* 1985/1986;2(4):27-35.
9.   Lloyd C. Vocational evaluation in a forensic psychiatric setting. *Canadian Journal of Occupational Therapy.* 1986;53:31-34.
10.   Holmes D. The role of the occupational therapist—work evaluator. *Am J Occup Ther.* 1985;39:308-313.
11.   A closer look at the changing workforce. *Kalamazoo Gazette.* March 31, 1996:46.
12.   Strong EK Jr, Campbell DP. *Strong-Campbell Interest Inventory,* revised ed. Palo Alto, Calif: Consulting Psychologists Press; 1981.
13.   Palmer F, Gatti D. Vocational Treatment Model. *Occupational Therapy in Mental Health.* 1985;5(1):41-58.
14.   Smith SL, Cunningham S, Weinberg R. The predictive validity of the functional capacity evaluation. *Am J Occup Ther.* 1986;40:564-567.
15.   Botterbusch KF. *Vocational Assessment and Evaluation Systems: A Comparison.* Menomonie, Wis: Materials Development Center, Stout Rehabilitation Institute School of Education and Human Services; 1987.
16.   Roberts JR. *Pennsylvania Bi-Manual Worksample,* 2nd ed. Circle Pines, Minn: American Guidance Service; 1969.
17.   Paul S. Test-retest reliability study of the Pennsylvania Bi-Manual Worksample. *Am J Occup Ther.* 1992;46:809-812.

18.   Houston D, Williams SL, Bloomer J, Mann, WC. The Bay Area Functional Performance Evaluation: Development and standardization. *Am J Occup Ther.* 1989;43:170-183.

19.   Bhambhani Y, Esmail S, Brintnell S. The Baltimore Therapeutic Equipment Work Simulator: Biomechanical and physiological norms for three attachments in healthy men. *Am J Occup Ther.* 1994;48(1):19-24.

20.   Jacobs K. *Occupational Therapy: Work-related Programs and Assessment*, 3rd ed. Boston, Mass: Little, Brown; 1991.

21.   Biernacki SD. Reliability of the worker role interview. *Am J Occup Ther.* 1993;47:797-803.

22.   Stauffer DL. *Treatment of the Chronic Schizophrenic Patient.* New York, NY: Hawthorne Press; 1986:31-49.

BIBLIOGRAPHY

Anthony WA, Jansen MA. Predicting the vocational capacity of the chronically mentally ill in research and policy implications. *American Psychologists.* 1984;39:537-544.

Asher IE. *An Annotated Index of Occupational Therapy Evaluation Tools.* Rockville, Md: American Occupational Therapy Association, Inc; 1989.

Matheson L, Ogden LD. *Work Tolerance Screening.* Trabuco Canyon, Calif: RISC Publishing; 1983.

Nelson RR, Condrin JI. *Evaluation and Treatment of Adults: A Vocational Readiness and Independent Living Skills Program for Psychiatrically Impaired Adolescents.* New York, NY: Hawthorne Press; 1987.

Radonsky VE, Haffenbreidel J, Harper C, Kligman K, Timms C. Occupational therapy in vocational readiness. *Occupational Therapy in Mental Health.* 1987;7:83-91.

Richert GZ. Vocational transition in acute care psychiatry. *Occupational Therapy in Mental Health.* 1990;10(4):43-61.

8

Performance Assessment of Self-Care Skills

Margo B. Holm, PhD, OTR/L, FAOTA, ABDA
Joan C. Rogers, PhD, OTR/L, FAOTA

The Performance Assessment of Self-Care Skills (PASS), version 3.1, is a performance-based observational tool. It is designed to assist therapists in the documentation of status and change in the performance of functional mobility (MOB), personal care activities of daily living (ADL), and instrumental activities of daily living (IADL). The tool enables therapists to rate the performance of each MOB, ADL, and IADL task from the perspective of three separate concepts—independence, safety, and task outcome. The PASS is also designed to assist therapists in treatment and discharge planning by identifying the type and amount of assistance required for successful task performance, as well as for risks to safety and the specific point of task breakdown. The purpose of this chapter is to describe the PASS in terms of its rationale, structure, and scientific properties.

THEORETICAL BASE

Interactive, or dynamic, assessment[1-3] is one theoretical base for the design and structure of the PASS. The creator of the interactive assessment approach is considered by most to be Vygotsky (1896-1934), a Soviet psychologist.[4] Vygotsky described a zone of proximal (potential) development, as the difference between a patient's independent performance on a test and the performance when the patient was assisted or guided on a test.[4] Interactive assessment consists of establishing the level of performance without assistance, the type and amount of assistance required for improved performance, and the outcome of the mediation on later task performance.[5]

The second theoretical base used in the design and structure of the PASS is graduated prompting.[6-7] Graduated prompting incorporates a hierarchy of prompts that are used only when there is a breakdown in task performance, and then only in a specific sequence. Hierarchies can be based on the power of the assist,[8] the cost of the assist based on the interventionist's time, or the level of intrusiveness to the prompt recipient.[7]

All 26 PASS task items consist of criterion-referenced subtasks, which the therapist uses to rate performance. The patient is given standardized directions, and standardized task materials are presented in the clinic. In the home, however, patients use their own task materials. Independence in task performance is rated, using an interactive assessment approach. When a patient is no longer able to proceed independently with a task (point of task breakdown), the therapist uses a 9-level system of graduated prompts to facilitate initiation or continuation of task performance. The type and number of prompts are recorded by appropriate subtask, to identify the patient's potential for task performance, and the type or number of assists that enable successful task performance. This blending of interactive assessment and graduated prompting yields a profile of patient performance that identifies the exact point of task breakdown, the type and number of assists that the patient needed for successful task performance during the assessment, and the types of assists that support the patient's potential task performance. In addition, the profile of assists identifies the specific types of assists that are beneficial to a patient, in other words, those that enable improved or successful task performance. These data are critical for efficient intervention planning and discharge planning in today's health care environment.

HISTORICAL DEVELOPMENT

The initial version of the PASS was developed by Rogers[9] and consisted of a performance test involving ADL/IADL situations. The original PASS was used with patients with probable Alzheimer's disease and with normal elderly.[10-11] A revised instrument was developed in 1988 by Rogers and Holm[12] for use in clinical practice and research and included two versions, PASS-Clinic (PASS-C) and PASS-Home (PASS-H). The PASS 3.1 is used for clinic and home assessments[13-17] and is also being used currently in two large federally funded clinical research projects.

DESCRIPTION OF THE INSTRUMENT

Format of the Instrument

The PASS consists of 26 tasks—five functional mobility (MOB), three personal self-care (ADL), and 18 instrumental activities of daily living (IADL) (Table 8-1). Because the instrument was designed to assess which types of assistance are necessary for a patient to return to the community (PASS-C) or remain in the community (PASS-H), the instrument has a disproportionate emphasis on IADL. Both versions of the PASS include the same tasks and subtask criteria, and the same directions. Only the task materials differ, with task materials being provided in the clinic and with patients using their own task materials in the home.

Task Materials and Equipment

Common household items are used, and specifications are listed in the manual. Items are purchased by the therapist to develop the kits. The PASS-Clinic kit requires more items than the PASS-Home kit, including some adaptive equipment (lighted magnifying glass, large LCD calculator), which may already be present in a clinic. It is recommended that the kit for the PASS-Home be transported in a small rolling suitcase.

Conditions and Instructions

Each PASS item includes directions for assessment, *Conditions and Instructions*. *Conditions* includes context for the item, eg, kitchen, bathroom, stairway, the materials and equipment and how they are to be arranged, and the position of the patient, eg, seated at a table, positioned next to the foot of the bed. *Instructions* includes the standardized wording for the instructions to be given to the patient, as well as cues to the therapist, eg, wait for response.

Table 8-1

Items in the PASS-Clinic and PASS-Home

Task	Focus	PASS Item
1	MOB	Bed Transfers
2	MOB	Stair Use
3	MOB	Toilet Transfers
4	ADL	Oral Hygiene
5	MOB	Bathtub and Shower Transfers
6	ADL	Trimming Toenails
7	ADL	Dressing
8	IADL	Money Management: Shopping
9	IADL	Money Management: Bill Paying by Check
10	IADL	Money Management: Checkbook Balancing
11	IADL	Money Management: Mailing Bills
12	IADL	Heavy Housework: Bending, Lifting, Carrying Out the Garbage
13	IADL	Telephone Use
14	IADL	Medication Management
15	IADL	Heavy Housework: Changing Bed Linens
16	IADL	Current Events: Obtaining Critical Information from the Media (Auditory)
17	IADL	Current Events: Obtaining Critical Information from the Media (Visual)
18	IADL	Home Maintenance: Small Repairs
19	IADL	Home Maintenance: Sweeping
20	MOB	Indoor Walking
21	IADL	Environmental Awareness: Home Safety
22	IADL	Leisure: Playing Bingo
23	IADL	Meal Preparation: Oven Use
24	IADL	Meal Preparation: Stovetop Use
25	IADL	Meal Preparation: Use of Sharp Utensils
26	IADL	Light Housework: Cleanup After Meal Preparation

Rating and Scoring

Each PASS task item is subdivided into critical subtasks for rating purposes. This allows the therapist to identify the specific point or points in the task sequence where breakdown occurs, and to record the type and number of assists necessary for safe and successful task completion. Critical subtasks are noted further, for rating purposes, by delineating which aspects of the subtasks are rated for *Independence*, and which are rated for *Outcome* (process of task performance, and the quality of the task product when appropriate).

On the rating form, under *Independence* data, for each subtask, a grid of hierarchical assists is presented for the therapist to check off for each type of assist given for the patient to accomplish a critical subtask. The assist hierarchy includes nine levels of graduated prompts. When a task cannot be performed independently, the therapist provides the minimal type and amount (frequency and duration) of assistance to facilitate task performance, safety, and an acceptable outcome. The types of assistance, beginning with the least assistive and progressing to the most assistive are: 1) verbal supportive, 2) verbal non-directive, 3) verbal directive, 4) gestures, 5) task object or environmental rearrangement, 6) demonstration, 7) physical guidance, 8) physical support, and 9) total assist. The grid is left blank if the patient performs the subtask independently.

Performance *Outcome* data are also gathered during task performance, and the rating form includes a grid for noting problems in the quality of subtask performance and the process of subtask performance. For each subtask criterion, sample quality standards are provided. Process outcome data are linked to task actions and are rated for the precision, economy of effort, and completeness with which a subtask is performed. Each time an assist is provided, the therapist must note whether the assist was given to improve the quality or the process of task outcome, or for task *Safety*.

Task *Safety* data are also anchored to each subtask. The therapist checks the grid opposite the subtask if any risks to safety are observed during task performance or if the therapist is required to intervene because of a risk to patient safety. Therefore, the PASS helps to identify the specific aspect of task performance where safety concerns were evident.

PASS items yield three distinct category scores—independence, safety, and outcome. Each category is scored on a predefined 4-point ordinal scale (Table 8-2). Independence for a PASS item consists of the mean of all subtasks item scores. Safety is scored considering the data from all subtasks, from the viewpoint of total task safety. Outcome is also scored for the total task, using the combined safety and outcome data. For outcome, if quality and process yield different scores, the lower of the two scores is used so that the patient is not put in a situation of risk through overestimation of outcome.

Since the PASS is criterion-referenced (the patient is rated according to established performance criteria), it may be given in total, or selected items may be used alone or in combination. Items chosen for administration can thus reflect the referral, and appropriate data can be gathered for making intervention plans or decisions regarding discharge disposition.

POPULATION

The PASS is designed for use with adults in the occupational therapy clinic or in the home. Although originally designed for a psychiatric population, the PASS has been administered to over 500 adults from various diagnostic populations. In addition to the well-elderly, it has been used with patients from the following diagnostic populations: dementia, depression, schizophrenia, mental retardation, traumatic brain injury, arthritis, cardiopulmonary disease, multiple sclerosis, cerebrovascular accident, spinal cord injury, and macular degeneration.

RELIABILITY AND VALIDITY

Reliability

Test-retest reliability was established by administering the PASS to 20 older adults, four well-elderly, and four subjects from each of the following diagnostic populations: arthritis, cardiopulmonary disease, dementia, and depression. Following clinical practice, the PASS-C was administered first, with retest occurring 1 day later; the PASS-H was administered 3 days later, with retest likewise occurring

Table 8-2
PASS Rating System for Summary Scores

Score	Independence	Safety	Outcome	
			Quality	Process
3	No assists given for task initiation, continuation, or completion	Safe practices were observed	Acceptable (Standards met)	Subtasks performed with precision and economy of effort and action
2	No Level 7-9 assists given, but occasional Level 1-6 assists given	Minor risks were evident but no assistance provided	Acceptable (Standards met but improvement possible)	Subtasks generally performed with precision and economy of effort and action; occasional lack of efficiency, redundant or extraneous actions; no missing steps
1	No Level 9 assists given; occasional Level 7 or 8 assists given, or continuous Level 1-6 assists given	Risks to safety were observed and assistance given to prevent potential harm	Marginal (Standards partially met)	Subtasks generally performed with lack of precision and/or economy of effort and action; consistent extraneous or redundant actions; steps may be missing
0	Level 9 assists given, or continuous Level 7 or 8 assists given or unable to initiate, continue, or complete subtask or task	Risks to safety of such severity were observed that task was stopped or taken over by the therapist to prevent harm	Unacceptable (Standards not met)	Subtasks are consistently performed with lack of precision and/or economy of effort and action so that task progress is unattainable

1 day later. PASS-C test-retest reliability was Independence, $r = .92$; Safety, 89% agreement; and Outcome, $r = .82$. PASS-H test-retest reliability was Independence, $r = .96$; Safety, .90% agreement; and Outcome, $r = .97$.

Interrater reliability was established by administering the PASS to 25 older adults from the same diagnostic categories. A total of five different therapists participated in dyads. Percentage agreement between 21 raters for the PASS-C was Independence, 92%; Safety, 93%; and Outcome, 90%. PASS-H interrater agreement between 26 raters was Independence, 96%; Safety, 97%; and Outcome, 88%.

Validity

Content validity of the PASS is based on the interview schedules of the OARS Multidimensional Functional Assessment Questionnaire—Activities of Daily Living,[18] the Comprehensive Assessment and Referral,[19] the rating scales for Physical Self-Maintenance and Instrumental Self-Maintenance,[20] and the Functional Assessment Questionnaire.[21] MOB/ADL/IADL categories, tasks, and task specifications explored in these instruments were delineated. Performance test items were then developed for each category, excluding transportation, incorporating as many of the task specifications as possible.

Evidence of the construct validity of the PASS is gleaned from four investigations. In the first study, the IADL scores of patients with primary degenerative dementia were found to be proportionally lower and to have more variability than ADL scores. In the second study, control subjects exhibited the highest level of performance, followed by patients with depression, then those with dementia. These results are consistent with the hierarchy of ADL and IADL and expected differences in level of ADL/IADL disability based on diagnosis and impairment severity.[10] In the third study, of 119 elderly females over 75 years of age (M=79.82, SD=4.32), the overall mean score on the PASS-C was highest for well-elderly (n=44, M = 2.84), followed by patients with depression (n=18, M = 2.80), cardiopulmonary disease (n=18, M = 2.77), osteoarthritis (n=33, M = 2.77), and dementia (n=6, M = 2.41). ANOVA indicated that the dementia group performed significantly worse than all other groups (df = 4, F = 7.66, $P < .001$), LSD = .106 ($P < .05$) and that the cardiopulmonary and osteoarthritis groups performed significantly worse than the well-elderly group (LSD = .106, $P < .05$). Conceptually this makes sense, because the dementia group exhibited more disabilities with the more complex IADLs, and the cardiopulmonary and osteoarthritis groups exhibited more disabilities with the MOB and ADL items, and the IADLs that included lifting, carrying, walking, and standing. In the fourth study, with the same subjects in their homes, the overall mean score on the PASS-H was highest for well-elderly (n=44, M = 2.91), followed again by patients with depression (n=18, M = 2.84), cardiopulmonary disease (n=18, M = 2.80), osteoarthritis (n=33, M = 2.80), and dementia (n=6, M = 2.30). ANOVA indicated that the dementia group again performed significantly worse than all other groups (df = 4, F = 8.74, $P < .001$), LSD = .123 ($P < .05$), and that both the osteoarthritis and the cardiopulmonary groups performed significantly worse than the well-elderly group (LSD = .123, $P < .05$). Again, this makes conceptual sense, because the dementia group exhibited more disabilities with the more complex IADLs, and the cardiopulmonary and osteoarthritis groups exhibited more disabilities with the MOB and ADL items, and the IADLs that included reaching, lifting, carrying, walking, and standing in the home. Since the PASS-C and the PASS-H test capability, it is internally consistent that the depressed subjects would perform second to the well-elderly, for theirs is not a problem of task performance, but rather of impaired motivation to initiate MOB, ADL, and IADL tasks.

SUMMARY

The PASS is a criterion-referenced, performance-based observational tool that helps therapists to distinguish among three aspects of MOB, ADL, and IADL performance—independence, safety, and outcomes. The use of critical subtasks under each task item helps the therapist to identify the exact point of task breakdown as well as task disabilities due to deficits in independence, safety, or quality of task outcome. The PASS also assists therapists in the identification of those tasks that patients can perform independently, safely, and with precision and economy of effort. Since the PASS is criterion-referenced, it may be given in total, or selected items may be used alone or in combination. The tool is quickly learned, even by novice therapists, and the data derived from the tool can be immediately used for intervention planning or discharge planning.

REFERENCES

1. Fuerstein R, Rand Y, Hoffman MB. *The Dynamic Assessment of Retarded Performers: The Learning Potential Assessment Device—Theory, Instruments and Techniques.* Baltimore, Md: University Park Press; 1979.

2. Missiuna C. Dynamic assessment: A model for broadening assessment in occupational therapy. *Canadian Journal of Occupational Therapy.* 1987;54:17-21.

3. Tzuriel D, Haywood HC. The development of interactive-dynamic approaches to assessment of learning potential. In Haywood HC, Tzurial D. *Interactive Assessment.* New York, NY: Springer-Verlag; 1991:3-37.

4. Vygotsky LS. *Mind in Society: The Development of Higher Psychological Processes.* Cambridge, Mass: Harvard University Press; 1978.

5. Haywood HC, Tzuriel D, Vaught S. Psychoeducational assessment from a transactional perspective. In Haywood HC, Tzurial D. *Interactive Assessment.* New York, NY: Springer-Verlag; 1991:38-63.

6. Gold MW. Stimulus factors in skill training of the retarded on a complex assembly task: Acquisition, transfer, and retention. *Am J Ment Def.* 1972;76:517-526.

7. Lent JR, McLean BM. The trainable retarded: The technology of teaching. In Haring NG, Schiefelbush RL. *Teaching Special Children.* New York, NY: McGraw-Hill; 1976:197-231.

8. Gold MW. *Try Another Way Training Manual.* Champaign, Ill: Research Press; 1980.

9. Rogers JC. *Performance Assessment of Self-Care Skills.* Pittsburgh, Pa: Unpublished performance test; 1984.

10. McCue M, Rogers JC, Goldstein G. Relationships between neuropsychological and functional assessment in depressed and demented elderly. *Rehabil Psychol.* 1990;35:91-99.

11. Shook J, Beck C. Caring for cognitively and physically impaired nursing home residents: Is there a difference in the assistance needed from staff? *Gerontologist.* 1989;29:293A.

12. Rogers JC, Holm MB. *Performance Assessment of Self-Care Skills* (3.1). Pittsburgh, Pa: Unpublished performance test; 1988.

13. Holm MB, Rogers JC. Functional performance differences between the health care setting and the home. *Gerontologist.* 1990;30:327A.

14. Rogers JC, Holm MB. In-home safety for persons with cognitive impairment. *Gerontologist.* 1990;30:217A.

15. Holm MB, Rogers JC. Functional assessment outcomes: Differences between settings. *Arch of Phys Med Rehabil.* 1990;71:761.

16. Goldstein G, McCue M, Rogers JC, Nussbaum PD. Diagnostic differences in memory test based predictions of functional capacity in the elderly. *Neuropsychol Rehabil.* 1992;2:307-317.

17. Rogers JC, Holm MB, Goldstein G, Nussbaum PD. Stability and change in function assessment of patient with geropsychiatric disorders. *Am J Occup Ther.* 1994;48:914-918.

18. Pfeiffer E. *Multidimensional Functional Assessment: The OARS Methodology.* Durham, NC: Center for the Study of Aging and Development; 1976.

19. Gurland B, Kuriansky J, Sharpe L, Simon R, Stiller P, Birkett P. The Comprehensive Assessment and Referral Evaluation (CARE). *Int J Aging Hum Dev.* 1977-78;8:9-42.

20. Lawton MP, Moss M, Fulcomer M, Kleban MH. A research and service oriented multilevel assessment instrument. *J Gerontol.* 1982;37:91-99.

21. Pfeffer RI. The Functional Activities Questionnaire. In McDowell I, Newell C. *Measuring Health: A Guide to Rating Scales and Questionnaires.* New York, NY: Oxford Press; 1987.

PART IV:
ASSESSMENTS BASED ON THE
OBJECT RELATIONS THEORY

9

The Use of Expressive Media as an Assessment Tool in Mental Health

Margaret Drake, PhD, OTR/L, ATR-BC, FAOTA

Almost anything humans do can be included in the definition of expressive activities. As a discipline that prides itself on being holistic, occupational therapy considers the entire body, mind, and spirit all as important parts of the expressive system. When a therapist thinks of expression, the need to consider all aspects of how people express themselves is important. Some people are expressive through travel, others through managing their money. Any human act is indicative of the way a person thinks and feels and is, therefore, an expression of that person. For the purposes of assessment in occupational therapy, the definition needs to be narrowed. One purpose of this chapter is to give a brief history of the development of expressive assessments and how they came to be used in occupational therapy. Another goal is to present the current drawing and expressive assessments used by occupational therapists.

DEFINITION OF EXPRESSIVE MEDIA

The *Uniform Terminology for Occupational Therapy*, Third Edition, defines the term self-expression as "using a variety of styles and skills to express thoughts, feelings, and needs."[1]

Expressive modalities, or media as they are sometimes called, include art, dance/movement, and language activities, such as journaling, poetry, or drama. Traditionally, occupational therapists have considered expressive media to be painting, drawing, sculpture, or collage, but they include much more. They include all the ways in which people are able to express themselves. For example, dressing and costume also are forms of expression, as are photography and video.

In an expressive assessment, the occupational therapist is trying to help the patient recognize the emotions, self-concept, self-awareness, self-in-relation-to-others, communication skills, and the modes of expression he or she prefers. The occupational therapist is attempting to determine the degree to which expressive media affect feelings, cognition, and behavior. Expressive media give the patient the opportunity to think visually. During this process, cognition also is assessed.

Expressive assessments are used in other areas as well. When used by psychiatrists and psychologists, they are referred to as "projective tests." In this case, the therapist is trying to gain access to the patient's unconscious or pre-conscious thoughts and feelings.

When occupational therapists use expressive or projective tests with patients who have physical problems, the therapists are attempting to see how function is affected by the disability, rather than what the patients are thinking and feeling. The expressive language of stroke and brain-injured patients and of children who are developmentally delayed may be affected. Expressive assessments, such as the Copy Flower House Test, help uncover perceptual problems experienced by stroke patients.[2] Drawing can assist in the discovery of body scheme disorders and difficulties with spatiality.[3] This is one way of assessing patients that can bypass cultural restrictions and unconscious censoring.[4,5]

BEGINNINGS IN PSYCHOANALYSIS

Freud was interested in imagery, but was most interested in dream imagery.[5,6] The basic theory was that the dynamic struggles within a person's mind provide the energy for motivation to action. Carl Jung also felt that humans communicated their unconscious feelings through dreams. However, Jung additionally examined the content of art and considered it to be indicative of intrapsychic events.[7] Freud and Jung's early work coincide with the advent of modern art in the early part of the 20th century. Modern art attempted to express what went on inside humans, rather than the simplistic realism that had dominated the world previously. This occurred in the dance and drama worlds as well. These ideas which were revolutionary only a century ago seem mundane now, in what some call "the post modern era."[8]

LATER DEVELOPMENTS: EGO PSYCHOLOGY AND OBJECT RELATIONS

Ego Psychology

Freud first discussed the ego in the book, *The Ego and the Id, and Inhibitions, Symptoms, and Anxiety*, published in 1927.[9] The idea about the ego evolved over time and focused on what was considered to be the person's main defensive unit of personality. In the theory, illness resulted when a person was no longer able to balance the demands of ego, super ego, and id. Freud's daughter, Anna, carried these ideas even further in her 1942 book *The Ego and Mechanisms of Defense*.[10] From these beginnings came what is now known as "ego psychology."[11]

Object Relations

Object relations theory is derived from Freud's ideas about how individuals relate to their environment. The word "object" refers to either human or non-human things. This theory includes many of the same ideas as ego psychology, and for most occupational therapists can be considered in the same category.[12,13]

Robert Assagioli, MD was one of Freud's followers. Parallel to the development of other branches of psychoanalysis and psychodynamic approaches, Assagioli began to outline the theories of transpersonal psychology and psychosynthesis. Psychosynthesis uses a variety of playful techniques between therapist and patient that incorporate important aspects of an individual, such as religious experiences, intuition, and aesthetics. Projective techniques, such as free drawing, music, and movement, are employed to help patients understand the power of unconscious symbols. This was considered part of the body-mind-spirit synthesis.[14] These more spiritual ideas have been incorporated into occupational therapy assessment.

HISTORY OF DRAWING IN ASSESSMENT

Florence Goodenough

Some European researchers preceded Americans in recording their observations of children's drawings. However, American scholars were the first to use sufficient subjects to obtain data that could be scientifically analyzed. Goodenough, an American psychologist,[15,16] published a drawing intelligence test in 1926. When it was first published, the editor pointed out that drawing was a more accurate assessment of immigrant children's intelligence than psychological assessments that used a language unfamiliar to those children.[17]

Karen Machover

Machover, a Canadian psychologist, began publishing research findings in the 1940s. She focused on affective content, unlike Goodenough who focused on intelligence testing.[18] Machover used the term "projective" to describe this methodology. The first projective technique, known as the Inkblot Test had been developed in 1921 by a Swiss psychologist, Herman Rorschach.[19]

Dale B. Harris

In the early 1960s, Harris revised the original Draw-a-Man test that had been standardized by Goodenough. Harris included some additional ideas, such as concept formation, ability to abstract generalize learning, and to elaborate on the term "mental capacity," which was first used by Goodenough.[16]

OCCUPATIONAL THERAPY BATTERIES USING EXPRESSIVE MEDIA

The first references in occupational therapy literature to projective techniques, now called "expressive" techniques, was in the late 1950s and early 1960s.[20,21,22] In the decade of the 1960s, when psychologists began refining the use of drawings in assessment, occupational therapists also began to formalize the use of artistic media in the assessment process.[23]

Fidler Battery

Gail Fidler wrote about the occupational therapy assessment processes in an article, "Psychological Evaluation of OT Activities," in a 1948 issue of the *American Journal of Occupational Therapy*. However, this article focused on evaluating the activity, rather than on the patient.[24] In the following year, Jay Fidler, a psychiatrist, wrote an article that included advice about evaluating psychiatric patients. The intention of the assessment was to help the therapist understand the patient's response. The task attempted was to assist the therapist in analyzing self-behavior.[25]

Gail Fidler's 1957 article "The Role of Occupational Therapy in a Multi-Discipline Approach to Psychiatric Illness" discussed the value of the projective assessment in occupational therapy. The author mentioned such things as "color, form, and movement" as well as behavioral and relationship responses.[26]

The Fidler Activity Laboratory, which evolved from the 1959 "Diagnostic Battery" uses five activities done in a group setting and takes up to 5 1/2 hours.[27] The Diagnostic Battery consists of only three activities—clay, drawing, and finger painting—followed by a request for comments from the patient. The five activities in the Fidler Activity Laboratory are:

1. Stencil cutout for coloring with a crayon
2. Finger painting
3. Collage with fabric and objects
4. Obstacle course
5. Circle ball tag game

This assessment attempts to look at the entire spectrum of emotions, attitudes, interpersonal, cognitive, and sensorimotor skills.[27]

Azima Battery

Fern Cramer Azima started her research in Canada in 1959. She has coauthored with her husband, psychiatrist Heller Azima, and the couple taught at McGill University in Montreal. They considered art therapy and play therapy as functions of occupational therapy.[21] The Azima Battery had four segments:

1. Free pencil drawing
2. Drawing of a person of each sex
3. Unstructured clay project
4. Finger painting

Some of the behavioral traits the assessment hoped to evaluate were ego defenses, mood, reality awareness, perceptions of the environment, and energy level. The value of knowing about this battery is to understand the process through which occupational therapy began to use formal assessments to document efficacy as a member of the treatment team. However, for most therapists today, it is too time-consuming to administer, so it is seldom used.

Goodman Battery

The development of this battery of assessments in 1967 was a direct outgrowth of the era of psychoanalytic therapy. This theory included the idea that the ego could be assessed by observing how the individual functioned. Some general aspects that were assessed throughout the four tasks included attitude and response to structured versus non-structured occupations.

The tile task portion of the evaluation looks at cognitive aspects, such as organization, discrimination, sequencing, spatiality, problem solving, and abstract thinking, as well as at interpersonal skills, such as independence.

In the second task, a spontaneous drawing attempts to determine patients' psychosexual stage, which details are omitted, response to lack of structure, and individual style in application of pencil to paper, such as pressure and continuity of line. Themes and object relations also are assessed, and verbalizations during this part of the assessment are analyzed for their dysfunctional qualities.

The third task, figure drawing, asks the patient simply to "draw a person." Upon completion of the drawing, the patient is asked to discuss what he or she was thinking about as they drew, then the patient is asked to describe what was drawn. This segment of the assessment studies ego boundaries, organization, emotional overlay, capability to do reality testing, and self-esteem.

The last activity is the clay task, which again attempts to determine the patient's psychosexual stage, use of tools, ability, and need for control, and constructive/destructive needs.[28]

BH Battery

In the early 1970s, Hemphill began work on the BH Battery.[23] At that time, occupational therapists in mental health were attempting to learn more about the inner workings of patients and were looking at functional behaviors and neuro-behavioral responses to the environment.[29] This assessment has two tasks with a rating scale for each—mosaic tile and finger painting.

These two tasks have structured administration methods, with specific placement of containers for materials, instructions, and timing of the activity. Both tasks have specific criteria for analyzing the patient's responses as well as the products. The administration and scoring of the BH Battery is detailed in chapter 10.

The connection with psychoanalytic theory is made when the patient is asked to tell a story about the finger painting. This assessment made it much easier to try to verify interrater reliability. The reduced administration time was an asset because, during the 1970s, therapists began to charge insurance companies for occupational therapy assessments. The insurance companies' response was to require more accountability. To be accountable, it became necessary to show baseline functional behavior and the changes that resulted from occupational therapy treatment.

Assessments and treatment planning became more refined. The BH Battery was helpful in more specific treatment planning. More specificity in treatment planning was, in fact, a hallmark of the 1970s in the development of the occupational therapy profession.

Comprehensive Assessment Process: A Group Evaluation

The refining of assessment methods continued throughout the decade of the 1970s, as demonstrated in the Comprehensive Assessment Process.[30] Ehrenberg developed the Comprehensive Assessment Process to help therapists learn more efficiently about patients to facilitate better treatment planning. The projective, or expressive, segment of this assessment included a mosaic tile hot plate and a choice between a magazine collage, a group mural, or a hypothetical problem-solving experience.

The protocol gives specific instructions for explaining the process to patients. Patients are informed that they will be told the assessment results. Patients are further told that an explanation will be given as to how the results will be used to guide therapy.

This assessment includes documentation forms for the aspects of the patient's life. An initial interview form lists questions about background such as education, work, and recreation. Another form is used to ask the patient to make a daily schedule. A third form asks questions about activities of daily living. This assessment moved the profession's mental health occupational therapists further in the direction of an assessment tool that looked at all aspects of a patient, including intrapsychic phenomena.

The Magazine Picture Collage

The Magazine Picture Collage attracts many therapists in acute care psychiatry as well as in more long-term treatment settings. It is thought that patients are easily persuaded to do this assessment because the materials are familiar and it does not require the use of techniques that can be interpreted as artistic or difficult. It is also inexpensive, using old magazines, construction paper, and glue—materials that are available in almost any clinic.[31]

Patients are asked to find any pictures they like and to glue them to construction paper. The therapist observes the patients as they work, using scissors and materials. Each patient is asked to include their name, date, and collage title on the back. The therapist then asks the patients to discuss what their pictures mean.

Research on this assessment is ongoing. It has been subjected to interrater reliability studies and studies of which features are associated with dysfunction. The score sheet provides a structured way to observe patient occupational behavior, however, it does not provide a numerical score.

LIFE SPAN ISSUES IN EXPRESSIVE ASSESSMENT

Factors of age appropriateness are important to consider when choosing an assessment. Just as therapists consider a patient's strengths and weaknesses when deciding on an assessment, they regard the patient's stage of life as an important issue. The therapist may consider the important developmental tasks of a particular life stage, eg, teenagers are expected to consider the question, "Who am I?"

Pediatrics

Most children draw before they write, beginning with scribbles. Fine motor control is an important consideration for young children. Often, their drawings can be interpreted only by what they tell the examiner about them after completion.

Most children are at ease with art materials, and simpler materials often provide more information than more complicated techniques. Crayons, pencils, and large paper, such as 12-inch by 18-inch sheets, provide children with the size they need for their fine and gross motor capabilities.[32]

Issues of most interest to therapists who use drawing assessment with children are concentration, memory of previously used materials, attention span, and interpersonal relationships. Therapists also consider grooming and facial expression of the figures in the drawing as important indicators. Problem solving and creativity are considered less problematic than those issues just mentioned, but are still considered important.[33]

Adolescence

As in other areas of their life, adolescents are self-conscious about their skill and ability to provide realistic artwork.[34] In a drawing assessment this often results in many erasures and much time spent on elaborate detail. An assessment using collage and other media allows the teenager to focus on the task, rather than on drawing skill, which may elicit more cooperation in the end.

Adulthood

Themes that appear often in the expressions of young adults have to do with mating and choosing a social group.[35] The faithfulness of friends and partners is an important issue in the expressive work of patients in this age group. Drawings that focus on family and peer relationships are likely to predominate.

The therapist will facilitate patient cooperation in an expressive assessment by asking about previous exposure to the fine arts. If a patient's response indicates little or no exposure to art or music, it may be more difficult to achieve participation. The Magazine Picture Collage might be an appropriate choice for such a patient. As this is a time of life when creativity often relates to the community,[35] family, and work life, these themes predominate in the expressive work of many midlife adults.

Aged

With the elderly, an expressive assessment should include inquiries to determine their lifetime exposure to fine arts and to more popular arts and crafts, such as quilting or whittling. Awareness of this past experience will help the therapist choose an assessment that might be more palatable to an elderly person. If an older woman has done quilting, for example, a mosaic assessment, such as that in the BH Battery,[23] could be presented as a similar process to quilting because it requires planning a pattern from small pieces.

GENERAL GUIDELINES FOR USE OF
EXPRESSIVE ASSESSMENTS

Guidelines are sometimes helpful to a therapist who is trying a new kind of assessment with patients. Some general guidelines are listed below. They are meant to make a process easier. They are not laws; therapists can deviate from them. If a guideline does not seem reasonable, it should not be used.

1. Choose expressive assessments that will assist in setting patient goals.
2. Avoid relying solely on the findings of an expressive assessment. Corroborate it with more objective assessments or observations.
3. For documentation purposes, note whether it is a formal or informal assessment and the patient's general appearance, eye contact, concentration, attention span, interpersonal relationships, ability to solve problems in the art process, and creativity.
4. Do not rely on your interpretation without patient input. Ask the patient to tell about his or her own expressive product.
5. Before asking a patient to do an expressive assessment, think clearly about which aspect of the process being used is the main focus—intrapsychic phenomena, emotions, self-awareness, self-concept, self-in-relation-to-others, communication skills, fine motor control, spatial awareness, visual field deficits, or other skills and processes. Having the aspects to be observed clearly in mind will help the therapist focus and avoid being distracted by any bizarre behaviors or statements by the patient.
6. Administer the assessment to yourself before asking a patient to do it. In this way, the person administering the assessment will know how it feels to do it, and which problems might come up, such as where art materials should be placed for maximum accessibility.
7. Use expressive assessments for non-English speakers, mutes, or others who are unable to speak. Drawing assessments assist patients in overcoming language barriers.
8. Administer the standardized test the same way each time. Standardized tests use the same materials in the same environment and are administered with the same instructions each time.
9. Use assessments that fit the frame of reference being used. For example, the Kinetic Family Drawing measures family dynamics.[36] This is considered part of

the systems theory from which comes the occupational performance frame of reference. The Goodenough Harris Drawing Test measures the developmental level,[37] an important part of the developmental/spatiotemporal adaptation frame of reference.[38]

10. Choose an expressive assessment that the patient will not find boring or demeaning to repeat. Can the assessment be administered again at intervals to assess progress, or will the patient find it too repetitive?

SUMMARY

Human expression is one of our most important behaviors. Through expression, through the body, individuals communicate with others and with the inner self. Through human communication, emotions are shared and understood. Patients gain self-understanding through feedback and the possibility of viewing their inner workings, as they are mirrored on a paper or in a piece of clay. Expressive assessments are a way of keeping a record of intrapsychic processes. They add a dimension to occupational therapy that a functional assessment does not provide. Through expressive media, therapists and patients are able to examine their own thoughts, as they observe how others interpret their expressions.

REFERENCES

1.   The Terminology Task Force (1994) Uniform Terminology for Occupational Therapy, 3rd ed. *Am J Occup Ther*. November 1994; 48:1047-1054.

2.   Siev E, Frieshtat B. *Perceptual Dysfunction in the Adult Stroke Patient*. Thorofare, NJ: Charles B Slack Inc; 1976.

3.   Arnadottir G. *The Brain and Behavior: Assessing Cortical Dysfunction Through Activities of Daily Living*. Philadelphia, Pa: The CV Mosby Co; 1990.

4.   Hammer EF. *The Clinical Application of Projective Drawing*. Springfield, Ill: Charles C Thomas Publishers; 1985.

5.   Drake LM. *Black and White Children's Art: A Cultural Comparison*. PhD Dissertation, University of California at Irvine; 1985.

6.   Rothgeb CL, ed. *Abstracts of the Standard Edition of the Complete Psychological Works of Sigmund Freud*. Rockville, Md: US Department of Health, Education and Welfare, Public Health Service; 1975.

7.   Jung C, von Franz ML, Henderson JL, Jacobi J, Jaffe A. *Man and His Symbols*. New York, NY: Doubleday & Co Inc; 1969.

8.   Gergen KJ. *The Saturated Self: Dilemmas of Identity in Contemporary Life*. New York, NY: Basic Books; 1991.

9.   Freud S. *The Ego and the Id, and Inhibition, Symptoms and Anxiety*. London, England: Hogarth Press; 1927.

10. Freud A. *The Ego and Mechanisms of Defense*. London, England: Hogarth Press; 1942.

11. Edelson M. *Ego Psychology, Group Dynamics and the Therapeutic Community*. New York, NY: Grune and Stratton; 1964.

12. Early MB. *Mental Health Concepts and Techniques for the Occupational Therapy Assistant*, 2nd ed. New York, NY: Raven Press; 1993.

13. Mosey AC. *Three Frames of Reference for Mental Health*. Thorofare, NJ: Charles B Slack Inc; 1970.

14. Assagioli R. *Psychosynthesis: A Collection of Basic Writings*. New York, NY: Viking Compass; 1971.

15. Harris DB. *Children's Drawings as Measures of Intellectual Maturity*. New York, NY: Harcourt, Brace & World Inc.; 1963.

16. Kellogg R. *Analyzing Children's Art*. Palo Alto, Calif: Mayfield Publishing Co; 1969.

17. Goodenough FL. *Measurement of Intelligence by Drawings,* reprint ed. New York, NY: Amo Press; 1975.

18. Machover K. *Personality Projection in Drawing of a Human Figure.* Springfield, Ill: Charles C Thomas Publishers; 1949.

19. Tarczan C. *An Educator's Guide to Psychological Tests.* Springfield, Ill: Charles C Thomas Publishers; 1971.

20. Willard HS, Spackman CS. *Occupational Therapy,* 4th ed. Philadelphia, Pa; JB Lippincott Co; 1971.

21. Azima H, Wittkower ED. A partial field survey of psychiatric occupational therapy. *Am J Occup Ther.* 1957; 13:1-12, 35.

22. Azima H, Azima FJ. Outline of a dynamic theory of occupational therapy. *Am J Occup Ther.* 1959;13:215-221.

23. Hemphill BJ. *Training Manual for the BH Battery.* Thorofare, NJ: Charles B Slack Inc; 1982.

24. Fidler GS. Psychological evaluation of occupational therapy activities. *Am J Occup Ther.* 1948;2:284-288.

25. Fidler JW. The patient's view of occupational therapy. *Am J Occup Ther.* 1949;3:170-177.

26. Fidler GS. The role of occupational therapy in a multi-discipline approach to psychiatric illness. *Am J Occup Ther.* 1957;11:8-12, 35.

27. Fidler GS. The activity laboratory: A structure for observing and assessing perceptual, integrative, and behavioral strategies. In Hemphill BJ. *The Evaluative Process in Psychiatric Occupational Therapy.* Thorofare, NJ: SLACK Incorporated; 1982:195-207.

28. Evaskus MG. The Goodman Battery. In Hemphill BJ. *The Evaluative Process in Psychiatric Occupational Therapy.* Thorofare, NJ: SLACK Incorporated; 1982:85-125.

29. Hopkins HL, Smith HD. *Willard and Spackman's Occupational Therapy,* 5th ed. Philadelphia, Pa: JB Lippincott Co; 1978.

30. Ehrenberg, F. Comprehensive assessment process: A group evaluation. In Hemphill BJ. *The Evaluative Process in Psychiatric Occupational Therapy.* Thorofare, NJ: SLACK Incorporated;1982:155-167.

31. Lemer C. The magazine picture collage. In Hemphill BJ. *The Evaluative Process in Psychiatric Occupational Therapy.* Thorofare, NJ: SLACK Incorporated; 1982:139-154.

32. Drake M. *Crafts in Therapy and Rehabilitation.* Thorofare, NJ: SLACK Incorporated; 1992.

33. Cassity MD, Cassity JE. Psychiatric music therapy assessment and treatment in clinical training facilities with adults, adolescents, and children. *Journal of Music Therapy.* 1994;31:2-30.

34. Erikson EH. *Identity Youth and Crises.* New York, NY: WW Norton & Co; 1968.

35. Erikson EH. *Adulthood.* New York, NY: WW Norton & Co; 1967.

36. Burns RC, Kaufman SH. *Actions, Styles and Symbols in Kinetic Family Drawings (KFD): An Interpretive Manual.* New York, NY: Brunner / Mazel; 1972.

37. Goodenough FL, Harris DB. *Goodenough-Harris Drawing Test.* New York, NY: Harcourt, Brace & World Inc; 1963.

38. Kielhofner G. *Conceptual Foundations of Occupational Therapy.* Philadelphia, Pa: FA Davis Co; 1992.

10

How to Use the BH Battery

Barbara J. Hemphill-Pearson, MS, OTR, FAOTA

The BH Battery was originally developed and used at the Fort Logan Mental Health Center, a state institution in Denver, Colorado. It was developed at a time when the Fidler and the Azima batteries were the only evaluations available, and occupational therapists in mental health were primarily practicing analytical theory. This chapter deals with the administration of the BH Battery, which evaluates the psychological area of human function. There are occasions when occupational therapists need to examine such concepts as reality concept, body image, and the defense mechanisms. The BH Battery provides a structured instrument to record patients' projections in a systematic manner. In the past, projective content was analyzed for its symbolic meaning. Currently, the process by which an individual completes the projection is the basis for assessment. The theoretical framework for which goals are written includes the object relations theory.

RATIONALE

In 1959, the Azimas maintained that the psychic spheres in which projective tests gave data were: 1) the ego system, 2) the object relations, and 3) the body schema. The authors stated that projective material could be used to give data in all these spheres because: 1) it is unstructured; 2) it can be structured into a definite form; and 3) it brings into operation the tactile and bodily mode of objective relations that is absent in other standardized tests.[1]

Even though occupational therapists agreed as to which behaviors could be evaluated, the establishment of standardized procedures through which projections could be rated had not been developed. Rating scales that had been constructed were no more than lists of behavioral observations in which the authors proved interpretations, based on theoretical concepts.

The BH Battery is a projective assessment, designed for use in clinical occupational therapy for the purpose of assisting in diagnosis, evaluating task skills, evaluating level of psychological functioning, and assisting in treatment planning. The author chose finger painting and mosaic tiling activities because the following functions can be assessed:

1. Ability to follow direction and problem solve
2. Frustration tolerance
3. Perception of parts into a whole

4. Ability to abstract, make decisions, and follow through in logical sequence
5. Internal organization
6. Intrinsic gratification
7. Body concept
8. Use of structure and flexibility
9. Ability to handle limits or boundaries
10. Feeling tone.

REVIEW OF THE LITERATURE

Painting has been used by psychoanalytically-oriented workers for some time, but their primary interest has been in content rather than process. The content, in conjunction with the patient's case history, was valuable. None of the standardized projective tests allowed the occupational therapist to observe the patient manipulating the material. Fidler believed that the patient's process in completing a task was the basis for personality assessment in occupational therapy.[2]

The rating scales in the BH Battery are designed for use in clinical occupational therapy. The items were derived from studies in mosaic tiling by Wertham and Golden,[3] and the finger painting from Dorken, Kadis, Napoli, and Waehner,[4-10] and from clinical observations. The mosaic tiling was chosen because it measures the patient's ability to conceptualize a whole, and form a mental image that then will be placed on a Masonite board. Frank stated that the personality could be approached by inducing people to reveal their ways of organizing experiences by giving them a field with structure, in which they could build in accordance with the materials offered. In the pattern of the building, as in block-building or making a mosaic, the subjects would reveal the organizing concepts of their lives at that period.

People express themselves in movement patterns that are characteristic and that reveal personality unity. Allport and Vernon used the concept of expressive movement as their rationale for understanding the value of finger painting as a diagnostic tool.[11]

ADMINISTRATION OF MOSAIC TILING AND FINGER PAINTING ACTIVITIES

Equipment and Materials

Several materials are needed for each activity. These can be seen in Table 10-1.

Environmental Factors

For optimal performance, the environment in which the battery is to be given should be well-ventilated and well-lighted. The room should be equipped with running water, two tables with chairs, and a wastebasket. The subject's table should be placed against a blank wall and the administrator's table to the left, approximately 5 feet away. A chair should be placed at each table, and the wastebasket should be placed where it is convenient for the subject.

Table 10-1
Equipment and Materials

Mosaic Tiling
1. One 6-inch Masonite board
2. Glue—preferably white
3. A container of 7/8-inch square mosaic tiles in red, green, yellow, blue, black, and white
4. Mosaic tiling record form

Finger Painting
1. Liquid finger paint, preferably the type with body in its original form; in four colors: red, blue, yellow, and black
2. 16- x 22-inch finger painting paper
3. A pan of water
4. Paper towels
5. Newspaper
6. A 6-inch ruler
7. A stopwatch
8. A 16- x 22-inch template, made of plastic sheeting marked into 16 squares
9. Finger painting record form

PROCEDURES

Mosaic Tiling

The mosaic tiling is the first activity undertaken. Before the subject enters the testing situation, the mosaic equipment should be arranged on the table on which the subject will complete the task. The Masonite board should be placed in front of the patient, with the glue bottle to the right and the tile placed along the upper edge of the table.

Invite the subject into the testing room and ask him to be seated at the assigned table. Explain the task to the subject, including the reason for taking the test and the test's use. If the subject refuses to do the task, accept the explanation and record the refusal on the record form. If the subject complies, state, "Glue the tile on the board in any way, shape, or fashion, and take your time. Please tell me when you are finished. Do not begin until I tell you." If the subject asks for more direction, simply repeat the instructions. The administrator should go to the assigned table, obtain a record form, and state, "You may begin." The administrator should immediately start the stopwatch and record the time on the record form. The administrator should walk over to the subject and ask, "If you had a use for your tile, what would it be?" After recording the answer on the record form, the administrator should clear the subject's table and proceed to the next task.

Finger Painting

The second task to be completed is finger painting. The administrator should arrange the finger painting equipment around the subject's table. Newspaper should be placed on the subject's table where the subject will be seated, with the paper towels to the upper left corner of the table and a container of water to the upper right portion of the table. The finger paints are placed to the patient's immediate right.

After the equipment has been placed on the subject's table, the administrator should prepare the finger painting paper by rolling it lengthwise and placing it under a running faucet or in a container of water. After preparing the paper, the administrator should ask the subject to place it, with the shiny side up, on top of the newspaper. The administrator next should ask the subject to unscrew and remove the lids from the finger painting jars. The administrator then states, "Do a finger painting in any way, shape, or fashion, and take your time. Tell me when you're finished. Do not begin until I tell you to." If the subject asks for more direction, the administrator should simply repeat the instructions. Before asking the subject to begin, set the stopwatch back to zero. After obtaining the proper record form, the administrator should say to the subject, "You may begin." Immediately start the stopwatch and begin to record the subject's behavior on the record form. When the subject states that he or she is finished, stop the stopwatch, record the time, and walk over to the subject. Ask him or her to explain the painting and to determine its content. Record the subject's answer on the record form. Inform the subject that the test is over. The administrator should thank the subject before he or she leaves the room and give him or her an opportunity to wash the paint off his or her hands.

Procedure for Recording the Responses on the Record Form

This battery is designed to measure the approach to two different tasks—mosaic tiling and finger painting—that require no previous experience or further directions other than those provided. Each test is complete and separate as a subtest, but together they comprise a battery that can be administered in one setting.

Each subtest is scored in two ways: 1) observations during performance (process analysis), and 2) observations following performance (product analysis). It is important that the examiner be especially familiar with the process observations required in the protocol, so they are accurately rated, as defined. The administrator is to record phase 1 while the individual is completing each of the activities. When the subject is finished with the entire battery, the administrator is to record phase 2 of the activity. The administrator will need a copy of the rating scale.

PHASE 1: MOSAIC TILING

Observations During Performance—Process Analysis

Posture

There are two variables to check—feet and arms. (Standing comes under the category of feet.) This item requires a response for both feet and arms. The administrator should record the posture in which the subject spends most of the time.

Attitude

The attitude is the manner in which the subject approaches the mosaic tiling. Normal speed means the subject begins the activity and continues at the speed the administrator would consider normal. However, if the subject approaches the mosaic tiling test activity lazily, he or she begins the activity and proceeds in a very slow, lethargic manner. If the subject shows any of the previous characteristics, but stops the process by gazing around, the subject is considered to have paused. The subject may show any of the previous characteristics and then refuse to complete the activity. If the subject begins and then refuses, circle the appropriate number. The last variable in this item is refusal. If the subject completely refuses to do the mosaic tiling, simply mark the appropriate number and continue to the next task. Only one response is necessary.

Order

Order is when the subject is able to follow the administrator's instructions and complete the activity in a sequential fashion.

The first variable to observe in this item is "sequential." Sequential refers to a following of one part after another, leading to completion of an activity. The administrator is to observe the manner in which the subject places the tiles onto the Masonite board. It does not matter if the subject puts the glue on the board or on the tile, as long as the tiles are placed in a sequential fashion. Often, the subject will sort the tiles before placing them. If a pattern is completed before placing, it is considered to be arranging a pattern on the table. If the subject does not glue a pattern, but completes it on the board, then rearranges that pattern before gluing, the administrator should mark "rearranges tile on board." The next variable in this item is when the subject has glued the pattern onto the board and then begins to pull the tile off to rearrange it. The administrator should mark the variable "rearranges tile after gluing." The last variable to consider is "places tile chaotically." Chaotic refers to confusion or disorder in doing mosaic tiling.

The key to marking this item is to wait until the subject is almost finished with the activity. What may look like sequential, may turn out to be one of the other four variables.

Direction of Movement

The administrator should observe the direction in which the subject works. The subject can work left to right from top, left to right from bottom, right to left from top, right to left from bottom, away from self from the right, away from self from the left, toward self from the right, or toward self from the left. The subject may work circularly in all directions. If a subject works diagonally, two directions may be used. It is important to note that this item may have more than one response.

Characteristics of Verbalizations

The administrator should watch for and record these verbalizations during the activity:

Satisfaction: expresses pleasure or contentment concerning the mosaic tiling, eg, comments, such as, "I like this, don't you?" "I like the colors." "This is fun." "I like doing this."

Apology: expresses regret, fault, or failure of the mosaic tiling, eg, "I can't do this." "This is awful." "I'm sorry I can't do this."

Dissatisfaction: expresses anger about the performance, such as, "This tile won't fit." "Why do I have to do this?"

Boastfulness: expresses extreme pride in the mosaic tile, eg, "I think this is real good." "Can I hang this up?" "Look what I did."

When the subject does not express any of the previous characteristics and remains silent about his or her performance, the patient is considered non-verbal.

Verbalization About the Tile

This item is marked after the subject has finished. The administrator should then ask, "If you had a use for your tile, what would you use it for?" The subject's answer may reflect any one of the four variables. If the answer implies non-use for the tile, record the response as "no use."

Time

The stopwatch is turned off when the subject indicates he or she is finished. The actual time obtained from the stopwatch is entered in the last block of phase 1 in the mosaic tile rating scale.

Summary

There are seven items to observe during the performance of mosaic tiling: 1) posture, 2) attitude, 3) order, 4) direction of movement, 5) characteristics of verbalizations, 6) verbalization about the tile, and 7) time.

The items in the rating scale that indicate multiple responses may have more than one mark. All others should have only one mark.

After the administrator records phase 1 of the rating scale, proceed to the next task. When the subject has completed both activities, phase 2 of the mosaic tile may be completed.

PHASE 2: MOSAIC TILING

Observations Following Performance—Content Analysis

Color

The first category in phase 2 is color. It is a multiple response category that includes six colors: black, blue, red, yellow, green, and white. The colors the subject uses in the mosaic tile are recorded.

Texture

"Texture" means the amount of glue used in this activity. The glue is sufficient if the administrator can pick up the mosaic tile and turn it over without any of the tiles falling off.

After turning the project over, if any tiles do fall off, or if the tiles appear loose, there is not enough glue. "No glue used" simply means that the subject failed to glue the tiles onto the Masonite board. When glue is sticking out between the tiles of the finished product, the administrator should mark "profuse glue." Glue on top of the tile means that glue is oozing out between the tiles or that glue is actually all over the tiles.

Surface Coverage

In this item, the administrator simply counts the number of tiles used by the subject. The maximum number of tiles that can be used is 49. If any tile is 1/4 inch or more over the edge of the board, the response should be marked "beyond the edges," regardless of the number of tiles.

Overlapping

Overlapping is the placing of a tile over a previously laid tile, resulting in tiles piled on top of one another.

Distribution

The distribution tells the administrator where the tile is being placed on the Masonite board.

Number of Designs

The number of designs can be observed through the use of color and shape of the pattern. When deciding how many designs there are in a pattern, the administrator should first look for symmetry, a pattern that is identical on both sides of the axis in shape, size, or color. If no symmetry exists, the administrator looks for more than one design. Each design should stand on its own, as though the subject changed his or her mind and started a different pattern. If there is no pattern, as in the case of a scattered design, the administrator should leave the category unmarked.

Use of Space

The amount of space is measured and the position of the separate tiles noted. The use of space indicates how the space is used. In mosaic tiling, "compactness" indicates that all the pieces touch each other.

Position of Design

The variables in this item are designed to direct attention to the number of vacant edges in the subject's mosaic. The entire edge must be incomplete, as if an entire row of tiles were absent, to be considered vacant.

Design

The variables in this item require that the administrator to observe the pattern in the subject's mosaic tiling. The choices are: scatter design, plain design, random design, random design with border, simple checkerboard, simple checkerboard with obvious center, and complex checkerboard with obvious center design.

Symmetry

Symmetry is when three of the following conditions are fulfilled: the repeated form elements of each side of the middle axis are equally or approximately equally shaped, have approximately the same dimensions and size, or are of the same color. In the rating scale, symmetry is either present or absent.

Summary

Phase 2 of the rating scale in mosaic tiling is recorded when both tasks are completed. The color category is the only item that has a multiple response. There are 10 items to record in phase 2 of the mosaic tile rating scale. They are: 1) color, 2) surface coverage, 3) texture, 4) overlapping, 5) distribution, 6) number of designs, 7) use of space, 8) position of design, 9) design, and 10) symmetry.

PHASE 1: FINGER PAINTING

Observations During Performance—Process Analysis

As with the mosaic tile, there are items in finger painting that are recorded as the activity progresses. In most cases, the definition of the item in finger painting is identical to the one given in mosaic tiling. However, the items that are repeated are defined again in the order in which they appear in the finger painting rating scale. Before asking the subject to begin painting, the administrator should set the stopwatch to zero.

Posture

There are two variables to check: feet and arms. (Standing comes under the category of feet.) This item requires a response for both feet and arms. To record posture, the administrator should estimate the positions in which the subject spent the most time.

Attitude

The attitude is the manner in which the subject approaches the finger painting. "Normal speed" means the subject begins the activity and continues at a speed that the administrator considers to be normal. However, if the subject approaches the medium "lazily," the subject begins and proceeds in a slow, lethargic manner. If the subject shows one of the previous characteristics, but stops the process by gazing around, he or she is considered to have paused. Also, a subject may show one of the previous characteristics and then refuse to complete the activity. If the subject begins and then refuses, circle the appropriate number. To begin, means that the subject has spent more than 1 minute either placing paint on the finger painting paper or placing paint on the newspaper. If the subject refuses to do the finger painting, simply record the appropriate number and tell the subject that the battery is over. Only one response is necessary for this item.

First Daub

To record where the subject placed the first daub of paint, the administrator should think of the finger painting paper as divided into nine squares. First, the administrator should determine if the subject is in the top, middle, or bottom square. The administrator then should record in which quadrant the subject placed the first daub of paint. It should be noted that the administrator should not record the direction in which the subject is painting, but where he or she places the first daub of paint. This item requires only one response.

Parts of the Hand Used

The parts of the hand used is a multiple response item, and each variable is to be recorded individually. If the subject is using the whole hand, this means the subject's hand is flat on the paper. The fingers of the hand are not recorded separately when the whole hand is used. They are recorded individually, however, upon appearance in the finger painting process.

Motion

While observing the part of the hand that is being used, the administrator should note the type of motion involved. Each variable in this item is defined. This is a multiple-response item and any of the following motions can be recorded:

Smearing: unskilled, undirected movement of large muscles

Scrubbing: hard, rubbing motion up or down, left or right, or in circles

Scribbling: isolated finger movements used in pencil writing

Pushing: upward movements away from the body, with emphasis on the upper outward thrust

Pulling: downward movements, with emphasis on pulling in or downward motion

Patting: gentle, recurrent striking motion with the inner surface of the hand

Slapping: violent, recurrent striking with the inner surface of the hand

Scratching: violent movement down, left, or right that is made with the fingernails

Stubbing: short spring-like strokes made with the distal joints of the fingers held extended

Picking: caressing form of plucking, using the finger pads

Tapping: short, spring-like strokes made with the distal joints of the fingers flexed.

Order

Order indicates that the subject is able to follow the administrator's instructions and complete the activity in a sequential fashion. The variables in this item are descriptive rather than judgmental.

When a subject takes paint from a jar and places it on the table for the purpose of mixing two colors, it is the same as "takes paint from jars." "Starts over on same sheet of paper" means that the subject has completed an object on the finger painting paper, either concrete or abstract, then has blotted out the entire painting. He or she then changes the painting, either by using the same color or by using a different color.

If the subject "wants another sheet of paper," he or she wants to start over again, but if the painting appears incomplete, he or she should be encouraged to continue. Only when the subject insists that he or she wants to start again should the administrator terminate the activity. The rest of the procedure should be carried out by the administrator's asking the subject to explain the painting. If the subject agrees to continue, record "wants another sheet of paper." The last variable to consider in this item is "places paint in a chaotic manner." "Chaotic" describes a subject who appears confused or disoriented while finger painting.

Overlapping

"Overlapping" is placing paint over previously laid paint. The subject will overlap for three reasons: 1) he or she is starting over on the same sheet of paper; 2) he or she is placing paint in a chaotic manner; or 3) he or she is adding detail to the painting. Only when the subject appears to start over or places paint chaotically, should it be recorded as overlapping.

Strokes

A stroke, or line, is a single, complete movement made repeatedly by parts of the hand in one or more directions. Strokes vary from fine or narrow, to wide and are made by the fingernail, index finger, or palm, respectively. Strokes are angular, curved, 6 inches or more, and opened or closed. The direction may be vertical or horizontal.

This can be a multiple response item and should be recorded if the subject's painting consists of strokes. Strokes may be used to outline objects. When meaningless lines are drawn in a painting that contains objects, these lines are also defined as strokes.

Characteristics of Verbalization

The administrator should note any verbalizations by the subject while he or she is painting.

Satisfaction: expresses pleasure or contentment about the finger painting, eg, "I like this." "I like the colors." "This is fun." "May I have this?"

Apology: expresses regret, fault, or failure about the finger painting, eg, "I can't do this." "This is awful." "I'm sorry I can't do this." "I'm just not artistic."

Boastfulness: expresses extreme pride in the finger painting, eg, "I think this is real good." "Can I hang this up?" "Look what I did."

When the subject does not express any of the previous characteristics and remains silent, the subject is considered non-verbal. The administrator must direct attention to the subject's tone of voice to record the correct response.

Occurrence of Verbalization

The variables in this item are ranked according to when the subject verbalizes during the finger painting process. Because there are three variables, the data is dichotomous and is a multiple response item.

If the subject verbalizes from the time he or she enters the testing situation until he or she is asked to leave, all three variables must be recorded. To verbalize during the preparation means that the subject talked from the time he or she entered the testing situation until the time the administrator said he or she could begin. If the subject talked from the time he or she was instructed to begin until indicating that he or she was finished, "process" is recorded on the rating scale. To verbalize during clean-up means that the subject began talking after he or she was asked to leave the testing situation.

To verbalize means to make statements or ask questions either about the testing situation or about outside interests.

Type of Story

The theme of the subject's painting is reflected in the combination of the content and the subject's explanation of the painting. When asking the subject to explain the painting, the administrator is permitted to lead the subject by asking him or her to tell a story about the painting. The theme of the subject's painting may be any of the following:

- Fantasy story: exists only in the mind of the subject. An object in the painting may be symbolic to the subject, may appear to be real or true but does not exist, or may differ from what the subjects says it is, as is the case in an illusion.
- Fictional story: about imaginary people and happenings that appears factual in spite of its possible falsity.
- Factual story: concretely tells about the objects in the painting, which may be about people or events.
- Cultural story: about a given race or ethnic group.
- Mythological story: about a given religion.

Time

The actual stopwatch time is entered in the last category of phase 1 in the finger painting rating scale.

Summary

There are 12 items to observe during the performance of finger painting. They are: 1) posture, 2) attitude, 3) first daub, 4) parts of the hand used, 5) motion, 6) order, 7) overlapping, 8) strokes, 9) characteristics of verbalization, 10) occurrence of verbalization, 11) type of story, and 12) time.

After recording phase 1 of the finger painting rating scale, the administrator can ask the subject to leave the testing room. The administrator then records phase 2 of the mosaic tiling and finger painting.

PHASE 2: FINGER PAINTING

Observations Following Performance—Content Analysis

Color

The first category in phase 2 is color, a multiple response item. There are four primary colors: yellow, red, blue, and black. There also are mixed and muddy colors in this category. A mixed color is when two primary colors are combined to obtain a different color, eg, mixing blue and yellow to obtain green. Mud is the color arrived at by mixing too many colors together without any forethought, plan, or goal, thus ending up with a murky color.

Format

The format is the shape of the paper and the proportions of its sides—either horizontal or vertical. The patient can use the finger painting paper either way.

Surface Coverage

A template is used to measure the amount of surface covered with paint. The template is plastic sheeting that is the size of the finger painting paper—11 inches by 14 inches—divided by dark lines into 16 squares. The template is placed over the painting, and each square is counted. If half a square is covered by paint, it is counted as covered. The administrator simply counts the number of squares containing paint, and circles the number containing the appropriate interval. To record beyond the edges, any paint that is more than one quarter of an inch of the finger painting paper is recorded as "beyond the edges."

Texture

Texture is measured by the proportion of water to paint that results in a smooth painting. "Smooth and wet," with equal amounts of paint and water throughout the finger painting process, produces the ideal texture for paint. "Smooth and dry" results in small amounts of paint and water, resulting in a painting that dries before the subject is finished. "Little paint but very wet" happens when the amount of paint is small, but the amount of water is so great that it pools on the finger painting paper. "Lumpy and dry" is the opposite—the amount of paint exceeds the amount of water. The result is a painting that has lumps of paint because too little water was used. "Lumpy and wet" leaves behind pools of water and lumps of paint that cause the painting to crack and the flakes to flake off when the painting dries.

Width of Lines

A stroke is defined as a single complete movement made by parts of the hand in one or more directions. The lines are drawn by displacing paint, using fingernails, the index finger, or the heel of the hand. The paint that is displaced by the parts of the hand is measured to determine the width of the lines. Using the fingernails makes thin lines, and using the heel of the hand makes bold lines.

Pressure

Pressure is defined as the amount of force used to make a stroke. Pressure is measured by the amount of paint required to make a dark line and the amount of pressure needed to displace paint to make a medium or light white line.

A dark line is made when the subject scoops the paint out of the jar with the finger, then draws lines on the paper. This results in a solid paint line. A medium line is made with the finger to displace paint that has already been laid, resulting in a medium stroke. Pressure to displace already-laid paint by the finger is also a technique that is used to produce a light white line that is distinct and can be clearly seen. Note that the subject may tear the paper if he or she uses too much pressure.

Multiplicity of Strokes

If the painting does not contain strokes, the administrator simply records "no strokes." To record multiplicity of strokes, the administrator counts the number of lines in the finger painting and circles the number in the rating scale that contains the appropriate interval.

Shape and Length

There are seven kinds of strokes to observe: angular, horizontal, vertical, curved, zigzag, open, and closed. The length of the angular, vertical, and horizontal strokes are measured with a ruler. The administrator should pay special attention to long strokes. If the strokes are more than 6 inches long, the variable to circle is indicated on the record form. The reverse is true if the strokes are less than 6 inches long. The shapes of the strokes are recorded.

Detail

In this item, the administrator must judge the extent of detail in the subject's painting, and determine whether the detail is essential or non-essential to the painting. Detail is often used in scenic painting. The administrator records "few but essential" if the subject has appropriately used detail. When the subject has painted an object that requires no detail, such as something abstract or symbolic, "none but unessential" is recorded. A painting that has objects that, in the judgment of the administrator, require detail, such as a house without a door or windows, is recorded as having "no details." "Minute" means that the subject's painting, in the administrator's judgment, contains an overabundance of detail, such as a house's every brick or a tree's every leaf. "Unrelated detail" means that the subject scribbled unrelated marks on the painting.

Shape

When the administrator can barely identify the shape of an object, it is considered "vague." An object is "clear" if its shape can easily be distinguished. A light object surrounded by dark paint, or vice versa, is a "sharp" object. This item may have more than one response.

Size of Objects

To measure the size of the objects in the finger painting, the administrator should use a 12-inch ruler. The object's largest dimensions should be measured. When the painting contains objects of various sizes, "mixture" is recorded on the rating scale. If the painting contains one or more objects of the same size, the administrator records the measurement by circling the appropriate number on the rating form. When two objects measure differently, ie, one is 3 inches and another is 5 inches, the "smaller that 6 inches" variable is recorded. The largest object to be recorded will be 8 inches. When all the objects are smaller than 1 inch, circle the appropriate number on the record form.

Distribution of Objects

The distribution tells the administrator where the objects are placed on the finger painting paper. The objects can be "equally distributed," "slanted" (across the page from one corner to the other), "centered" on the page, or "across the center."

Symmetry

Symmetry is when three of the following conditions are fulfilled: the repeated objects on each side of the axis of the finger painting paper are equal or have approximately equal shapes, are of approximately the same dimension, are the same size, and are the same color. Symmetry is either present or absent.

Content

In this category, the administrator observes the content of the painting as a total picture. There are 14 possibilities: plain, repetitious, lettering, hand print, landscape, building, abstract, animals, people, plants, objects, religious, symbolic, and geometric. If the administrator is uncertain about the content, the patient is asked to interpret his or her painting. The number of objects contained in the painting is not recorded. This is an item that requires one response.

Time—Entire Activity

The time of each phase 1 activity is to be recorded in the last block of the rating scale, then added to obtain the total time. Then the total activity time for this category is recorded. Each variable has a 15-minute interval. The total time is recorded in the appropriate interval, ie, if the total time was 35 minutes, the number to circle is 4.

Summary

Phase 2 of the rating scale in finger painting is recorded when both activities have been completed. There are 14 items to record in phase 2 of the finger painting: 1) color, 2) format, 3) surface coverage, 4) texture, 5) width of lines, 6) pressure, 7) multiplicity of strokes, 8) shape and length, 9) detail, 10) shape of objects, 11) size of objects, 12) distribution of objects, 13) symmetry, and 14) content.

STATISTICAL STUDIES

Several studies have examined the interrater reliability and validity of the BH Battery over the past few years. In the first, 11 raters were randomly selected, with replacement procedures, from 91 known registered occupational therapists. A video training tape was used, and interrater reliability of the categories was examined by calculating the percentage of rater agreement. The stability of the battery was examined by showing the raters the video twice and comparing the responses with the correlation coefficient. The results demonstrated a 75% rater agreement of the entire mosaic tile scale and 73% of the entire finger painting rating scale. Stability of .73858 at .05 level of confidence was achieved. The study was repeated, using a training manual, that achieved identical results. A validity study was undertaken that compared the overall score of the BH Battery with the score of the Claudia Allen Cognitive Test. No significant correlation was achieved.

RESEARCH

Projections evaluated in the BH Battery need further research. Instead of comparing the score obtained from the BH Battery with the overall score of the ACL, the ACL needs to be compared with the individual variables of the BH Battery. Because the BH Battery provides a means to measure projections, it would be a simple process to compare the scores with other tests.

SUMMARY

The BH Battery is a projective test that evaluates the psychological area of human function. This test provides the therapist with the means by which to examine such concepts as level of psychosis, level of depression, decision-making process, self esteem, abstract thinking, and the mental health mechanisms. The test can be interpreted by consulting Chapter 8 of *The Evaluative Process in Psychiatric Occupational Therapy*.[12] The chapter also presents a complete literature review and discusses the meaning of projections. The interpretations are based on a literature review, patient reports, and the authors' experiences in conducting more than 200 evaluations. For a more current discussion of the use of projective testing, the reader is additionally referred to Chapter 9 of this textbook.

REFERENCES

1.   Azima H, Azima F. Outline of a dynamic theory of occupational therapy. *Am J Occup Ther.* 1959;13,1-7.
2.   Fidler G, Fidler F. *A Diagnosis and Evaluative Process. Occupational Therapy: A Communicative Process in Psychiatry.* New York, NY: Macmillan Co; 1963.
3.   Wertham F, Golden L. A differential method interpreting mosaics and color block design. *Am J Psychiatry.* 1941;98:124-131.
4.   Dorken H. The reliability and validity of spontaneous finger paintings. *Journal of Projective Techniques.* 1954;18.
5.   Kadis G. *Projective Psychology.* New York, NY: Macmillan Co; 1950.
6.   Napoli J. Finger painting and personality diagnosis. *Genetic Psychological Monograph.* 1946;34.
7.   Napoli J. Interpretive aspects of finger painting. *J Psychol.* 1947;26:22-23.
8.   Napoli J. A finger painting record form. *J Psychol.* 1948;26.
9.   Napoli J. Finger painting. In Anderson H and Anderson G, eds. *Introduction to Projective Techniques.* New York, NY: Prentice Hall Inc; 1956
10.   Waehner T. Interpretations of spontaneous drawings and paintings. *Genetic Psychology Monographs.* 1946;33.
11.   Allport G, Vernon P. *Studies in Expressive Movement.* New York, NY: Macmillan Co; 1933:171-182.
12.   Hemphill B. *The Evaluative Process in Psychiatric Occupational Therapy.* Thorofare, NJ: SLACK Incorporated; 1989.

11

Build A City:
A Projective Task Concept

E. Nelson Clark, MS, OTR/L, LCDR, USN, RET

Build A City is a projective task concept, based on empirical research in projective methods, materials, and clinical experiences. The purpose of the Build A City project is to describe a technique that can be used for task groups in the treatment of psychosocial disorders, present an evaluation method for the observation of small groups, and provide working definitions that can be employed in the projective task concept.

The first definition of the concept is a presentation of standardized raw materials from which patients fashion a product that reflects the conscious and unconscious aspects of themselves. Second, it is a method of studying the personality by confronting the subjects with a group situation to which they can respond, according to the significance of the task and the various levels of feeling when responding.

The concept is viewed as relevant to occupational therapy at a time when traditional arts and crafts are devalued as a practice,[1,2] shortened hospital stays require new approaches,[3] cultural and societal issues demand attention,[4] and treatment must be provided in a manner that can be measured in terms of functional outcomes, as measured by subsequent performance.[5-7] The task also is viewed as important to the philosophy of occupational therapy,[8] in that tools and materials are used in a constructive process that enables a therapist to participate in the observation and evaluation of occupational behaviors. The projective task group also supports the assumption that groups centered around an activity are more relevant to the communication process and the development of social skills than an oral group without a project.[9]

HISTORICAL DEVELOPMENT

The Build A City projective task concept was developed in 1975 and presented at the 1977 American Occupational Therapy Association Conference by the author and Nancy E. Dowey, MS, OTR.

As has often been said, "Necessity is the mother of invention." The project actually had naive beginnings out of the rubble of a stockroom, while attempting to provide a quick and meaningful group activity. Scrap materials of various media were gathered and placed on a table, and the group simply was instructed to build a city.

The process and product that followed left the therapists astonished and delightedly curious. Strong support by supervising physicians and peer approval from conference presentations gave encouragement to understand the dynamic process that was being observed, which was different from that of traditional arts, crafts, and activity groups.

Literature Review

The framework for the Build A City concept is built upon the classic definition of projective methods by Lawrence Frank,[10] play configuration studies,[11] constructed scene studies using preconstructed materials,[12,13] constructed village studies,[14] group concepts and techniques by occupational therapy theorists,[15,16,17] and the components of various frames of reference used by occupational therapists, as described by Mosey.[18]

PROJECTIVE METHODS

Projective methods are classified by the technique or manner used to evoke responses from the subject/patient. In his classic reference, *Projective Methods*,[10] Frank classifies methods to provide a working definition for projective materials. These categories are identified as follows:

- Constitutive Methods: This technique requires the subject to impose some structure or organization upon the unstructured, plastic-nature, materials, or a partially organized situation. Examples of psychological assessments are the Rorschach Ink Blot Test or free-form artistic productions.
- Constructive Methods: This method requires the subject to arrange materials having a definite size, shape, or pattern into a larger configuration, including the sorting of diverse objects, such as play therapy, using toys or puppets to create situations or drama productions.
- Interpretive Methods: This approach elicits from the subject an interpretation of past experiences or a composition in which the subject finds personal meaning or affective significance. Examples would be the Thematic Apperception Test, in which various pictures are shown to patients to elicit their responses, or a piece of literature or drama is read to evoke special meaning from the patients.
- Cathartic Methods: This method encourages patients to express their emotional or affective reactions to the immediate stimulus. This approach includes the patients' responses to virtually all tasks and activity.
- Reactive Methods: These methods are a study of the way patients alter or distort the conventional medium of communication, such as speech or handwriting, which can give clues to the subjects' personality process.

Frank emphasized that the subjects bring to the group or testing situation, a set of unique values and experiences.[10] Thus, the essential feature of a projective method is to evoke from subjects the expression of their private worlds and reveal the personality process in which they function.

Azima and Azima emphasized that therapists help patients bring their expressions into activities during the occupational therapy process by allowing a projection of their conscious and unconscious feeling into the task.[15] They also stressed that, despite how much a therapist may tend to ignore the issue, patients continue to bring their inner world and behaviors into their work. Fidler and Fidler further added that the creation of objects enabled patients to more easily accept their dynamics, and that visual and created objects keenly focus the patients' attention.[16] The patients are able to work through directed interpretations because of the presence of this visible indicator.

Visible indicators are central to the concept of Build A City. A wealth of information can be gleaned by assisting patients in telling their stories of how they chose certain items to construct, which skills were necessary to be successful, when it was necessary to gain assistance from others, and what was the outcome of their actions. As participants begin to view the constructed efforts, conscious or subconscious acts emerge that may be appropriate or inappropriate to the task. The occupational therapist then can observe these anxieties to determine if the resulting task performance and behavior is functional or destructive to the task process and patient interaction during the process.

Play Studies

In Erikson's clinical and statistical studies, children were provided with a selection of preconstructed toys and instructed to make an exciting scene of a movie.[11] Erikson observed that the inner lives, fantasies, dreams, and experiences of the children were projected onto the task. Erikson discovered that girls in the age ranges of 11 to 13 tended to construct different scenes and configurations than did boys in the same age group. Boys preferred action scenes, with tall buildings that often fell, while the girls built quiet scenes, often reflecting home or school. Erikson also observed that children with immature behaviors were observed to spread their creations about in a disorganized fashion, and that children with marked insecurities crowded their scenes into one corner. Although Erikson's work with children was recorded in the 1940s, similar observations have been noted in adult patient performance in Build A City.

Lowenfield's Build A World technique[12] and Mucchielli's Le Jeu Monde et le Test du Village Imaginaire,[14] with techniques and observations similar to those in Erikson's play configuration studies, used a multitude of preconstructed items to construct a world and villages to record behaviors and performance of patients and other groups.

Lowenfield's technique instructed patients to build in a sand tray that could be moistened and molded.[12] Three hundred toys, representing people, buildings, cars, trees, animals, etc, were given to the patients for use in further construction. These items were not projective in nature, as they were preconstructed replicas. The Lowenfield technique was used for all age groups, in collaboration with psychotherapy, in the ongoing diagnosis of individuals. Patients were often instructed to make sequential productions during their treatment.

In Mucchielli's study, villages were assembled from preconstructed materials.[14] The villages were classified according to pathological symptoms. In contrast to normal people building normal villages, Mucchielli discovered that disabled people built villages that revealed disorder. Some of the abnormalities observed by Mucchielli were empty villages, overcrowded villages, chaotic villages, rigidity, clustered, disassociated or split villages, empty town centers, no people in the village, fragmented or maze-like construction, a dominating or traumatic theme, and abnormal behaviors during the construction process.

Both Boyer and Buhler describe abnormalities in the world constructions that are similar to Mucchielli's abnormal villages.[12,13] These authors also describe the abnormal behaviors of patients who participated in the building of these worlds.

These abnormalities, as described by Mucchielli, Buhler, and Boyer, have been observed in the cities constructed in the Build A City concept. However, it must be emphasized that the studies of Erikson, Lowenfield, Buhler, and Mucchielli used pre-constructed materials (toys). In contrast to preconstructed toys, Build A City uses projective materials, those having no preconceived or identifiable form, and tools to enable the patient to manipulate and change the materials into identifiable objects to achieve similar visible productions as those previously cited.

The manipulation of tools and constructive behaviors demonstrated by the participants are viewed as vital to the occupational therapy process. This process is the doing part of the group activity. Doing is defined by Fidler and Fidler as "enabling the development and integration of the sensory, motor, cognitive, and psychological systems; serving as a socializing agent."[16] They added that this process of doing verifies competency.

Frames of Reference

The projective task concept is difficult to place in any one category of projective methods or in any one frame of reference. The use of projective techniques or activities traditionally implies analysis, which is the classic psychiatric approach. However, an investigation of the various frames of reference used in the practice of occupational therapy reveals several interesting factors in the makeup of a projective task.

Mosey states that in the analytical frame of reference, common referents of symbols are used in evaluation to assess the patient's problem areas, however, in the treatment process, no predetermined meaning can be assigned to symbols.[18] She further states that symbols are effected by the unconscious, and past and current life experiences. The context in which the construction of the symbol or object occurs is emphasized as being most important. Mosey notes that a free, plastic material encourages the making of a more symbolic and unconscious production.

However, Azima and Azima felt that a directed creation or production was more useful for diagnostic purposes because it limited the extent and scope of creation to a degree.[15] Thus, it allowed the therapist to concentrate more heavily on the exploration and interpretation of the created work. Azima and Azima further defined directed creation as a definite object of a medium chosen for the patient and that the patient was not restricted in the manipulation of it.

In the action-consequence frame of reference, Mosey gives examples of a shared task.[18] In a shared task, six to eight patients are evaluated in a group activity. The group is asked to participate in a simple activity that requires a collaborative interaction. Necessary tools and materials are provided, and the therapist does not participate. This format is similar to the methodology of Build A City.

The developmental frame of reference is evident in the final group production of the projective task. Comparing the results of various cities constructed by groups, ranging from chronic schizophrenics to normal adults, one can observe the developmental skills involved in the actual handling of the media during construction, the thought processes, and the group interaction skills. The processes and results of using Build A City with adult patients are similar to those observed by Erikson in his work with children.

ADMINISTRATION OF BUILD A CITY

Materials

Build A City is a task that uses standardized projective building materials (Table 11-1). The materials were selected for their projective qualities and relatively low cost. Some of the materials can be used repeatedly, saving some costs. The styrofoam should be replaced when the patients have imposed identifiable form on the blocks, ie, carved a structure that can be identified as a church or a fast food restaurant, thereby eliminating the projective potential of the styrofoam block. Materials should be replaced, as necessary, in order to provide an ample supply.

Tools

The tools provided to construct Build A City (see Table 11-1) were selected for their safety and function. The common table knife should have a rounded tip and non-sharpened edge. The wooden clay tools are provided for modeling clay structures. The small finishing nails are included as fastening devices—these are more easily manipulated and safer than straight pins.

Procedure

Before the group comes to the clinic or space where the project is to be completed, the therapist should assemble all materials and tools in the center of a table that will accommodate a group of four to eight people comfortably.

After the group arrives, the therapist thanks the group members for attending and, without describing the task at hand (most often the group members have several curious questions), gives the standard instructions.

The task requires the following standard introduction/instructions to the group: "I would like all of you, as a group, to build your ideal city. You may use only the tools and materials provided on the table. You have 30 minutes in which to complete your ideal city. Are there any questions?" The therapist may repeat all or portions of the above directions. During the course of the task, the therapist may announce the amount of time left to complete the task. No other directions are to be given. The therapist then assumes the role of one who observes and evaluates.

EVALUATION OF THE GROUP PROCESS

Azima and Azima outline four steps in order for a projective task to be considered a legitimate evaluation tool in occupational therapy.[15] Preparation is the first step. The approach to the task, ie, administration, must be followed in the same manner each time. Production, the second step, must be performed by the patients without any form of assistance or guidance by the therapist. In the third step, the association or story that the patients reveal about their creation and their group interactions must be accepted as the patients' true perception of events. The final step, interpretation, occurs when the therapist and or other members of the health care team use the creation, and the patients provide explanations, leading to an evaluation of the dynamic processes of the patients.

As previously discussed, the structure imposed on the task assists in the diagnostic capabilities of the performance. The group is instructed to build their ideal city, instructed to use only the tools and materials they are provided, and given a 30-minute time limit to complete the task. The therapist is then free to observe.

In the freedom of observation, it soon became evident that an observation checklist, rating scale, or some other form of evaluation tool would be necessary to record the quick events that occur during the production of the city. The writing of longhand notes was definitely not suitable for this activity.

BUILD A CITY GROUP RATING SCALE

A Bales Type Category System[19] was modified to observe and record positive or negative patient interactions. A rating scale of this nature enables the observer to quickly identify and record behaviors. The structure of this scale also assists in eliminating some of the observation anxieties that therapists may have in trying to remember patient performance. During the course of research, other scoring systems were considered but abandoned due to the need for having a scale that could quickly be identified and recorded (see Build A City Performance Rating System on page 171).

The rating form has five columns available for a group session. In the event that the group has more than five members, subsequent columns can be added. At the beginning of the session, the therapist places the initials of each group member at the top of the column. During the course of the activity, the therapist then records a category letter (A,B,C, or D) and the number of the behavior within that category. For example, if a patient suggests to the group how to construct a street for the city, the therapist would record a B1 in the column under the patient's initials. If the same patient then criticized another group member because he or she did not like that person's suggestion, the therapist would place a D3 in the same column, underneath the previous B1 recording.

In this manner, a running record is kept of patient interactions. On the rating form, 17 individual blocks are available for patient interactions. Depending on the functional level of the patient group, varying numbers of blocks may be needed. A severely regressed patient may need only a few blocks, while a manic individual may need several. However, 17 blocks have been found to be sufficient to give an accurate representation of a patient's participation over the course of 30 minutes.

Upon completion of the group task and the recording of each member's performance during the session, the therapist can sum up the individual responses. For example how many A1s, A3s, D3s, or B2s, etc, did the individual or group have? The total for each behavior may then be graphed on the reverse of the rating form by placing a dot on the number of the behavior and the number of responses in the graph box. For example, a patient may have five A2 behaviors, three B6s, two A3s, and one D1. The rating of this patient would indicate that the session was a relatively positive one in the estimation of the rater. A group score can be tabulated in a similar manner by summing up all like behaviors and plotting the score.

The ability to quickly track an individual over the course of the group task, without recording in longhand, is a useful tool. In this manner, feedback can be provided to the patient, not only by group peers during the group and post-group sessions, but also by specific interactions noted on the rating sheet. A further suggestion would be to videotape the group (use privacy act statements and permission if appropriate), and show the group the reasons for specific behavior ratings. The rating form can also be used with similar task groups to help evaluate behaviors.

The City Symptoms by Mucchielli, as previously discussed, and the Build A City Component Checklist, to follow, provide useful assessment and post-discussions of

---

Table 11-1
Tools and Materials for Build A City

Tools/Description
1. Scissors: two pairs of blunt-nose that can cut construction paper easily
2. Blunt table knife: one round-edge, non-serrated table knife
3. Clay fettling tool: to be used for forming clay if needed

Materials/Description
1. Styrofoam: 2 sheets 36" x 24" x 2" (standard size sold in craft stores), with sheets cut into a variety of block sizes up to 6" x 12"
2. Construction paper: 12 sheets of assorted colors
3. String: approximately 12 feet (a small ball)
4. Brads (finishing nails): 50 that are 3/4" or 1" in length (a small pack)
5. Clay: 12 ounces (the approximate size of a tennis ball) of one color (neutral color—grey or blue)
6. Pipe cleaners: 2 dozen of one neutral color (light tan, grey, light blue, etc)

Author's note: Tools and materials must be kept standard and neutral to remain projective. The minimum number of tools are recommended to examine sharing and asking behaviors.

---

the actual city. Discussion of the inclusion or absence of certain components often provides individual or group insight, and can often be fun and entertaining. However, since the city is a projective work, not all components can be interpreted the same way for each group.

Therapists are advised to be cautious when commenting on various structures of the city. Commenting on the quality of construction is only a value judgment on the commentator's part. The therapist must remember that patients have a certain amount of self-esteem projected into their work.

THE PROJECTIVE TASK AS A DIAGNOSTIC TOOL

The question of whether to use a projective task for diagnostic purposes appears to lie within the comparison of traditional standardized projective tests and the properties of projective tasks. Again, Azima and Azima believed that on many occasions, non-directive productions of objects could be used as projective test materials.[15]

The differences between projective tests and projective tasks offer some advantages for projective tasks. Although some of the following projective tests may not be used for clinical diagnosis as in years past, the following comparisons are made for educational interest.

Projective tests have a systematic mode of administration for standardization. Although the projective task is also introduced in a standard manner, once the activity begins, the patient assumes a non-systematic mode of constructing the activity. Because many behaviors can emerge during the task process, administration of the project has to be performed many times with various patients to gather valid interpretations. Although standardized tests also require extensive data gathering and interpretation, a projective task would tend to yield a certain amount of new and unpredictable projective behaviors and varying information due to interpersonal interactions and the group process. This systematic data gathering was noted in the Erikson, Lowenfield, and Mucchielli studies.[11-14] On the positive side, these unpredictable situations could enhance therapist observation and provide clues to the patient's personality.

Projective tests have form constancy, ie, the test appears the same way each time for precise interpretation. A projective task presents general constancy in the initially presented materials, but once the group begins interaction, materials change in form, such as the altering of paper, clay, or other building materials, and in meaning. The negative aspect of this characteristic is the attempt to systematically categorize the created objects. For example, in one Build A City creation, lines (strings) that connect buildings may be interpreted by the patient as filling the construction's need for communication (telephone lines). Another patient, in another city, may provide lines between buildings and interpret them as places to hang clothes. The positive aspect is the patient's individual construction process and his overall contribution to the group process. This gives the therapist an invaluable opportunity to observe patient behavior through a patient's interactions with the rest of the group. The patient's contributions can also stimulate conversation about the object's constructed use and its meaning.

Aside from the previous examples of differences between projective tests and a projective task, the projective task can provide data in the same areas as psychiatric tests. For example, the Rorschach Ink Blot Examination[20] can give insight into an individual's ego systems, while a task can identify an individual's ego function within a group process. The Thematic Apperception Test reveals how an individual relates to objects.[21] The task definitely reveals how one uses tools and materials. The patient is free to relate his experiences, views, and cognitive skills during the group process and construction of the task. Body schemes, as observed in the Human Figure drawing,[22] are also noted in the constructed figures within the task. In reference to body schemes, a significant difference between the test and the task is that the task brings into operation tactile and bodily responses that are absent or neglected in projective testing. To the trained occupational therapist, these bodily responses are advantageous in the observation of sensory-motor performance.

A distinct advantage of a projective task is that it can be used repeatedly with the same patient, whereas a projective test should not be. The lack of perceptual clues in projective tasks does not provide the external reference that produces a practice and learning effect. Frank, as referenced earlier, also felt that these aforementioned differences were advantageous.[10] The author stated that "any kind of situation can be utilized as a projective method if the subject's performance is treated not as a product to be rated, but as personality indicators to be interpreted."[10]

Azima and Azima specified that, for diagnostic purposes, direct interpretations are not to be given to a patient.[15] As in projective testing, the patient is not given an immediate interpretation of their answers or remarks. However, in post performance discussion of the projective task, the group members are encouraged to give their interpretations of construction and interactions. The therapist should facilitate these discussions to encourage the patients to explore their task-performance outcomes and to compare these behaviors with their behaviors in previous task groups, either in the clinic or in their normal societal work groups.

EXPECTED OBJECTIVES AND OUTCOMES OF INTERVENTION

Objectives

The occupational therapist should provide a working laboratory in which the Build A City task group can:

1. Demonstrate and identify communication and work skills within a task group.
2. Stimulate a sense of self in a community.
3. Assess the dynamic operation of a city/community and its components.
4. Identify symbolic content, as therapeutically appropriate.

In a study of Lowenfield's Build A World project, Bolgar and Fischer found that six areas of reactions to the task emerged.[23] The patients reactions were categorized into choice, quantity, form, contents, behavior, and verbalization.

At the beginning of each creation, a patient or group must make fundamental choices, such as whether or not to participate or which actions to take. Choices can also be influenced by a variety of factors, such as group pressures and mental status.

The group members then address issues of quantity—how much material to be used, how big, and how many. Again, quantity reflects the decision-making abilities of the individuals.

The content of the production deals with the subject or focus of the group. Normal subjects tend to build real communities with real streets, while regressed or abnormal subjects tend to build themes or scenes, as in the Erikson studies with adolescents.

The behavior of the patients includes the willingness of individuals to participate, whether their work is spontaneous or planned, and any other notable occupational performance characteristics. Although speaking has been noted to increase initially during planning stages, conversation drops during actual construction. In the Build A City post-groups, group members discussed their participation more than is observed with traditional activities. The increased oral response is attributed to the visible indicators (construction) and the structured observation checklist, which encourages communication.

ROLE OF THE OCCUPATIONAL THERAPIST

Frank remarked that "no matter how objective or quantitative a test may be, the use of the findings will call for clinical experience and judgment. The extent will be made on the conceptual scheme of the therapist."[10]

The historical role of the occupational therapist in group work is well-documented.[24] The expertise of the occupational therapist is to observe and analyze behaviors of an individual during the performance of a task. Azima and Azima write that during this task process, regardless of how much a therapist may tend to ignore the issues, the patient continues to bring his inner world and behaviors into the work situation.[15]

Therapists who are aware of patients' emerging anxieties and their performance as a result of those behaviors can help them examine behavior and reduce non-functional behavior. However, therapists who fail to interpret, or even deny, the patients' projected anxiety in any task situation may experience a certain amount of anxiety in themselves. The unaware therapist can countertransfer this anxiety by keeping the activity at superficial levels or by viewing the craft as something patients just make as a hobby.[25]

The structuring of the activity process, observation, and interpretation may help alleviate therapist anxiety and aid the therapist in focusing on appropriate strategies for reducing anxiety in the patient.[26] The Build A City project uses the concept of structuring by giving both the patient and therapist instructions, standard materials, timed parameters, and a structured evaluation.

By using the structured group observation and rating form, the therapist can more accurately discuss the group's behaviors and accomplishments. The therapist should compliment the group on completion of the task and on each member's efforts, no matter how small. Therapists should be diplomatic/therapeutic about unusual creations, identify bizarre and symbolic content as appropriate and therapeutically experienced, and encourage the participants to explain the various creations or buildings.

Questions to ask the group include: "What is an ideal city?" "How does the ideal city differ from that of a real city?" "Which components make a city functional?" The therapist should stimulate conversation about how individuals contribute to the building and functioning of an ideal city.

The following component checklist can be used by therapists to observe inclusion or exclusion in the city construction:

1. Support systems: gas stations, food stores, merchandise stores, places for employment
2. Institutions: medical, educational, law enforcement, religious
3. Methods of control: stop signs, fences, roads, boundaries
4. Types of recreation: parks, movies, discos, playgrounds
5. Communications systems: telephone lines, mail boxes, streets, sidewalks
6. Human, animal, and plant life
7. Mechanical objects: cars, bicycles, airplanes, moving objects
8. Types of housing.

BUILD A CITY OBSERVATIONS

As stated previously, the product of the group task is the visible indicator of the performance of each patient and the group as a whole. For the therapist who observes this 30-minute task, the process can often be anxiety-provoking, exhilarating, sometimes incredulous, and always intriguing. Over the past 20 years, since the inception of the project, hundreds of Build A City tasks have been completed by patient and student groups and in professional workshops. The following are but a few of these examples.

The results of a city constructed by a group of regressed schizophrenics can be observed in Figure 11-1. Like Mucchielli's abnormal villages, this city can be observed to be empty, fragmented, and disassociated from each of the other buildings. Developmentally, this group could be viewed as lacking the skills to interact with each other and to actually construct a city with viable components that resemble a community. However, in the post-group session with this group, a most remarkable piece of verbalization emerged. One patient, who previously was essentially non-participatory in occupational therapy sessions, stated simply and hesi-

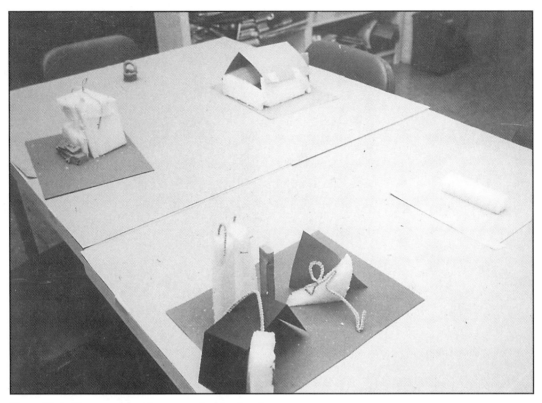

Figure 11-1. City constructed by regressed schizophrenics.

tantly that her creation was a library. When asked the significance of a library, she stated that her mother often took her there to read. According to the therapists, this was the most this patient interacted orally regarding her past experiences.

In Figure 11-2, a city constructed by hospitalized adult males, ranging in age from 18 to 28, was aptly named "King Kong City." Erikson described this scene in his study of adolescent boys as constructing tall buildings, action, destruction, and amorphous fashion.[11] In the illustration, we can see a clay figure that represents an ape climbing a building, while a scene of action and destruction is played out in the construction. In the post-group, the patients verbalized anger at their hospitalization and situations. Most notable was the individual who constructed the airplane. He was an airplane mechanic who was displaced from his work after he became disabled. He discussed his depression regarding his job loss and attempts at organizing his life. Post-group conversation was directed toward the result of anger and how it interfered with the construction of needed life-support systems in the construction. Similar cities that have been observed have dealt with anger. One city depicted an Old West scene, with an acting out of hanging various people in the town.

Figure 11-3 shows a city constructed by college students that can be viewed as a healthy community. Many components of a city are present, such as food provision, housing, places of employment, people, and recreation. However, upon closer examination, one might note that systems of control or authority are absent, such as police stations and stop signs. Control issues were voiced during the construction process and later in the post-group discussion. When probed further, the group revealed anger at feeling that they were not included in the selection of their fieldwork place-

Figure 11-2. King Kong City. Note the large clay figure (King Kong) and airplane on the pipe cleaner.

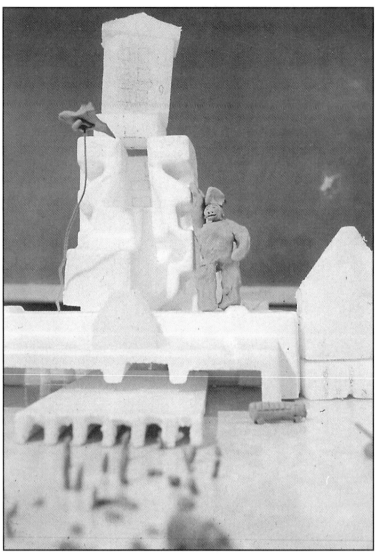

ment sites. Although this city appeared to be healthy in most respects, the materials and process allowed group members to impose their own conflicts on the situation.

SUGGESTIONS FOR CONCEPT IMPLEMENTATION

By building on the historical roots of occupational therapy and using constructive tasks to observe occupational behaviors, therapists are encouraged to employ the concepts described in Build A City. Although Build A City describes a specific group task, other group tasks could be constructed from the concept to gain insight into various cultural and societal settings, such as Build A Farm (Figure 11-4), Build A Park, Build A Factory, or Build A Neighborhood.

The materials could be different for each project, but they should be projective in nature, keeping with the concept. Metal foil, thin wood, leather scraps, wire, etc, are some examples of projective materials. Again, the importance would be to determine the materials, keep the materials standard, and follow the described protocols of Build A City.

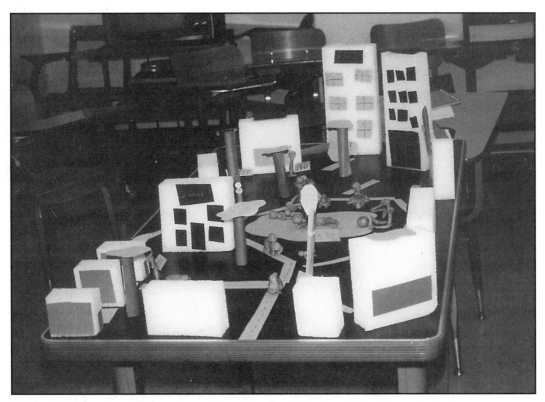

Figure 11-3. City constructed by college students. Note the park in the middle with people playing.

SUMMARY

Since the inception of Build A City, no two cities have been observed to be constructed alike. Some had similar characteristics, but they were not alike. One might surmise that, in the living laboratory of the occupational therapy clinic, the city constructed of projective materials would parallel the real cities of the world. Real cities are constructed by different groups of people, from different cultures, and with different agendas and problems. Each city of the world and each city in the clinic has its own personality. A city constructed by a regressed group, afflicted with disorders, are observed to be fragmented, sparse, and non-functional. Can the same be said of some the cities constructed by the modern day person or the decline of neighborhoods within cities?

Recent innovations, such as a computer simulation game, SIM City 2000[27], challenge the individual to construct cities by computer that could function as a real city. A highly sophisticated software program will assess the needs and construction of the city, and inform the computer uses as to its success. Although this type of simulation is far from the constructive and projective group nature of Build A City, it nonetheless gives validity to people's need to function within society and understand the components of a successful city.

The Build A City concept describes a group activity that 1) can be completed in 45 minutes, 2) provides a rating scale for evaluative measures, 3) communicates relevant social/cultural issues, 4) uses standardized projective materials, and (5) encourages the constructive, doing process that is valued in occupational therapy.

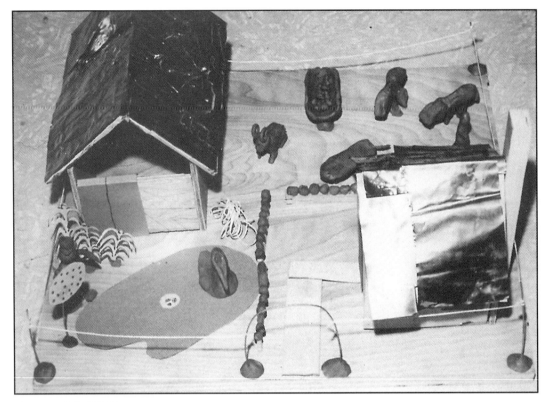

Figure 11-4. Build A Farm.

REFERENCES

1.   Shannon PD. The derailment of occupational therapy. *Am J Occup Ther*. 1977;31:229-234.
2.   Dickerson A, Kaplan SH. A comparison of craft use and academic preparation in craft modalities. *Am J Occup Ther*. 1991;45:1-17.
3.   Jackson G. Short term psychiatric treatment: How will occupational therapy adapt? *OTMH*. 1984;4:11-17.
4.   Dillard M, Andonion L, et al. Culturally competent occupational therapy in a diversely populated mental health setting. *Am J Occup Ther*. 1992;46:721-725.
5.   Robinson AM, Avallone J. Occupational therapy in acute inpatient psychiatry: an activities health approach. *Am J Occup Ther*. 1990;44:809-814.
6.   Rogers JC, Holm MB. Accepting the challenge of outcome research: Examining the effectiveness of occupational therapy practice. *Am J Occup Ther*. 1995;48:871-876.
7.   Foto M. Outcome studies: The what, why, how, and when. *Am J Occup Ther*. 1996;50:87-88.
8.   American Occupational Therapy Association. The philosophical base of occupational therapy. *Am J Occup Ther*. 1995;49:1026.
9.   DeCarlo JJ, Mann WC. The effectiveness of verbal versus activity groups in improving self-perceptions of interpersonal communication skills. *Am J Occup Ther*. 1985;39:20-27.
10.   Frank L. *Projective Methods*. Springfield, Ill: CC Thomas; 1948:2,4.
11.   Erikson E. Sex differences in the play configuration of preadolescents. *Am J Orthopsychiatry*. 1941;21:667-692.
12.   Bowyer L. *The Lowenfield World Techniques*. New York, NY: Pergamon Press; 1970.
13.   Buhler C, Kelly G. *A World Test: A Measurement of Emotional Disturbance*. New York, NY: Psychological Corp; 1941.

14.   Mucchielli R. *Le jeu du monde et le test village imaginaire*. Paris, France: Presses Universitaires de France; 1960.

15.   Azima H, Azima F. An outline of dynamic theory of occupational therapy. *Am J Occup Ther*. 1959;13:215-221.

16.   Fidler G, Fidler J. *Occupational Therapy: A Communication Process in Psychiatry*. New York, NY: Macmillan Co; 1963.

18.   Mosey A. *Three Frames of Reference for Mental Health*. Thorofare, NJ: CB Slack Inc; 1975.

17.   Fidler G. The task-oriented group as a context for treatment. *Am J Occup Ther*. 1969;23:43-48.

19.   Bales RF. *Interaction Process Analysis: A Method for the Study of Small Groups*. Cambridge, Mass: Addison-Wesley; 1950.

20.   Beck S. *Rorschach's Test. Basic Processes*. New York, NY: Grune & Stratton; 1961.

21.   Bellak L. *A Guide to the Interpretation of the Thematic Apperception Test*. (Rev.) New York, NY: Psychological Corp; 1951.

22.   Buck J. *The House-Tree-Person Technique*, revised. Beverly Hills, Calif: Western Psychological Services; 1966.

23.   Bolgar H, Fischer LK. Personality projection in the world test. *Am J Orthopsychiatry*. 1947;17:117.

24.   Howe MC, Schwartzberg SL. *A Functional Approach to Group Work in Occupational Therapy*, 2nd ed. Philadelphia, Pa: JB Lippincott Co; 1995.

25.   Horner AJ. *Psychoanalytic Objects Relations Therapy*. Northvale, NJ: Jason Aronson Inc; 1991.

26.   Clark EN, Cross M. The creative clay test. In Hemphill B. *The Evaluative Process in Psychiatric Occupational Therapy*. Thorofare, NJ: SLACK Incorporated; 1982.

27.   Haslam F, Wright W. *SIM City 2000*. Orinda, Calif: Maxis Software; 1993.

BIBLIOGRAPHY

Alt L, Bellak L. *Projective Psychology: A Clinical Approach to the Total Personality*. New York, NY: A Knopf: 1950.

Anderson H, Anderson G. *An Introduction to Projective Techniques*. New York, NY: Prentice-Hall; 1951.

Beck S. *Rorschach's Test: Basic Processes*. New York, NY: Grune & Stratton; 1961.

Bell J. *Projective Techniques*. New York, NY: Logmans Green; 1948.

Bellak L. *The Children's Apperception Test*. New York, NY: CPS Co; 1948.

Bellak L. *A Guide to the Interpretation of the Thematic Apperception Test*. (Rev.) New York, NY: Psychological Corp; 1951.

Bender L. *A Visual Motor Gestalt Test and Its Clinical Use*. Research Monograph: No. 3. New York, NY: Am Orthopsychiatric Assoc; 1938.

Buck J. *The House-Tree-Person Technique*, revised. Beverly Hills, Calif: Western Psychological Services; 1966.

Carr A. *Symposium on the Prediction of the Over Behavior Through the Use of Projective Techniques*. Springfield, Ill: CC Thomas; 1960.

Dennis W. *Group Values Through Children's Drawings*. New York, NY: J Wiley & Sons Inc; 1966.

Goodenough F. *The Measurement of Intelligence by Drawings*. Yonkers on Hudson, NY: World Book Co; 1926.

Hammer E. *The Clinical Application of Projective Drawings*. Springfield, Ill: CC Thomas; 1960.

Harris D. *Children's Drawings as Measures of Intellectual Maturity*. New York, NY: Harcourt Brace & World Inc; 1963.

Harrower M. *Personality Changes and Development as Measured by Projective Techniques*. New York, NY: Grune & Stratton; 1958.

Harrower M. *Creative Variations in the Projective Techniques*. Springfield, Ill: CC Thomas; 1960.

Kaplan B. *Studying Personality Cross Culturally*. Evanston, Ill: Row, Peterson; 1961.

Kellogg R, Scott O. *The Psychology of Children's Art. A Psychology Today Book*. New York, NY: Random House Inc; 1967.

Lindzey G. *Projective Techniques and Cross Cultural Research.* New York, NY: Appleton-Century-Crofts; 1961.

Machover K. *Personality Projection in the Drawing of the Human Figure; a Method of Personality Investigation.* Springfield, Ill: CC Thomas; 1949.

Murstein B. *Theory and Research in Projective Techniques; Emphasizing the TAT.* New York, NY: J Wiley & Sons; 1963.

Murstein B. *Handbook of Projective Techniques.* New York, NY: Basic Books; 1965.

Napoli P. Finger Painting. In Anderson and Anderson, eds. *An Introduction to Projective Techniques.* New York, NY: Prentice-Hall; 1951.

Personality Monographs: Vol 1. *Projective and Expressive Methods of Personality Investigation (diagnosis).* New York, NY: Grune & Stratton; 1950.

Phillipson H. *The Object Relationship Techniques.* London, England: Tavisto Publication; 1955.

Rabin A, Haworth M. *Projective Techniques With Children.* New York, NY: Grune & Stratton; 1960.

Schneidman E. *The Make-A-Picture-Story-Test.* New York, NY: Psychological Corp; 1949.

Torda C. Some Observations on the Creative Process. *Perceptual Motor Skills.* 1970;3:102-126.

Vernier C. *Projective Test Productions.* New York, NY: Grune & Stratton; 1952.

Zubin J. *An Experimental Approach to Projective Techniques.* New York, NY: John Wiley & Sons; 1965.

The author acknowledges significant work by Nancy E. Dowey, MS, OTR, in the formulation of the Build A City project.

Client initials ____ ____ ____ ____ ____

A. Emotionally Positive Responses
    1. <u>Shows solidarity.</u> Raises others
       status, gives help, rewards
    2. <u>Shows tension release.</u> Jokes,
       laughs, shows satisfaction
    3. <u>Agrees.</u> Shows passive accept-
       ance, understands, concurs,
       complies

B. Problem Solving Responses
    Answers
    1. <u>Gives suggestions.</u> Direction
       implying autonomy for other
    2. <u>Gives opinion.</u> Evaluation,
       analysis, expresses feeling, wish
    3. <u>Gives orientation.</u> Information,
       repeats, clarifies, confirms

C. Problem Solving Responses
    Questions
    1. <u>Asks for suggestions.</u> Direction
    2. <u>Asks for opinion.</u> Evaluation,
       analysis, expression of feeling
    3. <u>Asks for orientation.</u> Informa-
       tion, confirmation

D. Emotionally Negative Responses
    1. <u>Disagrees.</u> Shows passive re-
       jection, formality, withholds
       help
    2. <u>Shows tension.</u> Asks for help,
       withdraws
    3. <u>Shows antagonism.</u> Deflates
       others status, defends or
       asserts self

Notes:

Instructions for the Build A City Performance Rating System

1. Place the initials of each group member at the top of each column.

2. During the group process, annotate an individual's response/interaction by matching it with the closest behavior description. Example: Client #1 opens the group with a statement "I suggest we build streets for this project." Client #2 states "only an idiot would make such a statement." Client #3 makes an appropriate joke to relieve tension that is building. Rating: For these interactions, Client #1 would be given a "B1" (Gives suggestion), Client #2 would be given a "D3" (Deflates others' status), and Client #3 would be given a mark of "A2" for giving a tension release statement.

3. Continue rating each client's interactions, as they occur, down each column. There are 17 blocks available for interactions. Only a few ratings have been found necessary for a quiet, regressed group. On the other hand, a lively group might go beyond 17 ratings. However, 17 ratings will give a good representation of how the individual performed within the group in a 30-minute period.

4. Upon completion of the group, count the number of each response, i.e., all of the A1s', all A2s', etc. and plot in the graph space below. For each client distribution of behaviors, more graphs will need to be duplicated. However, only one graph will be needed if the total group is being illustrated.

5. The plotting of responses will indicate the number of behaviors and give indicators as to type of interactions given by the group or individual. R. F. Bales (1950) indicated behavior as "satisfied" "dissatisfied." If a client was high in agreement behaviors, he was termed satisfied. If a client illustrated negative behaviors or gave a lot of suggestions, he tended to be a dissatisfied individual in this particular process.

A1   Shows solidarity
A2   Tension release
A3   Demonstrates agreement

B1   Gives suggestions
B2   Gives opinions
B3   Gives orientation

C1   Asks for orientation
C2   Asks opinions
C3   Asks suggestions

D1   Disagrees
D2   Shows tension
D3   Shows antagonism

```
0        5        10        15        20
```

The Build A City Performance Rating System is a Bales Type Category System adapted from the following reference: Bales RF. *Interaction Process Analysis: A Method for the Study of Small Groups.* Cambridge, Mass: Addison-Wesley; 1950.

PART V:
ASSESSMENTS BASED ON THE
MODEL OF HUMAN OCCUPATION

12

The Role Checklist

Anne E. Dickerson, PhD, OTR/L, FAOTA

The Role Checklist was developed by Oakley[1] to operationalize a construct within the model of human occupation.[2-4] While the concept of this construct's roles has changed as the model of human occupation has evolved, the Role Checklist remains a viable assessment for determining participation in roles and the value of enacted roles. The purpose of this chapter is to present a brief overview of the concept of role, as it pertains to occupational therapy in general and to the model of human occupation[4] in particular. It will be followed by a description of the development of the Role Checklist, its clinical use, reliability and validity studies, and current research.

BACKGROUND

Role refers to the characteristic and expected behavior of an individual in a specific social position.[5] Roles serve as an organizing component for competence in daily life,[6] and role acquisition is often seen as one of the most important aspects of socialization.[7,8] Part of the development of self-identity is based on the groups to which one belongs, whether by chance (sex or culture) or by choice.[9] Dion[8] suggests that the core of personal identity in most adults is associated with major institutional roles, such as worker or parent, and that successful socialization can be measured by the individual's ability to perform well in roles.[5] Further, Gove and Zeiss found that although men and women experience roles differently, occupancy among major roles, such as spouse, worker, and parent, determine happiness.[10]

Throughout the life span, people acquire and relinquish roles. Some role changes occur suddenly, while others are more blurred and occur slowly over the life span.[11-12] Individuals prepare themselves for these known role changes through anticipatory socialization, whereby the individual explores new expectations associated with a new role.[11,13] After role change, resocialization may be needed, especially in adulthood, to alter self-concepts. The amount of resocialization depends on the difference between the previous role and the new one.[11,14] Any conflict between the two roles must be resolved, with the individual needing support in the new role.[1,15]

OCCUPATIONAL THERAPY AND ROLES

Occupational therapy primarily addresses the individual's occupational roles during treatment. Roles are seen as having an occupational dimension if they include play, leisure, or productive behavior.[3-4] Branholm and Fugl-Meyer[16] found a link between fulfillment of occupational roles and life satisfaction in both young and old individuals, while others have described role loss in the elderly and its link to decreased life satisfaction.[17-19]

Addressing role dysfunction has been recognized as an appropriate task for occupational therapists.[6,18,20-24] Disruption to role performance and life satisfaction is likely to occur when individuals acquire disabilities that necessitate unwanted changes in their lifestyles. Furthermore, people who experience sudden, traumatic injury or illness are also at risk for role dysfunction. Not only must they deal with an immediate change in their performance capacities, but they also must deal with an abrupt loss of one or more roles that constitute an important component of their self-image. For example, the young male surfer who becomes quadriplegic in an accident must deal not only with losing his ability to walk or perform activities of daily living, but also with losing his ability to participate in a major life role through which he often defined himself to others. Therefore, individuals with disabilities may lose their sense of self when they experience role loss. Role loss can undermine confidence, lead to depression and lack of motivation, degrade self-image, and, ultimately, block the rehabilitation process.[24]

Occupational therapy helps patients maximize their abilities by teaching them new habits and skills, so they can resume old roles or assume new occupational roles. Occupational role performance has been examined with specific groups including patients with psychiatric diagnoses,[25-26] bone marrow transplant survivors,[27] individuals with severe burns,[28] and adults with severe traumatic brain injury.[20] In all of these studies, significant differences were found in role performance. Specifically, individuals with these diagnoses participated in fewer roles or performed less productively in roles they did maintain. Results also indicate that these role losses can cause a decrease in the feelings of self-esteem and the quality of life experiences.

MODEL OF HUMAN OCCUPATION

Within the framework of the model of human occupation, roles are an important component of the habituation subsystem and are seen as a means to meet the needs of both the individual and society.[2,4] Roles within the model of human occupation are seen as providing the method for constructing competent social behavior.[4] Through interaction within the social system, an individual acquires a role, and learns the identity and behaviors associated with that role. That is to say, the individual internalizes the role.[4] Kielhofner refers to the internalized role as "a broad awareness of a particular social identity and related obligations which together provide a framework for appreciating relevant situations and constructing appropriate behavior."[4]

As people interact within the social environment, the ease and structure of those interactions are assisted by the fact that they interact within roles. The people who respond share a common idea of which behaviors roles prescribe. Therefore, roles facilitate appropriate action and interaction. These role behavior patterns are identified by the model of human occupation as *role scripts*.[4] Role scripts are "a collection of appreciative capacities that guide comprehension of social situations and expectations, and the related construction of action that enacts a given role."[4] In other words, role scripts provide behavior guidelines for specific situations within a social environment, without much conscious awareness. For example, while eating in a restaurant with my young son, I will enviably attempt to control his misconduct in my role as his mother. Role scripts do not prescribe exactly what I am going to say or do, but they facilitate a swift, intuitive reaction so that I can enact my role as mother automatically, thereby allowing my energy and concentration to be directed elsewhere. Others who observe my actions generally accept them as appropriate, for they, as members of my cultural group, are familiar with behaviors that are expected within the role of mother. They may indicate this acceptance with some acknowledgement, such as a nod or smile, that further reinforces my understanding and enactment in my role as a mother. Thus, an important function of roles is to direct and constrain behavior. Since society depends on its members to function within roles, certain role behaviors are expected and serve to maintain social order and cohesiveness of groups.[4]

The model of human occupation has identified three ways in which roles organize occupational behavior.[4] First, roles influence the manner and style of our interactions as well as the content. For example, in my role as mother to my son, my manner likely would be authoritative when telling him to not use his fingers while eating. While, in the role of spouse, I may be more appealing or humorous, suggesting to my husband not to use his fingers.

Second, roles influence the sets of tasks or performances that become part of our role-related routine. That is, roles will define certain tasks that are regularly used within an enacted role, such as discipline in the role of a mother.

Third, roles partition daily and weekly cycles into times when we ordinarily inhabit certain roles. For example, my mother role typically predominates early evening, when I am getting my sons ready for bed. This will differ from my spousal role later in the evening, when my husband and I may share the happenings of the day or spend some intimate time together. Thus, roles are tied to cyclical time or recurrences and, by occupying parts of our daily routine, give regularity to our occupational behavior.[4]

Finally, any given social role may have occupational, personal-sexual, or familial-social dimensions.[29] For example, the role of mother has occupational, personal, and familial dimensions. However, it is the occupational dimension that is of primary concern to the occupational therapist. As previously stated, the occupational dimension of a role is recognized when the role expresses play or leisure, or the role requires productive behavior.[4] The Role Checklist was developed to delineate occupational roles and to evaluate an individual's participation in and value of those roles.

ROLE CHECKLIST

Description
The purpose of the Role Checklist is to assess people's occupational role performances and indicate their role identification, as well as the value they attach to their roles. It is a written inventory that is appropriate for adolescent, adult, and elderly people with physical or psychosocial dysfunction.

Since the Role Checklist is based on the Model of Human Occupation and was designed to identify the occupational behavior of patients, the roles identified on the checklist are roles that provide opportunities to fulfill behavior within the occupational dimension. The 10 roles included in the checklist are student, worker, volunteer, caregiver, home maintainer, friend, family member, religious participant, hobbyist/amateur, and participant in organizations. Each of these roles is briefly described, including a reference to the frequency with which the role is enacted. These frequencies are included in the definition, as the model is concerned with how roles structure occupational behavior. Fulfilling the role should include doing something within the role, rather than merely being a relationship. For example, being a friend is a relationship and based on feelings, while doing something with a friend at least once a week shows enactment of occupational behavior. There is also an "other" category on the checklist for the individual to identify enacted occupational roles that are not listed.

The assessment is based on self-report. Usually it is completed by the therapist's interview of a patient; however, it can be completed independently by the patient. The instrument takes approximately 15 minutes to complete and consists of two parts. In addition, a summary sheet has been developed to view and interpret results more easily.

Part 1 asks the patients to consider whether they have performed each of the 10 roles listed on the checklist in the past, are presently fulfilling any of the roles, or anticipate fulfilling any in the future. The past refers to any time up until the preceding week. The present refers to the past week, or 7 days, including the day of the administration of the checklist. The future refers to tomorrow or any day thereafter.

Part 2 asks patients to indicate the value of each of the roles delineated in the checklist, regardless of whether they have fulfilled the role or not. The measure of the degree to which the individual values each role is indicated by three choices: not at all valuable, somewhat valuable, or very valuable.

CLINICAL USE OF THE ROLE CHECKLIST

Administration

Individuals with physical or psychological disabilities have been shown to have difficulties with role performance.[20,25-28,30-31] If role function is deemed to be a component in the domain of occupational therapy, as it is in the model of human occupation, it should be addressed by occupational therapists in psychosocial, developmental, and physical dysfunction settings. The Role Checklist is a convenient and easy assessment tool to gather initial information about role performance. It can be used with individuals from adolescence to older adulthood and is not specific to any diagnostic category. In addition to identifying problems with continuity of role performance, the Role Checklist can identify other problem areas. For example, it can illustrate concretely to people that they are attempting to fulfill too many roles and are overcome by the demands of each of the roles. Further, the assessment addresses the value of roles and, therefore, can be used to identify role loss, which may cause problems with self-identity and self-esteem. The checklist allows comparison of role participation and role value. People who participate in roles that are not highly valued or do not participate in roles that they do value may demonstrate frustration or lack of motivation. Contradictions between goals and current life situation or functional status may lead to occupational dysfunction. Most importantly, the com-

Table 12-1

Administration of the Role Checklist

The following set of directions has been developed to standardize the administration of the Role Checklist:

A. Instruct individuals to complete the demographic information at the top of the checklist.
B. Part 1
1. Ask the patient to read the instructions.
2. Inquire if the instructions are understood and answer any questions pertaining to the administration of Part 1.
3. Define the time frame as follows: "The present refers not only to today, but also includes the previous seven days. The past refers to the period of time up until seven days ago. The future is anytime from tomorrow on."
C. Part 2
1. When individuals have completed Part 1, ask the patient to read the instructions for Part 2.
2. Inquire if the instructions are understood and answer any questions pertaining to the administration of Part 2.
3. Define valuable as follows: "Valuable refers to the worth you place on each role—that is to say, how important or desirable the role is to you."
4. Remain with the patient until the checklist is completed.

pletion of the Role Checklist can provide a mechanism for further dialogue between therapist and patient about issues that are often difficult to articulate and define (Table 12-1).

The Role Checklist is a useful assessment tool for occupational therapists. It can be used in a variety of settings and should be presented in occupational therapy curricula as an important tool for the profession. Those therapists who are already using the checklist with a variety of patients provide anecdotal evidence that it is useful in occupational therapy treatment. Furthermore, it has been translated into several languages—Spanish, Portuguese, French, Arabic, German, and Swedish. Unfortunately, although there is documentation about the validity, reliability, and ability to identify role-functioning problems, research has yet to demonstrate how the Role Checklist can be used in therapy. That is, research is needed to demonstrate that once identified, role dysfunction can be resolved, based on the results of using the checklist within the framework of the model of human occupation.

RESEARCH STUDIES WITH THE ROLE CHECKLIST

Instrument Development

Following a review of the literature in social psychology, sociology, and occupational therapy, more than 20 roles, relating to family, work, and leisure activities, were identified.[1] To be considered for inclusion as a role on the checklist, each of the 20 roles was examined for its implication for productive or playful use of time. This preliminary list of roles was submitted to graduate students, faculty, and therapists. Their feedback supported the content validity of the proposed role taxonomy, but indicated a need to define each role, avoid sexual stereotyping, and include frequency criteria. From the feedback, a version of the instrument with 10 roles was used in a pilot reliability study. Seventeen undergraduate occupational therapy students were asked to indicate their perceptions of role occupancy in the past, present, and future. The median percent agreement between two administrations of part 1 of the instrument, given 2 weeks apart was 82 percent.

The instrument was also piloted in an inpatient psychiatric program. Clinical use revealed that wording the definitions in the present tense biased the instrument. In addition, the clinical testing also indicated it was insufficient to ask only about role incumbency; it was also necessary to determine the value attributed by the patient to each role. Thus, role definitions were reworded, without tense, and part 2 was added so that respondents could indicate how valuable and meaningful each role was to them.

Initial Test-Retest Reliability Study

Oakley, Kielhofner, Barris, and Reichler established initial test-retest reliability of the checklist with a normal population.[29] The checklist was administered to 124 normal adults on two separate occasions, either 1 to 4 weeks apart, or 5 to 8 weeks apart. This group consisted primarily of white, female, well-educated subjects. Approximately half of the subjects were between 18 and 30 years of age, and half between 31 and 65 years of age. Fifty percent of the subjects were married.

Kappa and percent agreement were computed to examine test-retest reliability. Both were used because each has desirable properties. Kappa is a measure of agreement that corrects for chance. Percent agreement is a familiar and widely used statistic that is easily understandable, but does not account for chance agreement. However, when observed agreement is close to perfect, kappa values are low since its calculations are based in part on the variability in responses.[32]

The estimate of kappa for each role is a weighted average of each of the estimates of kappa for the time categories of past, present, and future. Weighted kappa for each time category was also obtained by calculating an average of the separate estimates of kappa across the 10 roles. Guidelines developed by Landis and Koch[33] for interpreting the kappa statistic appear in Table 12-2.

In this study, the estimates of kappa for individual roles for a given time category ranged from slight to almost perfect agreement, with the majority being either moderate or substantial. The percent agreement for each category ranged from 73% to 97%, with the majority exceeding 88%. The estimates of weighted kappa for each role over the three time categories ranged from moderate to substantial, with the majority falling in the substantial range. The percent agreement for each role ranged from 77% to 93%, with an average of 87%. Finally, the estimates of weighted kappa for each time category over the 10 roles were substantial for the present, while estimates for the past and future were moderate. The percent agreement averaged 87%, with little appreciable difference noted between the time categories.

Thus, for part 1, the estimates of weighted kappas for all roles indicated substantial concordance, while the composite estimate of percent agreement was 87%. In general, there was a tendency for the measures of concordance to be stronger for adults 31 to 79 years of age than for the younger subgroup 18 to 30 years of age, and for the early retesting between 1 to 4 weeks, as opposed to later retesting between 5 and 8 weeks.

For part 2, the weighted estimate of kappa for all roles indicated moderate concordance for the value component of the checklist. The composite estimate of per-

Table 12-2
Guidelines for Interpreting Kappa Statistics

Kappa Statistic	Strength of Agreement
< 0.00	Poor
0.00-0.20	Slight
0.21-0.40	Fair
0.41-0.60	Moderate
0.61-0.80	Substantial
0.81-1.00	Almost Perfect

cent agreement was 79%. Again, older subjects appeared more consistent than younger subjects, and there was greater concordance with earlier retesting. Although it appears that the value of roles seems less consistent than the assessment of perceived incumbency of roles, it is more likely a reflection of the response categories. Three responses are possible for the role values, while the measure of perceived incumbency is binary. Measures of agreement tend to decrease as the number of possible outcomes increase.

For the role of religious participant, the data presented was based on an earlier version of the wording for this role. Therefore, the reliability of this role was not established in this study.

Other Reliability and Validity Studies

In an unpublished study, Pezzulli examined the test-retest reliability of the Role Checklist with depressed adolescents in a short-term psychiatric hospital.[34] The checklist was administered twice, 2 weeks apart, to 38 subjects in two groups, ages 13 to 15, and 16 to 18. Results for part 1 indicated that all roles, except the student role, achieved at least fair strength of agreement and most achieved at least moderate levels. For part 2, or role value, all roles achieved at least fair strength of agreement, with most reaching the moderate level of reliability.

A later study was conducted to establish the concurrent validity of the Role Checklist and provide further evidence its reliability.[35] The test-retest and interrater reliability were evaluated, using two methods of implementation—oral directions and written directions—by two administrators. A concurrent measure, the Activity Configuration was used to determine validity.[36] The Activity Configuration, as an overview of activities performed during a typical week, identifies whether the individuals actually engaged in the roles they indicated on the Role Checklist.

The subjects were 68 junior, senior, or professional master's degree occupational therapy students. The ages of the subjects ranged from 19 to 50 years, with the majority (81.8%) females between 20 and 23 years of age.

The percent agreement and the kappa statistic were again used to test for strength of agreement. For the reliability component of the study, data was analyzed for all subjects to determine the strength of agreement between the initial assessment and the retest 3 weeks later. The reliability was then determined to compare the written and oral administration methods and the two administrators. The reliability results of a control group were used to ensure that completion of the Activity Configuration had no effect on the reliability of other subjects.

The results for all subjects in part 1 of the checklist indicated that kappa statistics ranged from slight to substantially, with most percent agreements above 80%. Weighted kappas for all subjects across roles ranged from fair to almost perfect and showed moderate agreement across time categories. Comparisons between groups receiving written versus oral instructions on part 1 revealed few differences, since scores were mostly at the moderate and substantial levels for both groups. Comparisons between administrators revealed that the majority of results in both groups were at the moderate level or above, although one administrator had more fair responses, while the other had more substantial or almost perfect levels.

Comparisons of the written, oral, and control groups on part 2 of the checklist showed agreements among subjects as ranging from poor to substantial. However, when considered with percent agreements, some of the categories were likely 0 because of perfect agreement, rather than no agreement. The weighted kappa was moderate for the written and control group and fair for the oral group. The overall percent agreement for all three groups was similar (79-80%). Both administrators had weighted kappas of moderate and percent agreements of 80% on part 2 of the checklist, although the kappas and percent agreements for the individual roles differed from one administrator to the other.

To determine validity, the activities from the Activity Configuration that fit role descriptions on the Role Checklist were compared with the roles indicated in the "present" column on the Role Checklist, and a kappa statistic and percent agreement tests were use to compare agreement. The results are shown in Table 12-3.[35] The results ranged from fair to almost perfect (student role), with most falling at the moderate or substantial levels. Most percent agreements exceeded 80%. These results indicate that answers on the post-test category of the Role Checklist represented actual occupational role participation during the previous seven days, thereby supporting the validity of the Role Checklist.

Although this study has several limitations including the fact that the sample was a small, homogeneous group of students and that the Activity Configuration is not a standardized measure, it does support the reliability and presents at least initial concurrent validity of the Role Checklist. Further, from all indications, the role of religious participant seemed to demonstrate stable and appropriate reliability for the checklist.

Research Studies Using the Role Checklist

A substantial number of studies have used the Role Checklist since its development. In some studies, the Role Checklist was one of a number of instruments used to demonstrate the use of the model of human occupation with various populations.[17,25,26,31,37,38] In other studies, the Role Checklist was used to examine role performance with either a specific population[20,27,39-41] or in conjunction with life satisfaction.[16,42]

Most recently, the Role Checklist was used to compare the roles of community-living and patient populations.[30] The subjects included 1,020 community-living adults (CLW) with no major diagnoses of physical or psychosocial dysfunction, and 292 adults with physical or psychosocial dysfunction who had been referred to occupational therapy at the National Institutes of Health. All 102 of the psychosocial dysfunction subjects were inpatients; 129 of the physical dysfunction patients were inpatients; and 61 were outpatients.

Table 12-3

Kappa and Percent Agreement for Activity Configuration and Role Checklist Compared to Control Group

Activity Configuration and Role Checklist

Roles	Kappa	Percent Agreement
Student	0	100
Worker	.60	87
Volunteer	.65	96
Caregiver	.59	81
Home Maintenance	.29	62
Friend	.24	60
Family	.39	68
Religious	.75	91
Hobbyist	.56	79
Participant	.42	90
Other	.49	97
Weighted Kappa/ % Agreement	.41	78

The chi-square test was used to determine if there was a significant difference between expected and observed frequencies in role incumbency and role value categories. Three specific analyses were performed: 1) CLW versus entire patient group, 2) CLW versus patients with psychosocial dysfunction, and 3) CLW versus patients with physical disabilities. Based on the demographics of the patient groups, eg, age, and sex, random computer elimination was used to develop specifically matched CLW cohorts. Therefore, age, sex, and race (all subjects were white) did not differ significantly between the two groups for the three samples.

CLW Sample Versus Patient Sample

Table 12-4, on role incumbency, indicates that the CLW and total patient group had similar past roles.[35] Only the roles of worker and volunteer were significantly different between the two groups. Specifically, a lower percentage of patient subjects fulfilled a volunteer role in the past, whereas a higher percentage of them fulfilled the worker role in the past, when compared to the CLW sample. This was an unexpected finding, which may be idiosyncratic for this patient population, or it may be that the worker role, although important for the individual in many aspects, may not have been the "healthiest" role for these subjects.

More importantly, the groups differed significantly in all of their present roles. These results are due to the fact that, in each role, the patient sample had a higher percentage of no answers to the question of whether they were presently fulfilling that particular role. However, fewer significant differences were noted between the two groups in identification of future roles. The fact that patients saw themselves as fulfilling future roles as volunteers (no significant differences between the CLW and patient groups), but not as workers, students, or caregivers, does not seem surpris-

Table 12-4
Comparison of Role Incumbency of the Community-Living Well Sample and the Patient Sample

Community-Living Well+: n = 523
Patient: n = 259

	Roles[++]			x^2		
	Past %	Present %	Future %	Past	Present	Future
Student						
CL	92.0	29.1	46.9	1.3	55.9***	7.3**
PT	94.2	5.8	36.7			
Worker						
CL	76.7	72.3	70.9	28.4***	172.1***	10.3**
PT	92.3	22.8	59.5			
Volunteer						
CL	65.4	24.1	46.7	6.0*	10.1**	1.0
PT	56.4	14.3	42.9			
Caregiver						
CL	70.9	57.0	62.9	.7	74.3***	12.3***
PT	67.9	24.3	49.8			
Home Maintenance						
CL	83.0	90.4	82.2	2.0	124.1***	.3
PT	86.9	56.0	80.7			
Friend						
CL	84.7	83.9	79.4	.0	55.1***	.1
PT	84.9	59.9	80.3			
Family						
CL	85.5	85.7	82.0	.3	39.1***	.5
PT	86.9	66.4	79.9			
Religious						
CL	66.9	29.5	38.8	1.2	7.8**	.3
PT	62.9	20.1	40.9			
Hobbyist						
CL	80.1	65.6	71.9	.5	45.7***	3.2
PT	82.2	40.2	65.6			
Part Org						
CL	52.2	23.9	35.3	1.3	24.1***	1.5
PT	47.9	9.3	30.9			

* $P < .05$, ** $P < .01$, *** $P < .001$
+Whites only; random elimination of young and old subjects and more females than males from CL sample.
++ Numbers indicate the percentage of the sample that checked the past, present, future roles.
Note: CL = Community-Living Well Sample; PT = Patient Sample

ing. A person is often a student for the enhancement of his career, and because the worker role may be seen as unlikely in the future, the student role also may be seen as unlikely. Further, individuals with disabilities may be more likely to see themselves in the future in a care-receiving role, rather than a care-giving role, especially when considering chronic conditions like arthritis, lupus, schizophrenia, etc, which

Table 12-5
Comparison of the Value of the Roles of Community-Living Well Sample and the Patient Sample

Community-Living Well+: n = 523
Patient: n = 259

	Value of Roles[++]			χ^2	
	Not at All %	Somewhat %	Very %	NC %	
Student					
CL	5.3	20.9	72.9	1.0	37.20***
PT	17.7	25.5	55.6	1.2	
Worker					
CL	4.1	13.0	81.1	1.8	24.81***
PT	11.2	20.9	66.4	1.5	
Volunteer					
CL	11.4	50.6	35.4	2.6	8.04*
PT	18.5	49.4	29.7	2.3	
Caregiver					
CL	2.6	20.9	74.0	2.6	47.7***
PT	15.8	21.6	60.6	1.9	
Home Maintenance					
CL	5.5	35.2	58.1	1.2	2.05
PT	6.2	30.1	62.6	1.2	
Friend					
CL	1.0	21.9	76.6	0.6	20.44***
PT	5.4	14.3	78.8	1.5	
Family					
CL	1.8	7.7	89.0	1.6	7.78
PT	2.3	13.5	83.4	0.8	
Religious					
CL	22.8	40.0	33.9	3.4	.24
PT	24.3	39.0	33.6	31.0	
Hobbyist					
CL	4.9	41.1	52.8	1.2	13.68**
PT	12.0	34.8	51.8	1.5	
Part Org					
CL	25.6	50.6	19.5	4.3	5.44
PT	32.4	45.2	16.1	5.8	

* $P < .05$, ** $P < .01$, *** $P < .001$
+Whites only; random elimination of young and old subjects and more females than males from CL sample.
++ Numbers indicate the percentage of the sample that checked either "not at all valuable," "somewhat valuable," or "very valuable."
Note: CL = Community-Living Well Sample, PT = Patient Sample, NC = Not Checked.

were the subjects' diagnoses in this study. However, the fact that the patient subjects were as apt to view themselves in a future volunteer role as the CLW subjects may indicate that a volunteer role may fulfill the same needs as a worker role.

Table 12-5 shows that the patient sample valued the roles of worker, student, volunteer, and caregiver roles less than the CLW sample.[35] This may be positive, since role dysfunction may occur if people cannot fulfill roles that they highly value. Occupational therapy intervention is probably indicated in such circumstances to identify which roles are important to an individual and to facilitate fulfillment of those roles. Individuals who have fewer, but highly valued roles, are of less concern than individuals who have low or no value in any role. Rather than try to expand the number of roles, the therapist could help patients value the roles in which they can and will participate. Thus, the first step in therapy is to identify the occupational roles in which the individual wishes to engage and then facilitate the means to fulfill those identified roles to the person's satisfaction.

The finding that the CLW subjects differed from patient subjects regarding the hobbyist role in terms of role incumbency and value is of particular interest to occupational therapists. Hobbies, or avocational pursuits, are often seen as providing a balance to or replacing worker roles, as in the case of a retired individual. Those patients who do not see themselves in the worker role may need occupational therapy services to help them develop valued leisure pursuits. If the patient lacks the worker role, an important role for most adults, other roles need to become more important so as to not suffer decreased self-esteem or poor life-satisfaction.

CLW Sample Versus Psychosocial Dysfunction Sample or Physical Dysfunction Sample

The psychosocial dysfunction group differed significantly from the CLW group in all present roles, except for the volunteer role (Table 12-6).[35] However, this group was similar to the CLW group for both past roles, except for student and worker, and for future roles, except caregiver. A higher percentage of subjects in the patient group indicated fulfillment in the past roles of student and worker, but more subjects in the CLW group indicated they saw themselves returning to caregiver roles. This would seem positive in that patients are able to see themselves as being able to fulfill most of their future roles. As mentioned previously, it seems likely that a patient's present status as care receiver would influence the ability to see himself or herself as a future caregiver. Appropriately, the patient sample ascribed significantly less value to the caregiver role than the CLW group. Unexpectedly, they also valued the worker role less than the CLW group, although they see themselves as fulfilling that role in the future, as did the CLW sample.

The fact that the patient sample valued the roles of family and friends less than did the CLW subjects leads to several speculations. Due to the nature of psychiatric illness, family or friend interactions may be strained, causing stress on the patient and eliciting a less-than-favorable view of these relationships. It may be a matter of poor role taking by the patient or improper counter-role responses by family members or friends that make these roles difficult or undesirable. Further examination of these factors is needed before any assumptions can be made. Nevertheless, this finding suggests an area of intervention for the occupational therapist. Activities that focus on facilitating interpersonal interactions, clarifying values, or role-playing a family member or friend may highlight specific problem areas that warrant therapeutic intervention.

The results (Table 12-7) indicate that subjects with physical disabilities differed significantly from the CLW group in all present roles, except religious participants. [35]

Table 12-6

Chi-Square Value for Roles and Value of Roles for Community-Living Well Sample versus Psychosocial Dysfunctional Sample

Community-Living Well+: n = 473
Psychosocial Dysfunction: n = 95

		Role Incumbency			Value of Roles
		Past	Present	Future	
Student	$X^2 =$	5.59	33.10	.56	6.30
	$P =$	.018*	.001***	.454	.098
Worker	$X^2 =$	15.06	143.78	.01	10.27
	$P =$	.001***	.001***	.912	.016*
Volunteer	$X^2 =$	1.68	3.16	.24	5.11
	$P =$	.195	.075	.623	.164
Caregiver	$X^2 =$	2.46	61.95	6.05	36.22
	$P =$	.117	.001***	.014*	.001***
Home Maintenance	$X^2 =$	1.77	127.09	.00	2.85
	$P =$	.184	.001***	.970	240
Friend	$X^2 =$	.07	64.62	.03	17.89
	$P =$	.788	.001***	.860	.001***
Family	$X^2 =$	41	70.60	.00	12.42
	$P =$	524	.001***	.970	.006**
Religious	$X^2 =$	.05	6.27	.65	3.93
	$P =$	.305	.012*	.421	.269
Hobbyist	$X^2 =$	.42	20.58	.17	7.66
	$P =$	.516	.001***	.684	.054
Part Org	$X^2 =$	.51	17.33	.34	6.95
	$P =$	. 476	.001***	.561	.073

* $P < .05$; ** $P < .01$; *** $P < .001$
+whites only; elimination of all subjects over 64 years of age.

As with the psychosocially disabled subject sample, a higher percentage of subjects with physical dysfunction indicated that they will not fulfill the worker, student, caregiver, or hobbyist roles in the future, when compared with the well sample. Similarly, they indicated the caregiver, worker, and friend roles to be less valued. However, there are differences between the psychosocial dysfunction and CLW samples, and the physical dysfunction and CLW samples. For example, the subjects with physical dysfunctions differed additionally in their expectations that they would fulfill future roles of student, worker, and hobbyist, and also on their valuing of the roles of student, hobbyist, and participant in organizations. The student role may be easily explained by the fact that the sample with physically disabilities was older than the sample with psychosocial dysfunctional (all subjects under 25 years of age in the CLW sample were omitted, since the sample with physically disabilities was older). However, it is interesting to note that the subjects with physical disabilities do not see themselves returning to the worker or hobbyist roles. Three explanations come to mind as to why subjects with psychosocial dysfunctional predicted fulfillment of roles over subjects with physical dysfunctional. First, it may be that the physical capacities of subjects with physical dysfunction may pre-

Table 12-7

Chi-Square Value for Roles and Value of Roles for Community-Living Well Sample versus Physical Dysfunctional Sample

Community-Living Well+: n = 473
Physically Disabled: n = 144

		Role Incumbency			Value of Roles
		Past	Present	Future	
Student	X^2 =	.13	13.15	15.51	37.19
	P =	.721	.001***	.001***	.001***
Worker	X^2 =	14.57	85.71	16.29	15.66
	P =	.001***	.001***	.001***	.001***
Volunteer	X^2 =	4.29	5.31	2.55	5.48
	P =	.038*	.021*	.111	.140
Caregiver	X^2 =	1.16	33.06	9.19	39.02
	P =	.283	.001***	.002*	.001***
Home Maintenance	X^2 =	.19	55.74	1.09	5.18
	P =	.659	.001***	.297	.159
Friend	X^2 =	.00	13.93	.001	19.28
	P =	.956	.001***	.976	.001***
Family	X^2 =	.000	5.29	1.02	1.79
	P =	.987	.021*	.976	.616
Religious	X^2 =	1.12	2.81	.03	.93
	P =	.290	.094	.869	.818
Hobbyist	X^2 =	.24	32.91	7.09	11.22
	P =	.516	.001***	.684	.054
Part Org	X^2 =	1.79	7.20	1.69	10.65
	P =	.180	.007**	.193	.014*

* $P < .05$; ** $P < .01$; *** $P < .001$
+whites only; random elimination of young and old, more females than males.

vent their returning to these roles. Second, it may be that subjects with psychosocial dysfunction are denying the difficulty they will have fulfilling future roles, such as worker, and, therefore, their self-reported results are misleading. A third explanation may be that the focus of the occupational therapy treatment between these two groups is diverse and caused the difference. Typically, the treatment of the patient with physical disabilities is focused on functional restoration of the performance components used in daily living tasks. There is little or no focus on the non-tangible goals of specific role performance.[43] On the other hand, the treatment of patients with psychosocial dysfunction is focused specifically on these aspects. For example, leisure-skill training is frequently a focus with individuals who have psychiatric disorders. Although further research is needed to confirm this third explanation, it does suggest that attention to role dysfunction in those with physical disabilities is necessary to increase life-satisfaction.

A study by Vause-Earland supports this third explanation, that the focus of occupational therapy treatment between patients with psychosocial dysfunction and patients with physical disabilities caused the difference between future fulfillment of worker and hobbyist roles.[43] The author found that, although occupational therapists in physical disability settings believed that occupational role assessment was an important focus of occupational therapy, they had limited knowledge and understanding of the four standardized role assessment instruments developed by occupational therapists, and only 5% of the 236 respondents occasionally used role-assessment tools in practice.

Although this study had several limitations, including the fact that sample groups were not randomly selected, the patient populations may not be representative of all patient groups. Also including the fact that no interrater reliability studies were done, the results of the comparison groups strongly suggest that roles are significantly affected by disability, whether physical or psychosocial in nature. Patients are either not choosing or unable to fulfill their present roles, even though they fulfilled those roles in the past. If role participation is seen as part of the occupational functioning of the individual, this study underscores the need for occupational therapists to address role incumbency and role value with patients. Further, it supports the use of the Role Checklist as an occupational therapy tool for intervention.

SUMMARY AND IMPLICATIONS FOR THE FUTURE

This chapter describes the concept of role and role functioning specifically within the model of human occupation; the development, reliability, and validity studies of the Role Checklist; how it can be used clinically; and recent research using the Checklist. The Role Checklist was designed as a response to the need to assess the roles of occupational therapy patients efficiently and effectively. The written inventory identifies a respondent's perceived role participation along a temporal continuum in 10 roles, as well as the degree to which each role is valued. Information gathered from the instrument can be used to help in patient assessment in terms of role participation, valuation of roles, role balance, and future orientation.

Test-retest reliability studies on the Role Checklist have indicated that the instrument is satisfactorily stable with normal adults, including the role of religious participant. Additionally, the instrument seems to be reliable regardless of who administers the assessment or whether it is administered in written or oral format. Validity studies have also substantiated the use of the Checklist. Content validity was based on a review of social psychology and occupational therapy literature. Concurrent validity has been examined with the Activity Configuration, and the Checklist appears to be valid in identifying role participation. Finally, the Role Checklist appears to discriminate between patient populations and community living adults with no major physical or psychosocial dysfunction, and may be able to provide information as to how occupational therapy can address issues of role dysfunction.

Further research is needed, however. Reliability studies with patient populations are needed, as well as other concurrent validity studies with other role assessment tools or occupational performance instruments. Studies demonstrating the usefulness of the instrument with other groups of patients, including minority groups, are also needed. Finally, as mentioned previously, long term studies would be useful to demonstrate if using the Checklist in occupational therapy treatment does indeed predict future role performance or the preparation to enter roles.

The checklist format offers the therapist and patient a visual and concrete image of problems in role performance and discrepancies between role performance and role value. It is hoped that, through continued use and development, the Role

Checklist can continue to be a valuable tool that occupational therapists can use now and in the future.

REFERENCES

1. Oakley F. *The Model of Human Occupation in Psychiatry*, unpublished master's degree project. Richmond, Va: Department of Occupational Therapy, Medical College of Virginia, Virginia Commonwealth University; 1982.

2. Kielhofner G, Burke J. Conceptual framework and content, part 1. A model of human occupation. *Am J Occup Ther.* 1980;34:572-581.

3. Kielhofner G, Burke J. Components and determinants of human occupation. In Kielhofner G, ed. *A Model of Human Occupation.*Baltimore, Md: Williams & Wilkins; 1985, 12-36.

4. Kielhofner G. *A Model of Human Occupation: Theory and Application*, 2nd ed. Baltimore, Md: Williams & Wilkins; 1995:71-72.

5. Neugarten BL, Datan N. Sociological perspectives on the life cycle. In Baltes PB, Schaie KW, eds. *Middle Age and Aging.* Chicago, Ill: The University of Chicago Press; 1973, 710-717.

6. Heard C. Occupational role acquisition. *Am J Occup Ther.* 1977;31: 243-247.

7. Brim OG. Personality development as role-learning. In Iscoe I, Stevenson HW, eds. *Personality Development in Children.* Austin, Tex: University of Texas Press; 1966, 127-159.

8. Dion KK. Socialization in adulthood. In Lindzey G, Aronson E, eds. *Handbook of Social Psychology.* New York, NY: Random House; 1985, vol 3, pp 124-147.

9. Garza RT, Herrington LG. Social identity: A multidimensional approach. *J Soc Psychol.* 1987;127:299-308.

10. Gove WR, Zeiss C. Multiple roles and happiness. In Crosby FJ, ed. *Spouse, Parent, Worker.* New Haven, Conn: Yale University Press; 1987, 125-137.

11. Kimmel DC. *Adulthood and Aging.* New York, NY: John Wiley and Sons Inc; 1974.

12. Rosow I. *Social Integration of the Aged.* New York, NY: The Free Press; 1976.

13. Blau ZS. *Old Age in a Changing Society.* New York, NY: New Viewpoints; 1973.

14. Stryker S, Statham A. Symbolic interaction and role theory. In Lindzey G, Aronson E, eds. *Handbook of Social Psychology*, vol 3. New York, NY: Random House; 1985, 311-378.

15. Schurtz R, Rau MT. Social support through the life course. In Cohen S, Syne SL, eds. *Social Support and Health.* New York, NY: Academic Press; . 1985.

16. Branholm I, Fugl-Meyer AR. Occupational role preference and life satisfaction. *OTJR.* 1992;12:159-171.

17. Duellman MK, Barris R, Kielhofner G. Organized activity and the adaptive status of nursing home residents. *Am J Occup Ther.* 1986;40:618-622.

18. Gregory MD. Occupational behavior and life satisfaction among retirees. *Am J Occup Ther.* 1983;37:548-553.

19. Smith NR, Kielhofner G, Watts JH. The relationship between the volition, activity pattern & life satisfaction in the elderly. *Am J Occup Ther.* 1986;40:278-283.

20. Hallett JD, Zasler ND, Maurer P, Cash S. Role change after traumatic brain injury in adults. *Am J Occup Ther.* 1994;48:241-246.

21. Kielhofner G, Harlan B, Bauer D, Maurer P. The reliability of a historical interview with physically disabled respondents. *Am J Occup Ther.* 1986;40:551-556.

22. Matsutsuyu J. Occupational behavior—a perspective on work and play. *Am J Occup Ther.* 1971;25:291-294.

23. Rogers JC, Holm MB. Occupational therapy diagnostic reasoning: A component of clinical reasoning. *Am J Occup Ther.* 1991;45:1045-1053.

24. Versluys H. Remediation of role disorders through focused group work. *Am J Occup Ther.* 1980;34:609-614.

25. Barris R, Dickie V, Baron KB. A comparison of psychiatric patients and normal subjects based on the model of human occupation. *OTJR.* 1988;8:3-23.

26.   Ebb EW, Coster W, Duncombe L. Comparison of normal and psychosocially dysfunctional adolescent males. *OTMH*. 1989;9:53-74.

27.   Baker F, Curbow B, Wingard JR. Role retention and quality of life of bone marrow transplant survivors. *Social Science Medicine*. 1991;32:697-704.

28.   Cheng S, Rogers J. Changes in occupational role performance after a severe burn: A retrospective study. *Am J Occup Ther*. 1989;43:17-24.

29.   Oakley F, Kielhofner G, Barris R, Reichler RK. The role checklist: Development and empirical assessment of reliability. *OTJR*. 1986;6:157-170.

30.   Dickerson AE, Oakley F. Comparing the roles of community living well and patient populations. *Am J Occup Ther*. 1995;49:221-228.

31.   Pizzi M. The model of human occupation and adults with HIV infection and AIDS. *Am J Occup Ther*. 1990;44:257-264.

32.   Fleiss J. *Statistical Methods for Rates and Proportions*, 2nd ed. New York, NY: John Wiley & Sons Inc; 1981.

33.   Landis J, Koch G. The measurement of observer agreement for categorical data. *Biometrics*. 1977;33:159-174.

34.   Pezzulli TW. *Test-Retest Reliability of the Role Checklist With Depressed Adolescents in a Short-Term Psychiatric Hospital*. Unpublished master's degree project. Richmond, Va: Department of Occupational Therapy, Medical College of Virginia, Virginia Commonwealth University; 1988.

35.   Manos C. *Reliability and Concurrent Validity of the Role Checklist*. Unpublished master's degree thesis. Miami, Fla: Department of Occupational Therapy, Florida International University; 1994.

36.   Cynkin S, Robinson A. *Occupational Therapy and Activities Health: Toward Health Through Activities*. Boston, Mass: Little, Brown & Co; 1990.

37.   Barris R, Kielhofner G, Burch-Martin RM, Gelinas I, Klement M, Schultz B. Occupational function and dysfunction in three groups of adolescents. *Occupational Therapy Journal of Research*. 1986;6:301-307.

38.   Smyntek L, Barris R, Kielhofner G. The Model of Human Occupation applied to psychosocially functional and dysfunctional adolescents. *OTMH*. 1985;5:21-40.

39.   Bavaro SM. Occupational therapy and obsessive-compulsive disorder. *Am J Occup Ther*. 1991;45:456-458.

40.   Sepiol JM, Froehlich J. Use of the role checklist with the patient with multiple personality disorder. *Am J Occup Ther*. 1990;44:1008-1012.

41.   Stoffel VC. The Americans with Disabilities Act of 1990 as applied to an adult with alcohol dependence. *Am J Occup Ther*. 1992;46:640-644.

42.   Elliot M, Barris R. Occupation, role performance, and life satisfaction in elderly persons. *OTJR*. 1987;7:215-223.

43.   Vause-Earland T. Perceptions of role assessment tools in the physical disability setting. *Am J Occup Ther*. 1991;45:26-31.

The author would like to thank Dr. Gary Kielhofner and, particularly, Frances Oakley for their helpful advice on and assistance in editing the earlier drafts of this chapter.

Material for part of this chapter is from the *Role Checklist: Development and Empirical Assessment of Reliability* by F. Oakley, G. Kielhofner, R. Barris, and R.K. Reichler. Copyright 1986 by the American Occupational Therapy Foundation, Inc. Reprinted with permission.

Material for this chapter is also from *Comparing the Roles of Community-living Persons and Patient Populations* by A. Dickerson and F. Oakley. Copyright 1995 by the American Occupational Therapy Association, Inc. Reprinted with permission.

13

The Assessment of Occupational Functioning—Collaborative Version

Janet Hawkins Watts, PhD, OTR
Renee Hinson, MS, OTR
M. Jeanne Madigan, EdD, OTR, FAOTA
Patricia M. McGuigan, MS, OTR/L
Sandra M. Newman, MS, OTR

The Assessment of Occupational Functioning—Collaborative Version, or AOF-CV, was developed by Watts and Madigan[1] to provide a semistructured, self-report method of collecting assessment information on key components of the model of human occupation.[2] It can be administered as either a self-assessment with therapist follow-up or as an interview. It was designed to collect a broad range of qualitative information that may influence occupational performance and to identify where more detailed evaluation is needed. The AOF-CV provides a broad picture of complex, interrelated factors that contribute to or hinder occupational functioning and is, thus, recommended as an initial evaluation. The purpose of this chapter is to discuss occupational therapy interviews and self-report evaluations, followed by a presentation of the AOF-CV description, purpose and rationale, theory base, and its administration. Finally, AOF-CV development and research are presented.

REVIEW OF LITERATURE

Use of Interviews in Occupational Therapy

The AOF-CV is one in a series of occupational therapy clinical interviews that includes the Occupational History, Occupational Role History, Occupational Performance History Interview, Occupational Case Analysis Interview and Rating Scale (OCAIRS), and the original Assessment of Occupational Functioning.[3-8] The first three are history-taking interviews and the last two are for gathering information, primarily about current functioning.

The Occupational History and a screening version, the Occupational Role History, were introduced in 1969 and 1982, respectively, and were developed for use with psychiatric patients. A Modified Occupational Role History was developed in 1986 for use with patients with physical dysfunction. The Occupational Performance History Interview was developed in 1984; subsequent studies examined its reliability, and generic and model of human occupation formats were introduced. A revised version was published in 1998. The OCAIRS and the original AOF were developed in 1983 and were initially used in acute psychiatric care and long-term care, respectively. Because of similarities in their theoretical frameworks and formats, a comparison study was conducted in 1986.[9-13] Since introduction of the AOF in 1986, research and refinement have continued.

Self-Report and Self-Assessment Evaluations

Self-report, history, and direct observation all contribute integrally to understanding individuals' strengths, needs, and concerns. No one method is inherently better. Each serves different purposes, contributes unique and useful information, and has strengths and limitations. Thus, in good clinical practice, all are used and integrated when possible.

Self-report refers to evaluations in which recipients of care provide evaluation data orally or in writing. The evaluation may be a therapist-administered interview, questionnaire, or some form of self-assessment. Self-assessment refers here to a specific type of self-report in which care recipients complete an evaluation on their own, typically as a paper-and-pencil self-report. While not commonly acknowledged in occupational therapy literature, self-assessments are often used by many therapists to decrease the time required for evaluation, and to facilitate self-reflection and free expression concerns.

Self-report evaluation methods offer certain advantages over direct observation evaluations.[14-19] These include:

- Simplicity
- Time and cost economies, with the greatest realized in self-assessment
- Facilitation of active patient participation
- Coverage of a wide range of often complex functions (eg, not only basic activities of daily living, or ADL, but also instrumental ADLs and aspects of emotional, social, and mental functioning can be evaluated)
- Facilitation of self-reflection
- Self-perceptions of concerns relevant to care recipients
- Use in gathering subjective information on social adjustment, motivation, and stress
- Facilitation of collaboration, when used as an initial assessment
- Patient convenience, as they complete the form at their convenience.

There are, however, concerns about self-reports and self-assessments,[15-16,19-20] such as:

- Reliability and validity of data on functioning
- More subjective than direct observation
- Too dependent on people's perceptual and descriptive abilities
- Not likely to provide the most accurate information on those with certain cognitive limitations
- Non-readers unable to participate in self-assessment. [14-19]

Concerns about the validity of self-reports are addressed in the research. Morris and Boutelle demonstrated high agreement between self-administered evaluations and personal interviews on a multidimensional functional assessment of independent-living, well-elderly.[21] For that group, the more economical and easily available self-assessment method was of comparable value to the personal interview. Another study of self-ratings and provider-ratings of basic and complex self-care activities showed good agreement (84%-97%). Agreement on performance of household tasks, such as cooking and cleaning, was lower (77% and 64%, respectively).[22] Additionally, Harris, Jette, Campion, and Cleary found agreement between self-reports and observed performance to be excellent for basic activities of daily living and high for instrumental ADLs.[16]

Other writings suggest ways to maximize the advantages and minimize the disadvantages, ie, improve the accuracy, of self-reports. For example, a structured format and standardized administration can increase reliability and validity.[15,17,19] Some suggest that combining evaluation tools may yield the most accurate information.[15,19,23] Others note that cognitive impairment may be associated with overestimates of ability[23]; hence, screening for cognitive ability before administering a self-report or self-assessment should help identify people likely to give more valid responses. Orientation, oral communication, and reading and writing comprehension can be used to identify those patients who can complete self-report evaluations.[20,22,24] Research can help identify which information may best be obtained through self-report and self-assessment. Finally, supplementing self-report and self-assessment with direct and ongoing clinical observations is recommended.[19]

The collaborative assessment process using self-report and interview has the potential to reduce the time and cost, as well as enhance the relevance and value of yield. Additionally, anecdotal reports suggest that therapists frequently give paper-and-pencil evaluations to certain patients for independent completion. Since it often is not feasible to directly observe the many facets of performance about which therapists need information, a method that maximizes the value of the interview and self-report is appropriate. Thus, it makes sense to standardize this process and subject it to careful examination through research, with guidance from prior research.

AOF-CV OVERVIEW

Description

The AOF-CV is a semistructured, self-report screening instrument, based on the model of human occupation, that collects information about volition and habituation subsystem structure and occupational performance skills. It does not directly address underlying performance capacities, eg, musculoskeletal constituents, or environmental variables. The AOF-CV yields a general overview of the person's occupational status in the form of qualitative information and a numerical rating. Thus, it is recommended for use as an initial screening tool. Additional formal and informal observations and evaluations should be used to provide more detail about specific performance areas.

The AOF-CV incorporates refinements to the earlier version of the AOF suggested by clinicians to improve communication across cultures and permit optional self-administration with therapist follow-up. The instrument consists of a one-page administration protocol; a one-page cover sheet that asks for the recent employment work history and reasons for job changes; a 22-question interview schedule, coded to model components; and a 5-point rating scale. Typical interview items include, "Name at least five things you enjoy doing. Why do you like to do these things? What interests do you actively participate in now? How often do you do each thing?" A typical rating scale item asks, "Does this person demonstrate personal values through the selection of well-defined, meaningful activities?" All items are rated using the following scale: 5-very highly, 4-highly, 3-moderately, 2-little, 1-very little.

Purpose and Rationale

The AOF-CV offers a self-report assessment method, with established psychometric properties, that is clearly theory-based. It was developed as an initial screening tool to be supplemented with other history-taking and direct observation methods. It was designed to be as efficient as possible, while still yielding clinically useful information.

The AOF-CV may be administered as either an interview, or as a paper-and-pencil self-report with a follow-up interview. The self-assessment version combines self-administration with a follow-up interview. When used as a self-assessment with therapist follow-up, the evaluation can not only enhance accuracy over either interview or self-assessment used alone, but can also 1) permit more time for the patient's unpressured, uninhibited self-reflection; 2) integrally involve the patient in the therapy planning process; and 3) save time. The self-assessment with therapist follow-up has the potential to improve both effectiveness and efficiency of the assessment process.

Theoretical Base

Core Concepts

The model of human occupation provides the conceptual framework for this evaluation.[2] The model of human occupation uses principles from general, open, and dynamical systems theories to describe human occupational functioning.[2] Human behavior is flexibly assembled so that the person, the task, and the environment all contribute to behavior. Thus, the human system continually creates its structure through the ongoing interaction of the person, task, and environment. At any point in time, each of these can take the lead, contributing to behavior creation, depending on its relative importance.

Furthermore, the internal human system's organization is differentiated into subsystems that enable occupational performance. The volition, habituation, and mind-brain-body subsystems are related heterarchically. Kielhofner states:

> [Each contributes] toward the action to be performed by the person. The concept of heterarchy of subsystems emphasizes that the three subsystems each contribute different but complementary functions to the operation of the whole system. It also implies that the functional relationship of the three subsystems will change across time.[2]

Finally, occupational performance skills are the performance of motor, process, and communication/interaction skills, observed in the context of occupational performances. These skills differ from the mind-brain-body subsystem in that they are observable skills; whereas, the mind-brain-body subsystem refers to underlying capacities for performance whose status must be inferred from medical or diagnostic procedures.[2] While the model of human occupation incorporates much more complexity, these core concepts serve as the basis for discussing the AOF-CV.

Relationship of the AOF-CV to Its Theory Base

The AOF-CV relates to the model of human occupation in the following ways:
1. It deals with a group of core concepts, ie, aspects of the volition and habituation subsystems; occupational performance skills, not the entire model in its complexity.
2. It focuses on the person more than the task or environment.

3. It addresses structure more than process.

4. It provides screening level information, not detailed data about all model elements.

5. It was developed to systematically ask questions about the person's volition, habituation, and occupational performance skills, but not about the mind-brain-body performance subsystem constituents.

The AOF-CV assesses the structure of the volition subsystem by asking questions about people's: 1) beliefs about their abilities and sense of control, ie, personal causation; 2) convictions about occupations, beliefs about how time should be used, and related goals, ie, values; and 3) favorable dispositions toward certain occupations, ie, interests. The habituation subsystem's structure is assessed in the AOF-CV by examining aspects of roles and habits.[2]

Questions related to occupational performance skills are general, and yield information about how people perceive their performances of movement, dealing with processes, and social communication and interaction. These were originally conceptualized as part of a performance subsystem; however, in the recent revision of the model, these are reconceptualized as occupational performance skills. The mind-brain-body subsystem[2] consists of underlying capacities for performance, such as musculoskeletal, neurological, cardiopulmonary, and symbolic constituents, that can only be inferred from the use of medical and diagnostic procedures. The AOF-CV does not assess the status of this subsystem.

Administration

The AOF-CV can be used either for patient completion with therapist follow-up or for therapist administration. It should only be used with patients who are capable of responding thoughtfully to an interview. The interviewer should have good interview skills and knowledge of the model of human occupation.

For patient administration with therapist follow-up, the therapist simply asks the patient to complete the interview form. Then, the therapist reviews responses, uses probes or clarifications as needed, and rates the items. The probes and clarifications are indicated if the specified questions elicit either no reply, a request for clarification, an answer suggesting interviewee misunderstanding, a superficial response, or other indications of poor communication. No other questions, probes, or clarifications should be used.

For therapist administration, the therapist follows the interview format, using parenthetical probes or clarifications as needed. The responses are noted on the interview schedule and provide information needed to mark the rating form.

Interpersonal and communication skills are rated, based on either the therapist's experience conducting the entire interview, or on the therapist's review and use of follow-up questions to interview the patient.

AOF-CV DEVELOPMENT AND RESEARCH

The AOF-CV is the current version of the original Assessment of Occupational Functioning (AOF), which was carefully researched and refined, and for which reliability and validity estimates have been determined through systematic study.[1,8-13,25-29]

AOF Development and Research

The original AOF was developed as a semistructured interview and rating scale that provided quantitative as well as qualitative data. The AOF was developed in response to the needs of a therapist for a brief, comprehensive, theory-based evaluation that could help establish treatment priorities for physically disabled or aged residents.

Research on the original AOF,[8] involving 83 subjects, found that ratings corresponded with the model of human occupation components and provided estimates of test-retest and interrater reliability, concurrent validity, and the ability to discriminate between healthy and institutionalized elderly adults.

After research on the original AOF was completed, but not yet published, the first revision of the AOF was completed.[10] Changes were made to improve the instrument's suitability for interviewing, to provide more information on some model variables, and to refine the rating scale.

In a study by Watts, Brollier, Bauer, and Schmidt,[12] the AOF (first revision) was compared with a revised version of the OCAIRS.[4] Forty-one patients with schizophrenia were studied, and qualitative data were obtained from five registered occupational therapists who had used both instruments. Both instruments were found to be conceptually similar and clinically valuable, and suggestions for refinements were given. A concurrent validity study, using the Global Assessment Scale[30] with 39 of these same patients, established concurrent validity of the AOF and OCAIRS.[9] Quantitative and qualitative data obtained from 11 content experts established content validity of the AOF (first revision).[10] The yield from this study was used to develop the AOF (second revision).[13]

Morgan studied the ability of the AOF (second revision) to distinguish between 25 well elderly subjects living in a retirement home and 25 intermediate care facility residents.[28] The instrument's total score and component scores for personal causation, roles, habits, and skills differed significantly, while scores for values and interests did not. This adds further support for the AOF's validity and utility, when used with elderly people.

Research by Baber[25] supported concurrent validity of the AOF (second revision) in relation to the Quality of Life Index, or QLI,[31] through a study with 30 physically disabled patients who had recently completed rehabilitation. The researcher found moderate to strong correlations of AOF component scores for personal causation, interests, roles, and skills, with conceptually similar QLI items (there were no conceptually similar QLI habit items, and the values component correlation was not statistically significant). Viik, Watts, Madigan, and Bauer[29] established preliminary validity for use of the AOF (second revision) with an alcoholic population using the Alcohol Dependence Scale[32] in a study with 48 subjects.

AOF-CV Development and Research

After 1990 the AOF was slightly revised to 1) clarify communication among diverse English-speaking cultures, ie, Australian Aboriginal and non-Aboriginal populations; 2) simplify items; 3) expand space and rearrange the rating sheet; 4) add administration guidelines; 5) combine related questions; and 6) reword items for optional self-administration. This resulted in the AOF-CV, which is in a format for either patient completion with therapist follow-up or for therapist administration.

The most recent research on the AOF-CV has examined 1) content validity, 2) appropriateness of terminology across cultures, and 3) which patients could provide useful information through the collaborative administration.[26,27] Content validity was examined by surveying experts from several English-speaking countries, including Australia, Canada, New Zealand, and the United States, asking therapists to match AOF-CV items to the model components from which they were derived.[27] The resulting pattern of item matches to model components was similar to those established in previous research.[10] Qualitative yield suggested that while the language of the instrument seemed to pose no problems, there was a need to interpret items relative to cultural values. For example, one person commented on the cross-cultural difficulties of the item "Do you feel in control of your life?" because, with Maori and Pacific Islanders, the good of the group takes precedence over the good of the individual.

A study by Elliott and Newman explored the value of the AOF as a self-administered evaluation and identified predictors of patient ability to use the AOF in the collaborative format.[26] Twenty-seven psychiatric patients completed the AOF-CV as a self-administered questionnaire. Scores on the Mini-Mental State, or MMS,[24] and ratings of educational level and verbal skill were recorded. Results suggest that higher MMS scores, educational level, and verbal ability may indicate which patients can complete the AOF independently with limited follow-up. Patients who scored 27 or higher on the MMS answered at least half of the AOF-CV questions independently with useful information. Overall 89% of questions were answered independently with useful answers, and therapist follow-up required an average of 12 minutes. Therapists commented that patients gained useful insight from completing the self-assessment. They also noted that the AOF-CV collected information similar to information currently obtained using "homemade" evaluations. Thus, the study suggests preliminary evidence of the AOF-CV's utility, when used as a self-assessment with therapist follow-up.

CASE EXAMPLE: JACKIE

Background

Jackie, a married 52-year-old female, was hospitalized with an exacerbation of multiple sclerosis and transferred to the Intensive Rehabilitation Unit after a 2-week hospitalization. Diagnosed with multiple sclerosis 15 years earlier, she has had long remissions with minor exacerbations until 2 years ago, when her exacerbations became severe with minimal remission. She has received inpatient and outpatient rehabilitation. Jackie lives with her spouse of 30-plus years (no children) in a retirement community apartment that is accessible to wheelchair, scooter, and walker. She and her husband were teachers in large city schools until they moved to the retirement community 2 years ago. Jackie no longer works, and her husband is a substitute teacher.

Evaluative Findings

Values

Jackie reported deriving meaning from reading, talking to others, and cooking. She was unable to state goals, other than continuing her current activities. She feels that time is standing still and that "living the same way day to day" is the best she can do.

Personal Causation

Jackie has mixed feelings about control. She states that she makes choices and actively participates in her medical management. However, she feels that her illness has left her with few options and limited abilities. She also reports that her husband has had to look after her and has had to curtail his life and plans. He has increased his sphere of influence in her life and "tells" her "what to do all the time."

Interests

Jackie likes to cook, read, and play the piano. Unfortunately, her illness either limits or totally interferes with these activities. Her vision, coordination, sensation, and higher cognitive functions have been compromised, leaving her with little ability to pursue her interests. Thus, talking, television, and radio are her only currently pursued interests.

Roles

Jackie's roles are wife and daughter. She reports very diminished capacity in the wife role. Her parents died several years ago; therefore, the occupational role of daughter is no longer valid. With increased caregiving and homemaking responsibilities, her husband cannot pursue his interests. He also feels that his provider role is compromised due to the medical expenses and the decreased income, since he is only able to work part time because of caregiving for Jackie. Her husband is frustrated, and Jackie feels helpless and useless with her greatly reduced homemaker and spouse role involvements.

Habits

Jackie describes her routine as being "mainly in bed." She gets up with her husband and needs his help with morning self-care. Because of poor balance, proprioception, and trunk control, Jackie does not leave the bed alone. Thus, she returns to bed to watch television or listen to the radio until he returns from work. When her husband is home, she assists with meal preparation by watching and directing the sequences. She also attempts to stir, and wipe the counters and table. She states that her days are all alike and that most people think that she is a recluse.

Skills

Jackie has severe ataxia, poor proprioception, and very limited trunk control. She can walk short distances, using a rolling walker with her husband's help. She also has a scooter for the home; however, she does not own a lift, nor can she afford adaptations to the car, which would allow her to use the scooter outside the home. Jackie has a pediatric-design wheelchair that has to be pushed by a caregiver. Her husband would not consider a wheelchair that could be maneuvered by Jackie, because it is too heavy for him to lift and carry to the car. Jackie is beginning to experience cognitive deficits associated with MS, including confusion, memory loss, and higher cognitive impairments in mathematics, sequencing, and reading. Her vision is blurred at times.

AOF-CV Ratings

The following ratings were made, with 1 meaning "very little" and 5 meaning "very likely":

Values: meaningfulness—2; occupational goals—1, personal standards—3, temporal orientation—4.

Personal Causation: belief in control—2, belief in skill—1, belief in efficacy—2, expectancy of success—1.

Interests: discrimination—2, pattern—2, potency—1.

Roles: balance—1, internalized expectations—2, perceived incumbency—1.

Habits: degree of organization—1, social appropriateness—2, rigidity and flexibility—2.

Skills: motor skills—2, process skills—3, communication/interpersonal skills—3.

Treatment Implications

Even though Jackie is the patient, focusing on both she and her husband should enhance her quality of life.

Values: Set long- and short-term goals and related strategies.

Personal Causation: Provide means of control and successful experiences. Provide home adaptations, adaptive equipment, and caregiver education regarding enhancing her mobility in her husband's absence.

Interests: Provide means to pursue interests compatible with current skills as well as with expected debilitation. Consider relative strengths in temporal orientation, process skills, and communication skills. Explore affordable interests for Jackie and her husband.

Roles: Increase Jackie's role-related tasks, especially in the home and with others.

Habits: Enhance home mobility during husband's absence. Identify energy conservation techniques and safe but active routines. Provide daily planner.

Skills: Provide adaptations and modifications to enhance Jackie's ability to control her environment. Train her husband to safely assist Jackie.

Occupational Status

Jackie is beginning to feel helpless and hopeless, because of her increasing debilitation and the developing cognitive impairments that impact her judgment. Education, modifications, adaptations, and use of supportive resources are essential to reduce Jackie's feelings of dependence, and to enhance Jackie and her husband's life satisfaction. Educating her husband on the importance of maximizing Jackie's independence and environmental control may increase his time to pursue outside interests and roles. Providing Jackie with successful, purposeful activities to increase environmental control and to increase family involvement will maximize her use of her remaining role capacity. Identifying financial and multiple sclerosis supports can minimize stress.

SUMMARY

This chapter described the development and use of the AOF-CV. The instrument grew out of clinician need and has continued to develop, using therapist feedback on its clinical value. The current version is the result of systematic study and revision, following feedback from clinicians. It provides a theory-based, initial screening of people's volition and habituation subsystem structure and occupational performance skills in a flexible format for either therapist or self-administration with therapist follow-up. The psychometric properties are known and published. The AOF provides a flexible and standardized tool of known psychometric properties that collects information typically sought by therapists in initial screenings.

REFERENCES

1. Watts JH, Madigan JM. *Assessment of Occupational Functioning—Collaborative Version.* 1993. (Available from the author at the Virginia Commonwealth Department of Occupational Therapy Web site: http://views.vcu.edu/sahp/occu/)
2. Kielhofner G. *A Model of Human Occupation: Theory and Application,* 2nd ed. Baltimore, Md: Williams & Wilkins; 1995:34.
3. Florey LL, Michelman SM. Occupational Role History: A screening tool for psychiatric occupational therapy. *Am J Occup Ther.* 1982;36:301-308.
4. Kaplan K, Kielhofner G. *Occupational Case Analysis Interview and Rating Scale.* Thorofare, NJ: SLACK Incorporated; 1989.
5. Kielhofner G, Harlan B, Maurer P, Bauer D. The reliability of the historical interview with physically disabled respondents. *Am J Occup Ther.* 1986;40:551-556.
6. Kielhofner G, Henry A. *A User's Guide to the Occupational Performance History Interview.* Rockville, Md: American Occupational Therapy Association; 1988.
7. Moorehead LC. The occupational history. *Am J Occup Ther.* 1969;23:329-334.
8. Watts JH, Kielhofner G, Bauer DF, Gregory MD, Valentine DB. The Assessment of Occupational Functioning: A screening tool for use in long-term care. *Am J Occup Ther.* 1986;40:231-240.
9. Brollier C, Watts JH, Bauer D, Schmidt W. A concurrent validity study of two occupational therapy evaluation instruments: The AOF & OCAIRS. *OTMH.* 1988;8(4):49-59.
10. Brollier C, Watts JH, Bauer D, Schmidt W. A content validity study of the assessment of occupational functioning. *OTMH.* 1988;8(4):29-47.
11. Hopkins SE, Schmidt WC. *A Comparison and Concurrent Validity Examination of Two Evaluation Instruments Used With Psychiatric Patients.* 1986. Unpublished master's degree research project. Department of Occupational Therapy, Virginia Commonwealth University/Medical College of Virginia, MCV Box 980008, Richmond, VA 23298-0008.)
12. Watts JH, Brollier C, Bauer D, Schmidt W. A comparison of two evaluation instruments used with psychiatric patients in occupational therapy. *OTMH.* 1988;8(4):7-27.
13. Watts JH, Brollier C, Bauer D, Schmidt W. The assessment of occupational functioning: The second revision. *OTMH.* 1988;8(4):61-88.
14. Garbutt JS. An introduction to self-assessment. *British Journal of Occupational Therapy.* 1989;52(2):47-49.
15. Granger C, Gresham G. *Functional Assessment in Rehabilitation Medicine.* Baltimore, Md: Williams & Wilkins; 1984.
16. Harris BA, Jette AM, Campion EW, Cleary PD. Validity of self-report measures of functional disability. *Topics in Geriatric Rehabilitation.* 1986;1(3):31-41.
17. Jette AM. The Functional Status Index: Reliability and validity of a self-report functional disability measure. *J Rheumatol.* 1987;14(suppl 15):15-19.
18. Law M, Baptiste S, McColl M, Opzoomer A, Polatajko H, Pollock N. The Canadian Occupational Performance Measure: An outcome measure for occupational therapy. *Canadian Journal of Occupational Therapy.* 1990;57(2):82-87.
19. McReynolds P. Diagnosis and clinical assessment: Current status and major issues. *Annual Review of Psychology.* 1988;40:83-108.
20. Dzurec LC. How do they see themselves? Self-perception and functioning for people with chronic schizophrenia. *Journal of Psychosocial Nursing.* 1990;28(8):10-14.

21. Morris WW, Boutell S. Multidimensional functional assessment in two modes. *Gerontologist.* 1985;25:638-643.

22. Kivela S. Measuring disability: Do self-ratings and service provider ratings compare? *Journal of Chronic Diseases.* 1984;37(2):115-123.

23. Edwards M. The reliability and validity of self-report activities of daily living scales. *Canadian Journal of Occupational Therapy.* 1990;57(2):273-278.

24. Folstein MF, Folstein SE, McHugh PR. Mini-mental state, a practical method for grading the cognitive state of patients for the clinician. *J Psychiatr Res.* 1975;12:189-198.

25. Baber KP. *Construct Validity Inferences About the Assessment of Occupational Functioning for Persons with Physical Disabilities.* 1988. Unpublished master's degree research project. Department of Occupational Therapy, Virginia Commonwealth University/Medical College of Virginia, MCV Box 980008, Richmond, VA 23298-0008.

26. Elliott KR, Newman SM. *A Concurrent Validity Study of the 1991 Research Version of the Assessment of Occupational Functioning.* 1993. Unpublished master's degree research project. Department of Occupational Therapy, Virginia Commonwealth University/Medical College of Virginia, MCV Box 980008, Richmond, VA 23298-0008.

27. McGuigan PM. *Content Validity of the 1991 Research Version of the Assessment of Occupational Functioning.* 1993. Unpublished master's degree research project. Department of Occupational Therapy, Virginia Commonwealth University/Medical College of Virginia, MCV Box 980008, Richmond, VA 23298-0008.

28. Morgan R. *The Assessment of Occupational Functioning: Use As an Elderly Screening Tool.* 1988. Unpublished master's degree research project. Department of Occupational Therapy, University of Indianapolis.

29. Viik MK, Watts JH, Madigan MJ, Bauer D. Preliminary validation of the Assessment of Occupational Functioning with an alcoholic population. *OTMH.* 1990;10:19-33.

30. Endicott J, Spitzer R, Fleiss J, Cohen J. The Global Assessment Scale: A procedure for measuring overall severity of psychiatric disturbance. *Archives of General Psychiatry.* 1976;33:766-771.

31. Ferrans C, Powers M. Quality of Life Index: Development and psychometric properties. *Advances in Nursing Science.* 1985;8(1):15-21.

32. Skinner HA, Horn JL. *Alcohol Dependence Scale (ADS) User's Guide.* Toronto, ON: Addiction Research Foundation; 1984.

Research on the AOF-CV was partially funded by Fred Sammons.

14

The Role Activity Performance Scale

Marcia A. Good-Ellis, MS, OTR

The purpose of this chapter is to describe the development and current use of the Role Activity Performance Scale (RAPS) as an evaluation and research instrument used by occupational therapists in both short-term acute care and long-term rehabilitative care psychiatry. A current trend in psychiatry is toward more descriptive procedures for diagnosis and treatment, as seen in the American Psychiatric Association's continuous refinement of the *Diagnostic and Statistical Manual of Mental Disorders,* now in version DSM-IV,[1] and *The Functional Emotional Assessment Scale for Infancy and Early Childhood.*[2] Occupational therapists in mental health have a historical professional emphasis on treatment techniques designed to return patients to optimal levels of performance in their life roles in the community. Florey states that "occupational therapy must a) examine the life roles relative to the community, b) identify various skills that support them, and c) create an environment in which relevant rehabilitative behavior can be evoked and practiced."[3]

HISTORICAL DEVELOPMENT—RATIONALE

The RAPS was originally developed for use in a study of inpatient family intervention for patients diagnosed with schizophrenic and major affective disorders at the Payne Whitney Psychiatric Clinic of the New York Hospital-Cornell Medical College.[4-6] It has been used to investigate primary role activity skills in several other studies:

1. Standardization of the RAPS with reliability and validity testing of 15 patients diagnosed with schizophrenic or schizophreniform disorders, and 15 patients diagnosed with major affective disorders.[7]
2. Follow-up of 50 patients diagnosed with major affective disorders.[8]
3. A study of the RAPS 12 subscales validity in terms of the accuracy of the retrospective semistructured interview with time line rating methodology; and predictive abilities of the subscales with 15 outpatients diagnosed with schizophrenia and 15 outpatients diagnosed with major affective disorders.[9,10]
4. Use of some of the RAPS subscales as criterion variables to examine the empirical validity of the Model of Human Occupation.[11]
5. Baseline and follow-up data of 55 adult inpatients meeting DSM-IIIR criteria for personality disorders after hospitalization at the New York Psychiatric Institute.[12]

The Role Activity Performance Scale was developed to measure a broad range of role functioning (12 role domains). The RAPS can be used to gather historical role activity data applicable for diagnosis and treatment planning or as a research tool in treatment outcome studies. The RAPS is responsive to occupational therapy's need to become more skilled in determining and applying relevant outcome criteria that are measurable and explainable to consumers, other professionals, and payors. Foto said that "outcome studies designed to objectively evaluate appropriateness, effectiveness, and efficiency are urgently needed to justify continued funding for health care services."[13] While occupational therapists have traditionally evaluated performance of skills in life roles, the information may not have been gathered with the specificity necessary to evaluate outcomes of intervention. The RAPS provides a shared language and measurement methodology for role activity performance evaluation. For occupational therapy, instruments like the Role Activity Performance Scale are being developed to facilitate investigation of the effectiveness of its interventions and frames of reference.[7]

DESCRIPTION OF THE RAPS

The RAPS is a semistructured interview and rating scale, capable of assessing role activity performance history over a period of up to 18 months prior to interview. The RAPS assesses 12 role domains: Work or Work Equivalents, Education, Home Management, Nuclear/Extended Family Relationships, Mate Relationship, Parental Role, Social Relationships, Leisure Activities, Self-management, Health Role, Hygiene and Appearance, and Rehab Treatment Settings. Therapists can select role domains and adjust the assessment period length, according to their clinical evaluation or research requirements. One of the unique features of the RAPS is that it can be adapted for assessment periods from a 1-day point-in-time measure to as long as 18 months.[7]

The RAPS rating methodology takes role activity functioning information and allows the rater to group periods of similar functioning into time segments. Time segment scores are determined by rating level of role activity functioning, according to a 6-point operational definition scale provided for each role domain. This flexibility of time segment scoring methodology permits a standardized rating of role activity performance over the long or short term.

SEMISTRUCTURED INTERVIEW

The semistructured interview questions for each role domain are sequenced into sections as follows: a) background information about the place of the particular role in the patient's life and lifetime role functioning history; b) description of role environment and responsibilities during the time period under study; c) difficulties in functioning and changes in level of functioning during this period; d) description of patient's strengths, coping strategies, or adaption to difficulties; and e) the patient's and others' perspectives of how the patient performed in the role domain. Each role domain's semistructured interview section inquires about role activity performance history, using a series of open-ended questions. An example of one RAPS subscale interview, with a few sample questions from each section, is shown in Table 14-1.[7]

Descriptive role activity performance information can be gathered from multiple sources—the patient, family, significant others, medical record, and other members of the treatment team. The average time needed for an experienced interview-

---

Table 14-1

Sample of the RAPS Interview Format: Work or Work Equivalent Questions

Section A
The following questions relate to your life before the study period.
1. What type of work have you done or been interested in during your life? What work did you want as a child? As a teenager? As an adult?

Section B
The following questions relate to the specific type of work you were responsible for and participated in during the study period.
1. List job titles.

Section C
The following questions relate to changes, stresses, or difficulties with work.
6. In what way are certain work responsibilities difficult for you? Describe the task and explain all physical, emotional, and interpersonal problems. What are the most stressful parts of your job?

Section D
Your answers to the following questions will help me to understand how you handle problems or changes at work.
9. How do you solve technical, physical, emotional, or interpersonal problems at work?

Section E
The following questions relate to other people's views of how you are doing your work and how satisfied you are with your work.
15. What feedback have you received from your boss, co-workers, or others?

Note: Only one question from each section of the interview is shown. For Sections B, C, D, and E, a specific study period must be identified.

Good-Ellis MA, Fine SB, Spencer JH, DiVittis A. Developing a role activity performance scale. *Am J Occup Ther.* 1987;41;4:232-241. Copyright 1987 by the American Occupational Therapy Association, Inc. Reprinted with permission.

---

er to assess an 18-month time frame is 1 to 2 hours, depending on the availability of relevant information. This methodology of gathering information allows, not only for verification of the accuracy of information, but also for the patient and significant others to give their perspectives on the changes in the patient's role activity performance over time.

The RAPS interview can be an extremely rewarding experience for a patient or the patient's support network. Some patients and significant others reported that either filling out the evaluation or answering the interview questions was an experience from which they came away gaining insights about themselves or their significant others. Often patients reported that RAPS follow-up interviews gave them a chance to reflect on how they were doing in their role activity performance. Higher-functioning patients and outpatients reported that undergoing the RAPS interview was useful for reviewing their changes in role activity performance.

The RAPS' use of open-ended questions allows the therapist to learn the language, values, culture, and beliefs of patients and their networks of significant others. In reviewing research on factors influencing better patient recall during medical interviews, Lipkin reported that "affective skills found to be associated with better (patient) recall include expressing warmth and interest, conveying understanding, avoiding bias and threatening questions, pursuing verbal and nonverbal cues, and facilitating (patient) expression with open-ended questions."[14] Not only is patient recall of critical issues and events affecting role and activity performance aided by the use of open-ended questions, but additionally by the associated time line prompts and recording methodology. Corcoran, as quoted by Hettinger, stressed that occupational therapists need to understand the family perspective, since occupational therapy patients are discharged from hospitalization into home settings quickly.[15] The RAPS provides an open-ended interview structure that can be used during the initial contact with the patient, patient's family, and network of significant others, and can be the start of the treatment alliance formed with the occupational therapist.

The RAPS' emphasis on recording role activity performance history by specific time segments yields better information than a briefer cross-sectional instrument. The interview format prevents patients from glossing over difficulties or just presenting what they want the team to know, both by asking open-ended questions and by allowing verification from the patient's family or network of significant others, including members of previous treatment teams. This richness of role activity information greatly enhances the occupational therapist's ability to formulate treatment interventions and advise the interdisciplinary team regarding discharge planning. The team then may be able to make more appropriate discharge plans and help break cycles of continued rehospitalization.

SCORING

The scoring process is based on a 1 through 6 rating scale, with operational definitions for each point on the scale within each of the 12 role domains. An example of one role domain's operational definition anchor points is shown in Table 14-2. The rater identifies changes in level of functioning by dividing the historical information into time segments during which the level of functioning is consistent. Interviewers are required to make scoring decisions that are based on what is considered to be the most accurate information. These time segment ratings of level of functioning are recorded on a time line and can be broken down into assessment periods, ranging from 1 day to 18 months. The rating for each of these time segments is recorded at the appropriate point on a time line representing the entire period under study. These time segment scores also are averaged to provide an overall performance rating for each role domain's time period under study. The length of the overall period evaluated varies according to the needs of a particular study or the individual patient.[7]

The rating system provides an overall score, as well as a summary of the range of best and worst functioning and the frequency of change in level of performance. For example, in Table 14-3, an individual's work functioning over a given time frame, eg, 5 months, might be marginal on the average (overall score = 3), with a range from adequate (score = 2) at best, to limited (score = 4) at worst, and with a moderate number of changes (three).[7]

DISTINCTIVE FEATURES OF THE RAPS

It has been noted in psychiatric treatment follow-up research that changes in social functioning generally take 6 to 8 months to develop,[16] which makes change in role performance difficult to document and study, as most social adjustment measures evaluate 1 week to 2 months of functioning.[17,18] In view of the shortcomings of

---

Table 14-2
Self-Management

Functions inherent in the overall management of oneself: personal goals, financial planning, future orientation, adaptive capacities to stress (positive/negative), role balance.

1

Subject has excellent to good ability to pursue personal goals, organize finances and plan for the future. Handles stress in a manner functional for self and others.

2

Does well pursuing personal goals and organizing finances, but with minor difficulties, eg, setting priorities and future orientation. Handles stress well. If there are problems they are short term.

3

Has signs of impairment in caring for self, eg, problems with identification or pursuit of goals or with future orientation. Able to maintain role balance, but with problems in time management or handling immediate stress. Able to maintain finances, but with a lot of disorganization and lack of future planning. Problems affect monthly functioning.

4

Has a great deal of difficulty weekly with self-management, eg, unclear goals, virtually no future plans, or disorganized finances. Not able to maintain a balance of roles. May require assistance with stress.

5

Subject only minimally appropriately cares for self. Handles finances with poor goal setting and lack of future planning. Does not productively channel energy or anxiety to handle stress on a day-to-day basis.

6

Essentially does not function in role.

Table 14-3
Case Example of Scoring on the Work Role Subscale Over 5 Months

Score:	3	2	3	3	4
Month:	1	2	3	4	5

Average level of performance: 3 + 2 + 3 + 3 + 4 = 15/5 = 3
Best level of performance: 2
Worst level of performance: 4
Number of changes in performance level: 3

Good-Ellis MA, Fine SB, Spencer JH, DiVittis A. Developing a role activity performance scale. *Am J Occup Ther.* 1987;41;4:232-241. Copyright 1987 by the American Occupational Therapy Association, Inc. Reprinted with permission.

---

these shorter or "cross-sectional" assessments, the RAPS provides a more comprehensive assessment and, thus, for patients with variable functioning (including radical changes) for whom such variation is significant, a more valid assessment of their long-term course of role activity performance.[8] The documentation of problematic styles of role activity functioning that are long standing, with minimal variation or fluctuation, can be important for other patients, eg, those diagnosed with personality disorder. The parametric properties of the time line procedure provide a standard procedure for recording critical events and associated changes in level of role functioning over the long term. Thus, the longer term course of role activity performance can be identified and recorded for both adequate baseline measurement and careful follow-up of many patient groups. The time segment ratings on a time line allow for quantitative and qualitative assessment of how the long-term course of an illness affects role performance.

The 6-point ratings, with operational definitions as anchor points for each of the 12 role domains, combined with the time segment approach to rating role activity performance history, allow for documenting fluctuations in levels of role activity performance as accurately as possible, with a great deal of sensitivity to change. The RAPS methodology of time segment ratings of critical events and detailed anecdotal information, gathered from a semistructured interview format, allows for the measurement of rich descriptive information on an individual's role activity performance over time. The RAPS is unique in translating an open-ended interview of role activity performance format into measurable ratings associated with a time line for historical recording.

The RAPS methodology of assessment can be applied to both pre-treatment and post-treatment documentation, allowing for careful follow-up of short- or long-term role activity performance changes. The RAPS documents the efficacy of treatment strategies, as shown by a patient's role activity performance in the community environment. The gathering of substantive historical data, highlighting strengths and deficits in activities of role performance, greatly facilitates establishing intervention priorities, and short- and long-term treatment goals for occupational therapy. Foto stressed that, "outcome studies must...address the question, not only of how services reduce or compensate for disability, but also how they translate into a better quality of life, not just for an individual, but for a defined group of patients."[13] Outcome studies that can accurately document, with instruments like the RAPS, patients' ability to perform in identified activities of role performance in the community are increasingly important in the managed care environment.

ADMINISTRATION OF THE RAPS

The RAPS initially appears difficult to administer, but once an evaluator has become familiar with the evaluation, it no longer seems complicated. Evaluators (occupational therapists and research assistants) who have become familiar with the RAPS report finding it fairly easy to administer, although materials at first appear complex. Learning to administer the RAPS takes practice with approximately five evaluations, after having read the manual and becoming familiar with the semistructured interview and scoring sheets. Unfortunately, time pressure in most clinical centers tends to discourage in-depth interviews; thus, valuable and relevant information that can facilitate treatment and discharge planning is often lost.[7]

Scoring also initially appears complex, but is actually quite straightforward and is facilitated by a computerized scoring program. The computerized scoring is based on the Lotus 1-2-3 or Quattro Pro programs, and works in the same way as those spreadsheet programs. The computerized scoring system can accommodate point-in-time scoring or any number of months from 1 to 18. The program calculates subscale total score, high and low score, and number of changes in level of functioning for each role domain. The overall RAPS total is an average of all relevant role domains.[9] Using the computerized semistructured interview of the RAPS, while not any faster in terms of collecting information, can help in the record keeping of role activity performance information.

STANDARDIZATION

Interrater reliability was tested across two pairs of raters over 30 subjects for the RAPS interview and scoring system.[7] Validity was tested in four ways: 1) review by experts in the field of occupational therapy (see acknowledgments), 2) tests of discrimination between two psychiatric diagnostic groups, 3) comparison with other standardized measures of social role functioning,[7] and 4) retrospective validity of the semistructured interview.[9]

Measure of Reliability

Interclass correlation—the ratio of controlled variation to total variation across four raters—was selected as the method of estimating the reliability of the RAPS because it is a more conservative estimate of reliability than the Pearson correlation coefficient.[19] To assess interrater reliability, the RAPS was administered to each subject at two separate times, not more than a week apart. At each session, two experienced occupational therapists independently rated the subject, with one therapist serving as the main interviewer and the other as an observer. Data was gathered for the 18 months prior to admission. In most cases, the semistructured interview and medical records provided the information. Four subjects were unable to tolerate a semistructured interview; nonetheless, these subjects were included to test interrater reliability under the difficult circumstances that characterize an inpatient environment. Family members were available for information in only three cases.

For interrater reliability, two methods of calculating each subject's total score were used: a) taking the unweighted average of the primary role score (weighted average, in order of importance, of work, education, and home management) and the remaining nine roles, and b) taking a weighted average, giving more weight to the primary role score. The interclass correlation coefficients for all subscales were high (Table 14-4), and there was no advantage to weighting primary role subscales more than other RAPS subscales.[7]

Measures of Validity

Independent experts in the field of occupational therapy reviewed the RAPS interview questions and operational definitions to determine the extent to which the instrument reflects the roles being measured and its relevancy to occupational therapy. As a result of the experts' comments, the instrument was modified by placing greater emphasis on activity requirements, rather than on each role's affective components.[7]

Validity: Discrimination Between Diagnostic Groups

Another measure of validity is the scale's ability to discriminate between different patterns of role functioning in two diagnostic groups. Two groups' scores—those of schizophrenic and schizophreniform disorders and those of major affective disorders—were compared with individual RAPS subscale scores. For the analysis, t-tests were used on the mean ratings of four raters for subscale comparisons and separately for each rater for primary role scores.

Table 14-4
Interrater Reliability Coefficients Across Four Raters

Subscale	Intraclass Correlation	n
Work/Work Equivalent	.99	28[a]
Home Management	.95	30
Family Relationships	.88	30
Social Relationships	.96	30
Leisure Activities	.93	30
Self-Management	.91	30
Health Care	.87	30
Hygiene and Appearance	.82	28[b]
Primary Role	.98	30
Total Score	.98	30
Weighted Total	.98	30

[a] Two subjects had no work role.
[b] One rater did not rate two subjects on the Hygiene and Appearance subscale.

Good-Ellis MA, Fine SB, Spencer JH, DiVittis A. Developing a role activity performance scale. *Am J Occup Ther*. 1987;41;4:232-241. Copyright 1987 by the American Occupational Therapy Association, Inc. Reprinted with permission.

The expectation that the RAPS could distinguish between groups with respect to best and worst levels of functioning was confirmed for the best level of functioning, but not for the worst level of functioning (Table 14-5). For the lowest level of functioning, only the Work, Social Relationships, Health Care Role, and Rehabilitation Treatment Settings subscales differentiated the two groups. The lack of discrimination on the other subscales is explained by the fact that all patients in both groups had been admitted recently, with the lowest period of functioning just prior to admission. The inability of the RAPS to differentiate the two groups on the lowest level of functioning score, which is, in essence, a point-in-time score on the majority of subscales for this population, illustrates the weakness of point-in-time instruments during periods of acute illness.

Concept Validity: Comparison to Other Measures

Scales that measure similar constructs should correlate moderately well. To further evaluate the RAPS' validity, the RAPS and several accepted standardized measures of social functioning were administered and scored separately. These standardized measures were *Social Assessment Scale-II* (SAS-II),[17] the *Katz Adjustment Scale* (KAS form R2),[20] the *Global Assessment Scale* (GAS),[21] *DSM-III Axis V*,[22] and *Levels of Functioning Scale* (LFS).[23] A comparison of the RAPS with these measures is shown in Table 14-6. The RAPS scores correlated positively with scores on all the other evaluation measures during comparable time periods, further demonstrating the RAPS' concept validity.[7]

Retrospective Validity

A second study investigated the validity of the RAPS' retrospective historical interview by again comparing its ratings to the same accepted psychosocial rating scales as above, excluding the LFS.[9] Thirty outpatients (15 patients diagnosed with

Table 14-5
RAPS Scores Between Diagnostic Groups

Subscale	Level of Functioning	Group 1 X	SD	Group 2 X	SD	One-tailed t	p	df
Work/Work Equivalent	Worst	6.00	0.08	5.37	1.31	1.91	.039	26
	Average	5.12	1.06	2.61	0.90	6.78	<.0001	26
	Best	3.79	1.62	1.37	0.51	5.18	<.0001	26
Education	Worst							8
	Average	(Insufficient number of cases for analysis.)						8
	Best							8
Home Management	Worst	5.91	0.38	5.60	0.91	1.20	NS	28
	Average	3.72	0.83	2.91	0.89	2.57	.0008	28
	Best	2.78	0.93	2.05	0.95	2.11	.021	28
Family Relationships	Worst	5.37	0.81	4.87	1.19	1.36	NS	28
	Average	3.85	0.66	3.13	0.74	2.85	.004	28
	Best	3.07	0.76	2.44	0.67	2.40	.011	28
Mate Relationship	Worst							6
	Average	(Insufficient number of cases for analysis.)						6
	Best							6
Parenting	Worst							4
	Average	(Insufficient number of cases for analysis.)						4
	Best							4
Social Relationships	Worst	6.00	0.00	5.40	0.99	2.36	.026	28
	Average	4.46	0.96	2.96	0.64	5.03	<.0001	28
	Best	3.63	1.11	2.13	0.70	4.45	<.0001	28
Leisure Activities	Worst	5.29	0.69	5.02	0.52	0.83	NS	28
	Average	4.85	0.68	3.56	0.97	4.23	<.0001	28
	Best	3.31	0.89	1.69	0.84	5.10	<.0001	28
Self-Management	Worst	5.73	0.59	5.42	0.62	1.41	NS	28
	Average	3.92	0.63	2.88	0.64	4.50	<.0001	28
	Best	2.91	0.78	1.71	0.79	4.20	<.0001	28
Health Care	Worst	5.87	0.31	5.09	0.99	2.91	.006	28
	Average	3.60	0.61	2.52	0.68	4.58	<.0001	28
	Best	2.27	0.82	1.61	0.80	2.23	.017	28
Hygiene and Appearance	Worst	3.24	1.26	2.99	1.09	0.58	NS	28
	Average	2.50	0.44	2.18	0.74	1.40	NS	28
	Best	1.87	0.53	1.33	0.50	2.54	.004	28
Rehabilitation Treatment Settings	Worst							6
	Average	(Insufficient number of cases for analysis.)						6
	Best							6
Primary role		4.45	0.83	2.70	0.82	5.78	<.0001	28
Total score		4.18	0.64	2.81	0.65	5.86	<.0001	28
Weighted total		4.34	0.80	2.75	0.73	5.68	<.0001	28

Note: Assessment was based on functioning over the previous 18 months. NS=not significant.

Adapted from Good-Ellis M, Fine SB, Spencer JH, DeVittis A. Developing a Role Activity Performance Scale. *Am J Occup Ther*. 1987;41;2:232-241.

Table 14-6
Comparison of the RAPS With Other Standardized Measures of Social Functioning

Characteristic	Social Adjustments Scale-II (SAS-II)	Katz Adjustment Scale (KAS-Form R2)	Global Assessment Scale (GAS)	DSM-III Axis V	Levels of Functioning Scale (LFS)	Role Activity Performance Scale (RAPS)
Scale	Measures level of functioning in: six major role areas (work, household, school, extended family, marital, parental, social and leisure activities, personal well-being) and five global areas (work-g, home-g, family-g, social leisure-g, and general adjustment-g)	Represents a significant other's view of patient's functioning; measures role functioning in the community over 16 items.	Represents social functioning and symptoms in one global score.	Represents the best adaptive level of functioning; occupational, social, and leisure functioning are all considered together in determining the rating on the single scale.	Represents seven items of role, social, and symptom functioning; length of time without hospitalization, quality and quantity of useful work, number and quality of social relations, absence of symptoms, ability to meet own basic needs, fullness of life, overall level of functioning.	Measures functional capacities in 12 areas: work/work equivalent, education, home management, family of origin and extended family relationships mate relationship, parenting, social relationships, leisure activities, self-management, hygiene and appearance, health care, and rehabilitation treatment settings.
Time period assessed	2 months prior to interview	3 weeks prior to interview	1 week prior to interview	Best 3 months of adaptive functioning during year prior to interview	1 to 2 months of usual functioning	Flexible; from 1 week to 18 months prior to interview
Sources of information	Interview of patient	Questionnaire answered by significant other	Interviews of patient and significant other; clinical records	Interviews of patient and significant other; clinical records	Interview of patient	All relevant sources of information (psychotherapist, family, patient)
Length of time to administer	Approximately 30 min to 1 hr for interview and rating	Approximately 15 min for informant to complete questionnaire	Approximately 15 to 30 min to gather information and score	Approximately 15 to 30 min to gather information for scoring	Approximately 30 min for data collection and rating	From 40 min to 1 1/2 hrs for interview and rating
Rating system	5-point rating scale for role areas; 7-point rating scale for global areas	3-point rating scale for each item (overall score based on 16 items)	One rating scale from 0 to 100	7-point scale	5-point scale	6-point rating scale for each area; total score based on average of role areas
Reliability	Demonstrated	Demonstrated	Demonstrated	Demonstrated	Demonstrated	Demonstrated

a The role areas are based on 52 items in the SAS scale.

Adapted from Good-Ellis M, Fine SB, Spencer JH, DeVittis A. Developing a Role Activity Performance Scale. *Am J Occup Ther.* 1987;41:2:232-241.

Table 14-7

Role Activity Performance Scale Correlations with GAS, KAS, SAS-II, DSM-III at Time of RAPS Interview and Three Retrospective Points in Time

Pearson Correlation and (number of pairs)	Time 1 9 Months Prior	Time 2 6 Months Prior	Time 3 3 Months Prior	Time 4 RAPS Interview
RAPS Total				
DSM	.42 (30)	.51 (30)	.67 (30)	.62 (30)
GAS *	-.53 (30)	-.62 (30)	-.72 (30)	-.67 (30)
KAS *	-.57 (30)	-.68 (30)	-.63 (30)	-.73 (30)
SAS Gen'l Adjust (g)	.74 (30)	.80 (30)	.83 (30)	.80 (30)
RAPS Work				
SAS Work (g)	.93 (27)	.90 (27)	.95 (26)	.94 (27)
SAS Work	.86 (27)	.83 (27)	.80 (26)	.86 (27)
RAPS Home				
SAS Household (g)	.61 (30)	.63 (30)	.59 (30)	.41 (30)
SAS Home	.50 (27)	.64 (28)	.68 (28)	.70 (28)
RAPS Family				
SAS Family (g)	.56 (30)	.53 (30)	.53 (30)	.44 (30)
SAS Nuclear Family	.47 (18)	.69 (17)	.66 (17)	.69 (17)
SAS Extended Family	-.04 (29)	-.06 (29)	.08 (29)	.17 (28)
RAPS Social				
SAS Social/Leisure (g)	.73 (30)	.73 (30)	.69 (30)	.64 (30)
SAS Social	.43 (30)	.44 (30)	.39 (30)	.33 (30)
RAPS Leisure				
SAS Social/Leisure (g)	.63 (30)	.63 (30)	.59 (30)	.52 (30)
SAS Leisure	.29 (30)	.50 (30)	.42 (30)	.35 (30)
RAPS Self Management				
SAS Gen'l Adjust (g)	.47 (30)	.60 (30)	.61 (30)	.63 (30)
SAS Self Management	.38 (30)	.43 (30)	.52 (30)	.51 (30)
RAPS Health Care				
SAS Health Care	.28 (30)	.65 (30)	.50 (30)	.55 (30)
RAPS Hygiene/Appearance				
SAS Hygiene	-.01 (30)	.31 (30)	.10 (30)	.43 (30)

* Negative correlation indicates inverse scales.

The RAPS: Validation of the Retrospective Historical Interview and Proceedings of Mini Course. Assessing Adults: Functional Measures and Successful Outcomes v. Role Activity Performance Scale (RAPS). Copyright 1991 by the American Occupational Therapy Association, Inc. Reprinted with permission.

schizophrenic disorders; 15 with major affective disorders, by DSM-III criteria)[22] were interviewed. The RAPS' historical ratings were compared to actual instrument ratings, taken at 9, 6, and 3 months prior to the retrospective RAPS interview. Again, the RAPS showed acceptable correlations with other accepted psychosocial rating scales (Table 14-7), suggesting that the content validity of this instrument is strong and lending support to the validity of the RAPS' retrospective time segment scoring.

In studies of this nature, correlations of .60 or greater indicate a high degree of agreement between two measures of the same domain. Correlations of moderate strength (.30 to .59) indicate that a proportion of the variation between the scores can be attributed to three factors: 1) the two measures are not measuring exactly the same domain; 2) measurement variance, differences due to an alternative method of measuring a common domain; and 3) measurement error.[24] Because some subjects were not involved in all role domains, four subscales did not generate sufficient observations for interpretation—Education, Mate Relationship, Parental Role, and Rehab Treatment Settings.

For the retrospective validity ratings of the RAPS interview, the correlations were good (.50 or better) (see Table 14-7).[9] Notably, the Work Scale showed correlations in the .90 or greater range for times 1, 2, and 3, indicating a remarkable degree of measurement accuracy, with retrospective validity as far back as 9 months.

As might be expected, the correlations tended to be lowest for the most retrospective period, 9 months prior to the interview (see Table 14-7). There was a sizable drop in the magnitude of the correlations between time 2 and time 3 for five of the comparisons—SAS Home, SAS Nuclear Family, SAS General Adjustment, SAS Health Care, and SAS Hygiene. This suggests that the most accurate period for history taking of this type of information is up to 6 months prior to the interview.

Two of the scales showed poor content validity (concurrent at time 4) and poor retrospective accuracy. One was the RAPS Hygiene / Appearance with SAS Hygiene. Differences in hygiene anchor points were found, with RAPS having a greater middle range for scoring disheveled appearance, while the SAS goes from good appearance to reasonable appearance, responsibility borne by someone else. When comparing the RAPS Family with SAS Extended Family items, one of them, guilt, did not correspond to anything measured by the RAPS and had consistently low correlations (r < .30).

RAPS PREDICTIVE POWER OF GLOBAL FUNCTIONING

The predictive power of the RAPS subscales was investigated as part of a study validating the RAPS retrospective historical interview.[10] In this study (Figure 14-1), the Global Assessment Scale (GAS), was given every 3 months, while the RAPS was given only at the end (time T4). The RAPS evaluation involved a full review of the past 9 months, thus permitting an exploration of retrospective criterion validity. The RAPS' ability to predict global functioning was evaluated by comparing RAPS subscale scores to the GAS scores 3 months later.

RAPS subscale point-in-time scores were calculated for times T1, T2, and T3 and paired with GAS scores 3 months later at times T2, T3, and T4. Thirty outpatients (15 patients with schizophrenic disorders; 15 patients with major affective disorders, as diagnosed by DSM-III criteria), were recruited into the study at the Payne Whitney Clinic. A data set was organized that paired R1 with G2, R2 with G3, and R3 with G4. This provided 90 observations (three points in time for 30 subjects).

Using this data set in a stepwise regression,[25] with the GAS as the dependent variable, all 12 RAPS subscale scores were allowed to enter. With an alpha of .10 to enter and an alpha of .10 to remove, the Self-Management subscale score was the first to enter (r = .562), showing that the individual RAPS subscale with the greatest predictive power of the GAS was Self-Management. The second step added the RAPS Work subscale to the model (r = .615), showing that Self-Management and Work together accounted for more of the variance in the GAS. In the third step,

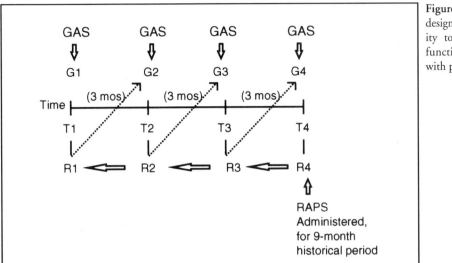

Figure 14-1. Study design for RAPS' ability to predict global functioning. (Used with permission.)

Home Management was added to the model (r = .644). The next step removed Self-Management from the model, leaving the Work and Home Management as the best combined predictors of the GAS and as the optimal solution, better than the three together. The final model was GAS = -.245 * Work - 4.13 * Home Mgmt + 82.15. With a squared multiple r of .396, approximately 40% of the variance in the GAS is predicted by the two RAPS subscale measures 3 months earlier.

While Self-Management was removed from the optimal solution, it appeared to be the role domain that was individually the best predictor of global functioning 3 months earlier. The RAPS overall definition of Self-Management is not activities of daily living—those skills are part of the RAPS Hygiene and Appearance role—but a unifying volitional construct, encompassing how one achieves life goals (see Table 14-2 for anchor points). This cluster of abilities suggests an underlying mechanism that arbitrates how one chooses to adapt to and process the full spectrum of life role choices or demands on a daily basis, and in relation to life goals and financial constraints.

SUBSCALE ROLE CLUSTERS ASSOCIATED WITH TOTAL RAPS SCORE

To evaluate whether some RAPS subscales had more predictive ability than others or contributed more to the RAPS total score, factor analysis methodology was used to identify subscale clusters and determine their influence on the total RAPS score. The data was gathered and analyzed from the same retrospective study of 30 outpatients (15 patients diagnosed with schizophrenic disorders, 15 with major affective disorders) described in the prior section. An assessment of the factor structure of the RAPS was performed using a principal components analysis with oblique rotation,[24] yielding three interpretable factors that together account for 88% of the variance in the RAPS Total Score. The three most influential factor/subscale combinations were:
1. Home Management and Nuclear/Extended Family Relationship
2. Work and Self-Management
3. Social Relationships and Leisure Activities.

These factor combinations were unexpected. Work, Home Management, and Education had previously been thought of as a grouping for primary role performance, but here they appeared in separate factors and grouped with subscales not previously expected to be closely associated.

Home Management and Nuclear/Extended Family Relationships

The first factor appears to represent a heart-hearth combination, meaning that the ability to carry out Home Management role functions is intricately related to Nuclear/Extended Family Relationships, and vice versa. This factor identifies the need for increasing awareness of family issues and active collaboration with team members, especially social workers, in coordinating treatment approaches. This data also supports recent trends in occupational therapy practice. Corcoran mentioned "a need to focus on the family environment" due to shortened hospital stays and a quick return to the home environment.[15] This RAPS factor suggests that more attention should be paid to family relationships and home environment, especially for assessing and intervening with home management skills.

Work and Self-Management

The second factor grouped Work and Self-Management roles. Here Self-Management appears to be an intrinsic underpinning to the primary Work Role. Self-Management, as described on the RAPS[10] (see Table 14-2), is oriented toward future planning—goal setting, financial planning, adaptive capacities in adjusting to stress (positive/negative), and role balance—all of which are often part of occupational therapy interventions. The necessity of maintaining a balance of work, play, and rest has been part of occupational therapy philosophy since 1922.[26] The association of these two scales lends further credence to the influence of self-management competencies on other life goals and the importance of integrating self-management role functioning into the planning and implementing of interventions directed at work and other primary role related goals. Thus, adaptive self-management functioning is likely to be necessary for individuals to succeed in the work role domain. For occupational therapy, this factor indicates that interventions that address RAPS Self-Management role domain skills may influence work role performance.

Social Relationships and Leisure Activities

The Social Relationships and Leisure Activities factor combination was less of a surprise, based on traditional occupational therapy treatment techniques.[27-30] This factor supports occupational therapy's use of social and leisure activities as the practice ground for improvement of role activity performance skills. Occupational therapy has often stressed the acquisition of or restoration of purposeful activity skills and socialization patterns needed to support the performance of patients in their life roles.[31] As Matsutsuyu reported, "Understanding the antecedent factors which evoke or sustain interest enhances the commitment process of the (patient) in reconstructing functional behaviors through adaption of old patterns or learning new or different modes of performance."[32] Occupational therapy often has stressed the dual acquisition or restoration of purposeful leisure and socialization skills as a means to improve performance in other life roles.[31]

These role domain clusters support King's call to occupational therapy to further develop knowledge of the adaptive responses that would enable an individual to acquire the necessary skills to meet life goals.[33] These clusters broaden occupational therapy's knowledge base of how role domain skills interrelate to achieve role activity functioning. This knowledge can be used to guide interventions when a patient has difficulties in one of these role domains.

RAPS RESEARCH WITH MAJOR AFFECTIVE PATIENTS

The findings discussed here are based on the Payne Whitney Inpatient Family Intervention Study, involving 50 patients (in follow-up at the time of this analysis).[6] There were 25 patients diagnosed with unipolar disorders and 25 with bipolar disorders, using DSM-III criteria. All were assessed using the RAPS at admission for an 18-month prehospital baseline level of functioning and at 6 and 18 months for follow-up. All received standard hospital treatment, including occupational therapy services, guided by the RAPS initial evaluation. Available treatment interventions included basic activities of daily living, goal setting, time management, and future planning, plus referral to recreational, dance, music, and prevocational services, as needed. The overall philosophy of treatment reflected an occupational behavior model.[34] The RAPS assessment emphasized both strengths and weaknesses, with treatment directed at improving innate and previously learned skills, as appropriate to individual role requirements.

USE OF THE RAPS TO IDENTIFY OCCUPATIONAL THERAPY IN- AND OUTPATIENT TREATMENT REQUIREMENTS

When considering post-hospital deterioration of role activity performance and rehospitalization after discharge, two patterns emerged[8]:

1. The data suggest that a RAPS total score of below 3 for patients with unipolar disorders and below 2.8 for patients with bipolar disorders provides cut points that can divide these patients into high- and low-functioning groups, with the low-functioning patients more vulnerable to further role performance deterioration post-discharge and the increased likelihood of rehospitalization. Thus, the initial RAPS assessment can help occupational therapists identify and prioritize patients in greater need of more targeted role activity performance treatment in hospital and post-discharge interventions, especially during the most vulnerable period of 0 to 6 months post-discharge.

2. The majority (62%) showed a prehospital/treatment pattern of lower Social Relationship functioning (higher RAPS subscale scores), either alone or combined with other lower functioning scores. This supports the reported conclusion that, with major affective disorder patients, the loss of social relationships can be associated with the onset of depression.[35,36] This finding suggests the use of a) the RAPS Social Relationship subscale post-discharge as an early indicator of the need for the renewal or addition of occupational therapy or other treatment interventions, and b) socially oriented activities in occupational therapy as a practice ground for patients to build up their social relationship "emotional tone" before testing their social skills in primary roles.[8]

Table 14-8

Association of RAPS Leisure, Social, and Family Role Functioning with Improved Primary Role Performance at 6 and 18 Months Follow Up

	6 Months Follow-Up	18 Months Follow-Up
Improved Primary Role	18	20
Improved Leisure Role	15 (83%)	16 (80%)
Improved Social Role	10 (55%)	11 (55%)
Improved Family Role	10 (55%)	10 (50%)

Adapted from *Quantitative Role and Performance: Implications and Applications to Treatment of Major Affective Disorders.*

USE OF THE RAPS TO IDENTIFY ROLE RECOVERY TREATMENT SEQUENCE PATTERNS

In assessing post-hospital improvement in role activity functioning (defined as at least one full level of change, eg, a score of 3 to 2 on the RAPS total score), a sequence of skill activation reoccurring within several RAPS role domains emerged over time (Table 14-8).[8]

Improved role activity performance was most strongly associated with concurrent improvement in the RAPS Leisure Activities subscale, starting at 6 months. The RAPS Social Relationship subscale improvement is moderately associated at 6 and 18 months follow-up. In all cases in which primary role improvement was delayed until 18 months, both social and leisure role improvement preceded primary role improvement. These data:

1. Support the traditional focus of occupational therapy regarding the relationship between work and play patterns (RAPS Leisure Activities).[29] The therapeutic value of using leisure or play activities, either social- or activity-related, as practice tasks leading to primary role competencies has often guided occupational therapy interventions with patients.[27-30]

2. Suggest a sequence of skill activation over time, with improvement in leisure activities and social relationships preceding and stimulating improved primary role performance. This sequence of skill activation can be based on a hierarchy of task demands, with improvement first occurring in the less complex demands of leisure and social skill role domains before improvement in the more complex primary role demands. Alternatively, this sequence can be related to leisure and social skills as being more immediately gratifying, providing reinforcement contingencies that activate role activity functioning more immediately and effectively.

3. Suggest that social relationships and "play" leisure activities can serve as practice tasks for the more formal discipline of primary roles. Motivation and the sense of competency can be more easily increased through the use of self-expression and self-gratification in social relationships and leisure activities.

In this study, it is significant that, within the bipolar group, there was more primary role improvement among patients in the family treatment group (46%) than in the comparison group (20%). As compliance to treatment and more complex medication regimens are especially important in bipolar patients, this study indicates that better family understanding and support assist in treatment compliance and concomitant improvement in role performance. This also suggests that incorporating the family or network of significant others as quickly as possible in a treatment alliance relationship leads to improved compliance and more positive outcomes.

CASE EXAMPLE

This case example (the material has been altered to protect confidentiality) illustrates the role recovery sequence in a major depressive unipolar patient.[31] The patient was a 42-year-old married female. For the previous 7 years, the patient had been functioning at a high level as a director of patient accounts in a large hospital. During these 7 years, she had experienced two episodes of depression and one psychiatric hospitalization. The RAPS baseline pre-hospital score of overall functioning was at a marginal level of 3.75 (total score), meaning performance on the role subscales was at marginal or below usual standard levels of role performance and often sporadic in nature (Table 14-9).

Anecdotal information from the RAPS, highlighting subscale performance changes during the follow-up period, illustrates the following sequence of improved role activity functioning:

1. Primary role performance had been quite variable—five changes in level of role performance—at baseline due to lack of interest, suicidal ideation, and suicide attempt. A 6-month follow-up showed a more stable and improved level of performance, with only two changes in level of performance, that continued through the next 12 months. At the 18 month follow-up, she reported that pre-vocational return-to-work group recommendations that she seek out and foster co-worker relationships had been significantly helpful to her performance at work.

2. The patient stated that family intervention and post-discharge marital therapy helped her to talk with her husband and "facilitated problem solving." She complied with individual, marital, and medication therapy during the full 18 months post-discharge.

3. The patient's leisure activities had consisted of reading alone in the pre-hospital period, and she stated that she "couldn't get started on anything and had no particular strengths for anything." From section A of the RAPS, long-term background history, she had reported enjoying music and being quite active in weaving. During her hospitalization, she was encouraged to try macrame as an easier, faster way to make use of her weaving skills. Thus, her interest, motivation, and confidence in completing short-term tasks was stimulated. She reported being able to continue working on small macrame and needlepoint projects post-discharge.

4. After the first 6 months post-discharge, the patient and her husband started doing some leisure activities together, improving RAPS role performance scores in Leisure Activities and Mate Relationships.

5. The patient was first able to improve on her completion of individual short-term leisure projects, then started to socialize minimally with co-workers, after which she included more social activities with her husband, and reactivated seeing two friends she had avoided prior to admission. Her Work RAPS subscale score improved following this sequence of events (see Table 14-9).

Table 14-9
Case Study Showing Primary Role Functioning and Total Subscale Scores from 18 Months Prior to Admission through 18 Months Follow-Up

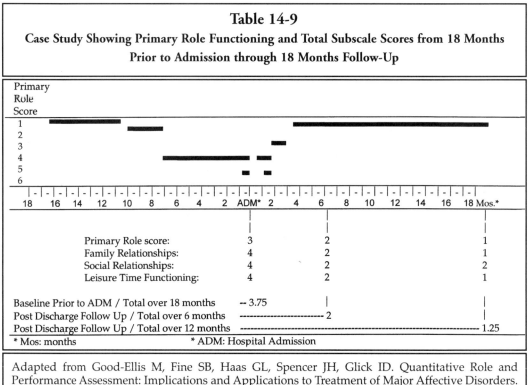

	18 months prior to ADM	ADM*	6 months	18 Mos.*
Primary Role score:		3	2	1
Family Relationships:		4	2	1
Social Relationships:		4	2	2
Leisure Time Functioning:		4	2	1

Baseline Prior to ADM / Total over 18 months   -- 3.75

Post Discharge Follow Up / Total over 6 months   ------------------------- 2

Post Discharge Follow Up / Total over 12 months   -- 1.25

* Mos: months   * ADM: Hospital Admission

Adapted from Good-Ellis M, Fine SB, Haas GL, Spencer JH, Glick ID. Quantitative Role and Performance Assessment: Implications and Applications to Treatment of Major Affective Disorders. Paper presented at Preconference to the American Psychiatric Association 38th Institute. *Depression Assessment and Treatment Update.* AOTA; 1986.

WORK IN PROGRESS

In a study in progress at the time of this writing at New York State Psychiatric Association,[28] patients meeting DSM-IIIR criteria[8] for Borderline Personality Disorder were evaluated with the RAPS at baseline and followed up with the RAPS subscales of Work Role, Self-Management, Education, Social Relationships and Leisure Relationships, at 3, 6, 9, and 18 months post-discharge. Preliminary findings for 15 of these patients support the sequence of role performance recovery discussed in this chapter. There is more data on approximately 55 patients with personality disorders, some of whom were followed up to 5 years post-discharge, but have not as yet been evaluated.

FUTURE RESEARCH

Any instrument needs continued development, validation, and conceptual and empirical improvement, which can only be accomplished by further research and sharing of research data. The RAPS has been developed and used within a fairly narrow set of populations, namely recently admitted and discharged psychiatric patients. It is important to recognize that the studies reviewed thus far are based on small sample sizes and research designs, limited by time and funding constraints. Although not tested to date, the RAPS would be an appropriate instrument with other psychiatric and non-psychiatric conditions, ie, geriatric, orthopedic, kidney dialysis, and organ transplant. Methods of prioritizing and ranking service needs based on the RAPS evaluation could be easily explored and extended to these and other conditions. To design or administer a shortened version of the RAPS, clinicians and researchers may want to consider the clustering of RAPS subscales reported earlier. Further evaluation of the relationship of RAPS Work subscale to the RAPS Self-Management subscale could potentially help refine vocational and prevocational rehabilitative treatment techniques. Further exploration of the use of RAPS Family subscales, primarily, though not exclusively, with Home Management, to establish rapport with patients and combined with their social supports, could refine goal setting for occupational therapists. The RAPS could be used to evaluate the efficacy of occupational therapy treatments. Education, Mate Relationship, Parental Role, and Rehab Treatment Settings all need retrospective validity testing. Documentation of specific skill or occupational therapy frame of reference variables, with RAPS overall role domain measurement, would better define skill variables contributing to role performance. More inclusion of exercise, therapeutic exercise, and dietary practices in the Health Role subscale or Leisure Activities subscale requires further development. It is hoped that this chapter will stimulate others to continue the ongoing research and development process for the RAPS.

SUMMARY

Interest in the functional outcome of treatment is not limited to psychiatry. Health care planners are currently predicting significant changes in all areas of practice, as the concept of successful treatment extends beyond the reduction of pathology and symptoms, to the individual's ability to function socially and economically in the community.[37] The RAPS evaluates the patient, not in terms of disease and symptoms, but in terms of how impairments or strengths affect role activity performance. The RAPS can assist in documenting and describing role activity performance changes that can be influenced by treatment interventions designed for a variety of subgroups of patients. Since functional behaviors and skills arise out of a person's life experience, evaluation instruments like the RAPS must be individualized and detailed to match patient characteristics with problem specific treatment.[38]

The RAPS provides an interview format for starting and continuing over time the occupational therapist's dialogue with the patient and the patient's network of significant others to facilitate the intervention process. Fidler has stated, "The artful skill(s) of enabling (the patient) to form a trusting, reciprocal relationship...are all integral aspects of occupational therapy practice."[39] Hasselkus, quoted in Joe, has found that "occupational therapy goal setting, whatever the diagnosis, needs to involve family caregivers and take into account their health and well-being, as well as those of the identified patient."[40] The RAPS methodology, including family or significant others' information, aids the occupational therapist in establishing treatment alliances with patients and their significant others. The factor analysis of the RAPS subscale role domains supports the hypothesis that the performance of home management skills are intricately associated and related to patients' relationships with family or significant others. The RAPS semistructured interview, with its open-ended questions, yields reliable valid role activity performance information that is important in setting realistic goals with the patients and their families or networks of significant others.

The need for precise historical data with which to analyze functional strengths and deficits has been identified by numerous occupational therapists over the years.

Strauss, et al have discussed the need for increased information on the evolution of psychiatric disorders.[41] The RAPS differs from other evaluations by covering a longer and potentially more useful period of time than most scales and provides a more meaningful picture of role domain functioning by using qualitative history taking combined with quantitative measurement. The RAPS offers a flexible time segment scoring system that can describe and quantify changes in levels of role activity performance functioning over time, thus allowing it to be not as greatly influenced by acute symptoms as other psychosocial rating scales. The RAPS' unique association of a semistructured interview format with time segment scoring allows for rating short or even point-in-time critical events as part of the longitudinal description of an individual's role activity performance.

The RAPS standardization studies described in this chapter indicate that it is a reliable and valid instrument, suitable for a variety of clinical and research tasks. Factor analysis of the RAPS role domain subscale structure indicates three main role performance combinations that contribute strongly to global functioning. The RAPS Nuclear and Extended Family Relationships provide important information about family and social supports, and are factorially aligned with the RAPS Home Management subscale. RAPS Self-Management aligned with the RAPS Work subscale and was also the best predictive index of global functioning. This finding suggests that interventions related to the Self-Management subscale, eg, goal setting, future orientation, role balance, adaptation to stress (positive/negative), and financial planning, may positively impact work and overall role activity functioning. RAPS Social Relationships aligned with RAPS Leisure Activities, supporting occupational therapy's constructs, to facilitate overall role functioning improvement. This data highlights the complexity of human performance and the need for occupational therapists to understand that goal attainment and community reintegration require a range of adaptive functioning and that responses cannot be simplistically tied to a single role-related goal or set of behaviors.[33]

When comparing post-discharge role performance patterns to the initial RAPS hospitalization total scores, several patterns of outcome role performance have emerged. Successful role functioning outcomes have helped support occupational therapy's sequence of treatment interventions, eg, the use of leisure and social relationship activities preceding and to stimulate primary role improvement. The analysis of deteriorating role functioning has suggested a means of identifying low-functioning patients, eg, 3.0 or greater for unipolar, 2.8 or greater for bipolar, and 3.5 or greater for schizophrenic disorders. Thus, a referral system for ambulatory occupational therapy services, based on these low-functioning cut points, could be useful to determine those in greatest need of occupational therapy and other services, especially during the vulnerable period 6 months post-discharge. While the shortcomings of the sample sizes presented here must be acknowledged, the initial findings on relationships between role domain patterns and overall functioning are significant for occupational therapy and deserve further validation.

Occupational therapists need to become more skilled in gathering, measuring, and using predictive and outcome data for their interventions, which, in turn, will be more clearly understood by consumers and payors. The RAPS is a highly relevant assessment instrument for role activity functioning, valid for establishing baseline levels of functioning, and, after intervention, useful in tracking outcome functioning through community and treatment environments.

REFERENCES

1. American Psychiatric Association. *Diagnostic and Statistical Manual of Mental Disorders*, 4th ed. Washington, DC: Author; 1994.

2. Greenspan SI. *Infancy and Early Childhood: The Practice of Clinical Assessment and Intervention With Emotional and Developmental Challenges.* Madison, Conn: International Universities Press; 1992.

3. Florey L. Service Delivery Model: Child and Adolescent Psychiatry. In Robertson SC, ed. *SCOPE Curriculum Manual.* Washington, DC: AOTA; 1986:113-116.

4. Glick ID, Clarkin JF, Spencer JH et al. A Controlled Evaluation of Inpatient Family Intervention: I. Preliminary Results of the Six Month Follow up. *Arch Gen Psych.* 1985;42:882-886.

5. Glick ID, Clarkin JF, Spencer, JH. A randomized clinical trial of inpatient family intervention IV. Follow-up results for subjects with schizophrenia. *Schizophrenia Research.* 1990;3:187-200.

6. Haas GL, Glick ID, Spencer JH. The Patient, the Family, and Compliance With Posthospital Treatment for Affective Disorders. *Psychopharmacology Bulletin.* 1986;22(3):999-1005.

7. Good-Ellis M, Fine SB, Spencer JH, DiVittis A. Developing a Role Activity Performance Scale. *Am J Occup Ther.* 1987;41:232-241.

8. Good-Ellis M, Fine SB, Haas GL, Spencer JH, Glick ID. Quantitative Role and Performance Assessment: Implications and Application to Treatment of Major Affective Disorders. Read before the preconference to the American Psychiatric Association 38th Institute. *Depression Assessment and Treatment Update.* (no longer in print) AOTA; 1986:36-43.

9. Good-Ellis M, Fine SB, Spencer JH. *The Role Activity Performance Scale: Validation of the Retrospective Historical Interview.* Unpublished AOTF grant report. Washington DC: AOTF; 1989.

10. Good-Ellis M, Havazelot L, Fine SB. *Assessing Adults: Functional Measures and Successful Outcomes V. Role Activity Performance Scale (RAPS).* (no longer in print) Read at AOTA conference; 1991.

11. Barris R, Dickie V, Baron KB. A comparison of psychiatric patients and normal subjects based on the model of human occupation. *Occupational Therapy Journal of Research.* 1988;8:3-23.

12. Havazelot L, Smith P, Rosnick L. *Follow-up Study of Inpatients Meeting DSM III R Criteria for Personality Disorder.* Read at the National Recreational Therapy Conference;1992.

13. Joe BE. Outcomes stressed in Foto speech. *OT Week.* 1996; 10 (11):12.

14. Lipkin M; Putnam S, Lazare A, ed. *The Medical Interview: Clinical Care, Education, and Research.* New York, NY: Springer; 1995:527.

15. Hettinger J. Ready, Willing and Able: Care That Fits the Family. *OT Week.* 1996;10 (11):14-16.

16. Henderson S. Social bonds in the epidemiology of neurosis. *British Journal of Psychiatry.* 1978;132:463-466.

17. Weissman MM, Klerman GL, Paykel ES, et al. Treatment effects on the social adjustment of depressed patients. *Arch Gen Psych.* 1974;30:771-778.

18. Endicott J, Spitzer R. A diagnostic interview: The schedule for affective disorders and schizophrenia. *Arch Gen Psych.* 1978;35:837-844.

19. Nunnally J. *Psychometric Theory.* New York, NY: McGraw Hill; 1978.

20. Katz M, Lyerly S. Methods for measuring adjustment and social behavior in the community: Rationale, description, discriminative validity and scale development. *Psychological Reports.* 1963;13:503-535.

21. Endicott J, Spitser RL, Fleiss JL, Gibbon M, Endicott J. Global Assessment Scale: for measuring overall severity of psychiatric disturbance. *Arch Gen Psych.* 1976:33:766-771.

22. American Psychiatric Association. *Diagnostic and Statistical Manual of Mental Disorders*, 3rd ed. Washington, DC: Author; 1980.

23. Carpenter J, Heinricks D, Hanlon T. Methodologic standards for treatment outcome research in schizophrenia. *Am J Psychiatry.* 1970;138(4):465-471.

24. Kerlinger FN. *Foundations of Behavioral Research,* 2nd ed. New York, NY: Holt, Rinehart & Winston; 1974.

25. Cronbach LJ. *Essentials of Psychological Testing,* 2nd ed. New York, NY: Harper & Row; 1970.

26. Meyer A. Philosophy of occupational therapy. *Archives of Occupational Therapy.* 1922;1:1-10. (Reprinted in *Am J Occup Ther.* 1977;31:639-642.)

27. Gray M. Effects of hospitalization on work-play behavior. *Am J Occup Ther.* 1987;41:232-241.

28. Hopkins H, Smith H, eds. *Willard & Spackman's Occupational Therapy,* 8th ed. Philadelphia, Pa: JB Lippincott Co; 1993.

29. Matsutsuyu J. Occupational behavior—a perspective on work and play. *Am J Occup Ther.* 1971;25:291.

30. Reilly M. *Play as Exploratory Learning.* Beverly Hills, Calif: Sage Publications; 1974.

31. Hinojosa J, et al. Position paper: purposeful activity. *Am J Occup Ther.* 1993;47:1081-1082.

32. Matsutsuyu J. The Interest Checklist. *Am J Occup Ther.* 1969;23:323-328.

33. King LJ. Towards a science of adaptive responses. *Am J Occup Ther.* 1978; 32:429-437.

34. Kielhofner G, Burke J. A Model of Human Occupation, part 1. Structure and content. *Am J Occup Ther.* 1980;34:572-581.

35. Beckham EE, Leber WR, eds. *Handbook of Depression, Treatment, Assessment and Research.* Homewood, Ill: Dorsey Press; 1985.

36. Klerman GL, Weissman MM. *New Applications of Interpersonal Psychotherapy.* Washington, DC: American Psychiatric Press Inc; 1993.

37. Tarlov AR. Shattuck Lecture: The increasing supply of physicians, the changing structure of the health-services system, and the future practice of medicine. *New England Journal of Medicine.* 1983;308:1235-1244.

38. Fine SB. Occupational therapy. In Karasu TB, ed. *The Psychiatric Therapies.* Washington DC: American Psychiatric Association; 1984.

39. Fidler G. *The psychosocial core of occupational therapy,* draft VI. AOTA, 4720 Montgomery Lane, PO Box 31224, Bethesda, Md, 20824-1220; 1994.

40. Joe BE. Caregivers on the frontline. *OT Week.* 1996;10 (11):14-16.

41. Strauss J, et al. The course of psychiatric disorder III. Longitudinal principles. *Am J Psych.* 1985;142:289-296.

The author acknowledges the support of American Occupational Therapy Foundation (AOTF), which funded the RAPS standardization studies and without which the development of the RAPS would not be as developed as it is today.

The author also acknowledges Susan B. Fine, MA, OTR, FAOTA, James H. Spencer, MD, and Gretchen L. Haas, PhD, who were the author's principal mentors as well as co-investigators and provided invaluable support in the completion of the RAPS and in preparation of the articles used in preparing this chapter.

In addition, the following people have contributed to the development of the RAPS (the author apologizes if anyone has been inadvertently left out): Robert Being, Jody Bortone, Barbara Bulay, Ann Conway, Karen Diasio Serrett, Anthony DiVittis, Mary Donahue, Stephen Ellis, Janet Falk-Kessler, Elaine Fondiller, Leora Havazelet Friedman, John Frings, Nedra Gillette, Judy Grossman, Kathy Kassebay, Carlotta Kip, Alfred Lewis, Lela Llorens, William C. Mann, Maralynne Mitchum, Ann Neville Jan, Grace Kaufman, JoAnn Leventhal, Karen MacDonald, Mary Palmeri, Ellen Rabinowitz, Anne Hiller Scott, Bettye Soppas, Joni Spitz, Elinor Smith, and Patricia Smith.

PART VI:
ASSESSMENTS BASED ON A
SKILL ACQUISITIONAL THEORY

15

The Kohlman Evaluation of Living Skills

Linda Kohlman Thomson, MOT, OT(C), FAOTA

The Kohlman Evaluation of Living Skills (KELS) is an evaluation designed to assess basic living skills. It is administered by using a combination of interview and task performance items. Setup, administration, and scoring can be completed in 30 to 45 minutes, which allows the occupational therapist to develop intervention plans and to assist in discharge planning in a timely manner. The KELS was originally designed to be used for evaluating people with psychiatric diagnoses on inpatient units, but it is applicable to a variety of populations. Research using small samples has been completed, but the development of the Kohlman Evaluation of Living Skills is an ongoing process. The purpose of this chapter is to describe the historical development of the KELS, administration and scoring procedures, and results of the research studies. A review of literature is included, as well as a discussion of the limitations of this assessment tool.

HISTORICAL DEVELOPMENT

The Kohlman Evaluation of Living Skills was first developed in 1978 at Harborview Medical Center in Seattle, Washington. At that time, the author was working on a locked inpatient psychiatric unit, and the tool was originally designed for that setting and population. From the beginning of its use, occupational therapists identified the applicability of the KELS to other settings and populations. Currently the KELS is being used throughout the United States and in some foreign countries, in a variety of settings and with many populations.

In 1978 the need to systematically assess basic living skills was present, but no appropriate evaluation tools were available. At that time each occupational therapist typically developed his or her own evaluation method to be used in each individual setting or facility. No consistency between facilities existed and questionable reliability existed within each setting. Most of the evaluations relied entirely on a written format. Therefore, it was difficult to know if a patient had a deficit in living skills, or in an area affecting the person's ability to complete a written test. The author identified that some of the patients with psychiatric diagnoses were unable to read and write, but were able to live alone in the community. Others had difficulty reading because of blurred vision due to the side effects of medications. It was important to have an evaluation that identified if a person could read or write, while not basing the assessment of living skills on those abilities alone. Therefore, the evaluation needed to include other methods besides solely a written format.

Time was another factor. The length-of-stay for inpatients was starting to decline in 1978 and has continued to decline. As is true today, many inpatient psychiatric units operated with high patient volumes and only one occupational therapist. With short lengths of stays and high patient caseloads, the occupational therapist has limited time available to assess patients. It is important to have an evaluation that takes a short period of time to administer and to score, yet generates an adequate database from which to develop intervention and discharge plans.

Another factor that was important to the author in developing the KELS was for the evaluation to be easy to administer. With limited resources of time and energy, the administration process needed to be efficient and not an energy drain for the occupational therapist. Competency also had to be achieved in a short period of time, with limited administration trials. It was likewise important for fieldwork students to be able to achieve competency in a short period of time.

Communication regarding a patient's status and progress occurs by verbal and written methods on inpatient units. The caseload for an occupational therapist can be very high, and frequently team conferences occur concurrently. Chart documentation may be the only means of communication available to the occupational therapist. Therefore, the score sheet needed to be easy to understand and short enough, so that staff members would attend to it and use the information.

During the entire development process of the KELS these factors have been retained to guide the item selection, administration, and scoring process. To summarize these characteristics are: 1) high interrater reliability, 2) evidence of validity, 3) short setup, administration, and scoring time, 4) easy administration process, and 5) competency in the administration process achieved in a short period of time.

After the development of the KELS for the locked inpatient psychiatric unit at Harborview Medical Center, other occupational therapists in the local area expressed an interest in the KELS and began to use it. The KELS was presented at two conferences, one of which was the National American Occupational Therapy Association Conference in 1979. After that time, many occupational therapists across the nation began to use the KELS with success. Since that time it has continued to grow in use across the country and is included in the curriculums of many occupational therapy schools. It is used in Canada and other foreign countries, although it must be noted that the items are based on the living skills for the United States, which is its primary intended audience.

Although the KELS was originally designed to be used in psychiatric settings, it has applicability to many populations and settings. It has proven particularly effective in assisting with discharge planning of geriatric patients in acute care settings. Some family practice physicians find it useful to evaluate whether people are able to remain in their homes or if additional services are needed in the homes. Rehabilitation units are using the KELS with a variety of patient diagnoses. Other patient populations for which the KELS is an effective measure are patients with developmental disabilities and those in special adolescent programs. In some states the KELS is being used as an effective tool to assist in determining gravely disabled or involuntary-treatment court cases. As health care has continued to move toward shorter hospital length of stays and as our geriatric population continues to increase, the Kohlman Evaluation of Living Skills has become more applicable to a variety of settings and populations.

REVIEW OF LITERATURE

The identification of an individual's performance in activities of daily living and the enhancement of that performance to optimal levels are focuses of occupational therapy intervention. Occupational therapy practitioners are involved with the successful integration of an individual into the natural environment[1] and with providing the individual with as much productive participation in society as is possible.[2] Since the deinstitutionalization trend of the 1960s and 1970s, treatment in mental health settings has been increasingly concerned with the integration of the mentally ill into the community as productive members.

The ability to perform is a factor that often causes people to seek psychiatric intervention. Clients or relatives present the problem in terms of an inability to do that which was once done or what is necessary within the environment. Being able to work, study, rest, play, and care for oneself or others is one of the barometers used to identify mental illness and health.[3]

There is an intrinsic need to deal with the environment.[4] As an individual learns to interact effectively with the environment, competence is increased. The individual learns about his or her relationship with the environment, which creates a feeling of efficacy and satisfaction. Motivation is believed to involve the satisfaction that occurs in successful experiences with the environment.[4] Motivation and satisfaction are barometers of mental health.

Activities of daily living are all methods by which an individual interacts and controls the environment. If an individual is unable to function and adapt to the environment, imbalances in work, self-care, and leisure activities occur; competence, satisfaction, and motivation are decreased; and the individual's health is impaired or threatened. In most health care settings today, the disposition or integration of patients into the community is usually a component of care plans. This is particularly true of people with chronic mental illness who frequently change living situations and have difficulty adapting to the environment. Occupational therapy practitioners have the skills to identify the level of function in daily living skills and facilitate successful performance and integration of individuals into the community. If a patient is placed in a living situation and has difficulty performing the necessary basic living skills for that situation, further stress is added to the individual's tenuous adjustment, and this actively interferes with integration into the community.[5] There is a need to place individuals in living situations that match their ability to perform daily living skills to increase the possibility of successful integration into the community.[6]

Occupational therapists have used informal evaluation procedures since the inception of the profession.[7] In the 1960s, occupational therapists began to be concerned about developing formal assessments. At that time there was an increasing concern with obtaining baseline data from which to plan interventions.[7]

In the area of living skills, there were no standardized assessments that met the needs of a short-term psychiatric setting to determine levels of function. In the 1970s the most commonly known assessment of living skills for psychiatric patients was the Comprehensive Evaluation of Basic Living Skills.[8] The authors identified it as an 8-hour assessment that was not intended for use with acute patients, in crisis intervention, or in short-term psychiatric facilities.[8] It was also an unstandardized assessment. The Functional Life Scale was another living skill assessment, but it was not developed by occupational therapists.[9] It was also a lengthy evaluation for long-term patients and did not meet the needs of occupational therapists in short-term settings. The Independent Living Skills Evaluation[1] was directed toward evaluating clients in a semisupervised apartment-living program. It took 2 ½ hours to administer and did not have reliability and validity data. Another living skill assessment was the Community Living Skills Assessment Inventory,[10] which focused on people in institutions and included many items related to people with physical disabilities. These items were not appropriate for people with psychiatric diagnoses, and the assessment was too detailed and lengthy for use in short-term care settings.

In gerontology there are some living skill assessments, but none adequately meet the needs of psychiatric patients. Some of these are the Geriatric Functional Rating Scale,[11] the Functional Activities Questionnaire,[12] the Functional Assessment Inventory,[13] and the Self-Evaluation of Life Function.[14] The assessment closest to meeting the needs of psychiatric patients is the Geriatric Functional Rating Scale,[11] which is designed to determine the need for institutional care. Its limitations are that it is based only on a self-report interview, with limited items of a global nature.

Frequently, patients with mental illness use several health care facilities, both inpatient and outpatient. In this process, continuity of care is difficult to maintain and repetition of care can occur. Donaldson stated that most rehabilitation facilities have an activities of daily living (ADL) evaluation form, but there is not one such form that is widely accepted and used.[15] This situation is true in most mental health facilities with living skills evaluations. There has been a continuing need for a unified standardized evaluation that has applicability to many settings. A unified evaluation more objectively measures change; increases communication between therapists, professions, and facilities; and decreases repetition in patient care. The KELS has steadily increased in distribution and use, and is intended to be a unified evaluation in a variety of health care and community settings.

ADMINISTRATION

The Kohlman Evaluation of Living Skills assesses 17 living skills categorized under five main areas. These areas include: 1) self-care, 2) safety and health, 3) money management, 4) transportation and telephone, and 5) work and leisure. The KELS may be given by an occupational therapist, or occupational therapy assistant under the supervision of an occupational therapist. Interview and task performance procedures are used to assess the living skills of the patient. All the questions tasks and supplies are designed to simulate the local environment of the patient. In the administration section of the manual, the method (task or interview), the necessary equipment, the administrative procedures, and the specific scoring criteria for each item are given. Separate sections for scoring and equipment are also included in the manual. Examples of completed KELS score sheets are located in the appendix of the KELS manual.[22]

Instructions are included to assemble the list of equipment, such as a bar of soap, a bill, and local phone number cards. Four pictures to be used in the Safety and Health section are included in the manual and are essential in the accurate administration and scoring of the KELS. Other necessary supplies are the local telephone books and a telephone. All of the equipment and forms, except for the telephone supplies, will fit in a three-ring binder so that it is easily transportable. Instructions are included in the manual to assist in constructing a KELS kit for your local area. The forms are included in the manual, and may be copied if intact and the copyright is retained on the form. It may be put into a computer documentation system, provided that the form includes the exact information and format of the one in the manual and the copyright is also included.

In the administration section of the manual, specific instructions are given for each item. This includes how to present the equipment and the statements to be made by the evaluator. These must be stated as given (in bold in the manual), and feedback regarding the client's performance is not to be given until the end. The instructions are to be followed precisely, or the results may not be valid or reliable.

SCORING

Independent and Needs Assistance are the two scoring categories for the KELS. The specific scoring criteria are given for each item of the assessment. The scoring criteria are designed to indicate the minimum standards required to live independently in the community. Independent is defined as the level of competency required to perform the basic living skill in a manner that maintains the safety and health of the individual without direct assistance of other people.[16]

For special situations in which the patient does not score within the scoring criteria given, the terms Not Applicable and See Note are used. These terms should be used as infrequently as possible. When they are used, explanations need to be stated on the KELS Scoring Sheet.

To score the results, each section marked Needs Assistance, excluding Work and Leisure, is counted as 1 point. Needs assistance scores under Work and Leisure are counted as only 1/2 point. Independent, See Note, and Not Applicable are counted as 0 points. A score of 5 1/2 or less indicates the person is capable of living independently, and a total score of 6 or more indicates the person needs assistance to live in the community. On the KELS Score Sheet (Figure 15-1), it is recommended that the score for each item be blackened in to facilitate reading and comprehending the results. At a minimum a large, bold X should be used. At the bottom of the KELS Score Sheet, a short summary note is written. In the summary, the overall results are discussed and recommendations for appropriate living situations are included. If further occupational therapy intervention is needed, it is included in the summary.

When giving the KELS, additional information is obtained about the patient's skills and abilities. Although reading and writing is not scored, the evaluator is able to determine if the patient has these abilities. With the Safety and Health pictures, of which some are purposefully designed to be dark, the patient must demonstrate figure ground skills to determine what is safe in the pictures. This skill is very important in ambulating safely and for maintaining a safe environment. Throughout the KELS, there are many opportunities to assess the client's cognitive abilities, such as memory, attention span, and comprehension. The evaluator also learns about the patient's judgment and if the patient is in touch with reality. In the Work and Leisure sections, information about the patient's time use is obtained. The additional information gathered during the evaluation is not scored, but is tremendously valuable in making treatment plans with the patient. This important additional information should be included in the summary note at the bottom of the KELS Score Sheet.

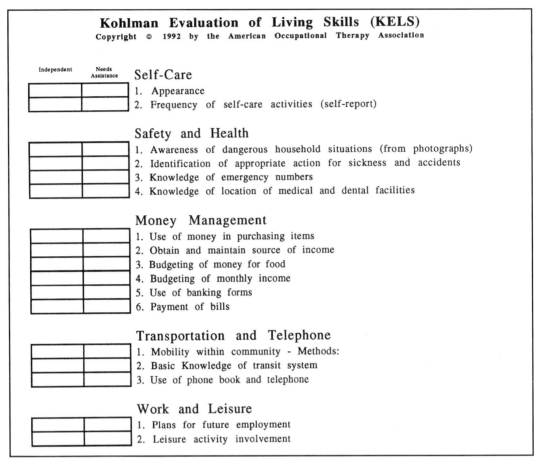

Figure 15-1. The KELS Score Sheet. (From Thomson LK. *The Kohlman Evaluation of Living Skills* (3rd ed). Copyright 1992 by the American Occupational Therapy Association, Inc. Reprinted with permission.)

Morrow created the Community Support Scale[17] as part of a master's degree thesis project. It is a tool designed to assist in determining the actual type of assistance a patient would need for each KELS item to remain living alone in the community. The research project in which it was used is discussed further in the Research section, and the tool is included in the KELS manual. This scale may be helpful in determining specific recommendations for a patient, but because of the lack of research using this scale, it is only appropriate to use it as a guideline. The scale is also included in the manual.

LIMITATIONS

As with any assessment, the KELS has its limitations and problems that may be encountered in the administration and scoring. At times a patient will give a partial answer, and the evaluator must ask additional questions to obtain a complete answer. Since this is a clinical decision-making process that cannot be controlled in the administration, there may be variations in the judgment of partial answers and the subsequent questions asked. Therefore, it is possible that a patient might be scored higher or lower by a different evaluator. It should be noted that research has demonstrated high reliability scores.

One limitation of the KELS is that some items are knowledge-based versus performance-based. This was done in the design and selection of items to make the total administration and scoring time both practical and short in length. Therefore, in some cases the occupational therapist may not have the confidence that the patient will actually be able to perform the living skill, even if the knowledge is present. In those cases, the occupational therapist may need to do additional performance-based assessments beyond the scope of the KELS. It is strongly encouraged that occupational therapists use the KELS as one type of living skill assessment and not view it as the only living-skill assessment available. Supplemental assessments, such as a kitchen screening, need to be completed at the discretion of the individual evaluator. The Milwaukee Evaluation of Daily Living Skills[18] (MEDLS) is another assessment that dovetails well with the KELS when more information is needed and time is available to do further testing. The MEDLS is performance-based, and individual items may be tested as needed.

If the KELS is going to be used in a multidisciplinary setting, it is essential to educate other professionals as to how the items are assessed and how to interpret and use the results. Without education, misinterpretation of results can occur. Education by a variety of means, such as individual contacts, written materials, and inservices, may be effective. Periodic re-education of staff is important to maintain communication and understanding regarding the KELS.

Another problem that can occur in the administration and scoring is that some evaluators feel a patient should score all items in the Independent category to be considered "normal." The term "Needs Assistance" should not be viewed as being abnormal or negative. Many people function very independently in the community and receive some assistance in daily living skills. An example is the wife who manages the home and whose husband manages the money. The woman would probably score Needs Assistance for Obtain and Maintain Source of Income and for Budgeting of Monthly Income. In the overall score, the woman might be able to live alone, but in the present home, assistance would have to be provided in those specific areas.[16] The KELS was not designed with the intent that a score of Independent should be scored in all areas in order to live independently in the community. The circumstances and daily living environment of the patient must be considered.

It is also important to recognize that the KELS is an assessment that is rarely, if ever, used as the sole determinate of a client's living situation. The KELS is used to provide specific information regarding a client's ability to function in basic living skills. This information is only one aspect of the decision-making process of a multidisciplinary team in determining discharge plans with a patient. The KELS is not meant to be used in isolation, but to be a valuable, contributing factor in assisting the team to make discharge plans that will allow the patient to function as independently as possible in the community.

RESEARCH

A variety of research studies have been completed on the KELS. All were done on relatively small samples, but each helped to establish the reliability and validity of the KELS. Most of these studies were done as theses in master's degree programs. As the KELS grew in use, more studies were conducted. Unfortunately some of the results are unknown to the author. To continue to document the effectiveness of the

KELS, more extensive research, using larger sample sizes and examining more variables, needs to done.

An interrater reliability study was completed in 1981 by Ilika and Hoffman[19] in Minnesota. This was an unpublished study in which the authors reported that the interrater correlations were significant at $P < .001$, with a variance from 74% to 94% agreement. The study involved psychiatric patients, but the exact research design is unknown. Since this study, minor changes have been made in the administration, and the percentage of agreement for reliability was higher in later studies.

Ilida and Hoffman[20] also completed a concurrent validity study in 1981. This study was also unpublished and was conducted in a psychiatric treatment setting. The KELS score was compared to the Global Assessment Scale scores. Results indicated correlations of .78 to .89, with significance at $P < .001$. These results were favorable, since both tests examine dysfunction in psychiatric patients but evaluate different factors.

In 1982 Kaufman[21] completed a concurrent validity study. This study, with psychiatric inpatients, compared scores on the KELS with scores on the Bay Area Functional Performance Evaluation (BaFPE). The total BaFPE test score correlated with the KELS test score at -.84 ($P < .0001$). The negative value is a result of the test scores varying in opposite directions. These results helped establish the validity of the KELS because both tests are designed to evaluate function and dysfunction in psychiatric patients, but do evaluate different indicators.

Tateichi[22] also completed a concurrent validity study in 1984. This study compared 20 subjects living in a halfway house (congregate care facility or CCF) and 20 living independently (N = 40). The primary hypothesis was that clients living independently are more likely to have lower scores on the KELS than clients living in a sheltered setting. A low score on the KELS indicates greater independence. When the scores were compared, using the Mann-Whitney U Test, results were significant (U = 47, $P < .001$), with subjects living alone scoring lower on the KELS than subjects living in the sheltered setting. Tateichi also looked at whether the cut-off score of 5 differentiated between the two groups. Unfortunately, a score of 5 1/2 should have been used to be consistent with the administration instructions. According to the results, the cut-off score of 5 was statistically significant, ($P < .05$), but with a high incidence of false negatives. In this study a false negative occurred when a person scored more independently in living skills (ie, less than 5) than the setting required. Of the clients living in the sheltered setting, 45% scored greater than 6 and were accurately identified, while 55% scored less than 5. This could be expected because people live in halfway houses for a variety of reasons. A deficiency in living skills is only one possible reason. Of the clients living alone, 90% scored less than 5 and were accurately identified, while 10% scored greater than 6.

There is concern for this 10% of the clients who scored greater than 6 and who were, in fact, living alone in the community. To determine what problems there are with the KELS, it would be important to analyze other variables between the two groups (the 90% and the 10%), eg, what assistance the patients were actually receiving, how long the patients had been living alone, whether the patients were still living alone 4 to 6 months later, and the hospitalization rate. Without additional information, it is difficult to know if changes need to be made to make the KELS more valid. Prior to the testing in the study, interrater reliability was established on three consecutive trials, with the percentages of agreement at 84%, 94%, and 94%.

In 1985 Morrow[17] completed a predictive validity study. The KELS was administered to 20 inpatients on a geriatric unit. These predischarge KELS scores were compared to actual living situations 40 to 60 days after hospital discharge to determine if the KELS could accurately predict placement. Thirteen subjects were discharged to community living and seven subjects were discharged to nursing homes. A Community Support Scale was designed as a supplemental scoring scale to the KELS. If a patient scored "Needs Assistance" on an item in the KELS, the Community Support Scale defined specifically what assistance the patient needed to remain in the community and an adjusted KELS score was calculated. In predicting which geriatric individuals would succeed in community placements 40 to 60 days post discharge, both the KELS and the adjusted KELS scores were 100% accurate. For those individuals with KELS scores greater than 5 1/2 and had been recommended for nursing home placement, 50% were actually living in the community. Using the adjusted KELS score improved the positive predictive value to 72% with this group. One problem with this study's interpretation is that nursing home placement is not recommended for all patients scoring greater than 5 1/2. The KELS cut-off score of 5 1/2 is actually meant to be interpreted that an individual with a score greater than 5 1/2 would need assistance to live in the community. The Community Support Scale did create a systematic scoring method to help the occupational therapist determine the kind of assistance needed in order for a patient to remain in a community living setting. This Community Support Scale is helpful in quantifying the assistance needed and in reducing discharge planning time for the treatment team. The Community Support Scale is discussed in the Scoring section and is included in the appendices of the KELS manual. Interrater reliability was calculated on two consecutive trials prior to the study, and 100% agreement was achieved in scoring the KELS and the adjusted KELS.

In 1987 McGourty (now Thomson) completed a predictive validity study.[23] The purpose of the study was to determine if the KELS could predict successful independent living 40 to 60 days after discharge from the hospital. The subjects were 50 psychiatric inpatients who were discharged to live alone in the community. Each subject was administered the KELS in the hospital, and the treatment team that made disposition plans were not given the results. Forty to 60 days after discharge a follow-up contact was made to determine if the subject was still living independently. The percent of agreement, calculated for interrater reliability, was 98%. The validity results were much less favorable. Several major problems were identified in the research design after the data was collected. One was the extreme variance in the size of the two groups. Two patients scored greater than 5 1/2 and 44 scored 5 1/2 or less (predicted to be able to live alone). Therefore, very few patients were discharged to live alone who were predicted to not have the necessary living skills to be able to live alone. The staff of the treatment teams had been using the KELS to assist with discharge planning for more than 2 years. It was felt that the occupational therapists during those 2 years had been very effective in educating the staff to look for critical factors for successful independent living. Therefore, the staff did an excellent job in discharging patients to live alone who would have scored well on the KELS (5 1/2 or less). This created an unexpected problem for the research study in that not enough patients scored greater than 5 1/2. In the future it is recommended that the staff not be familiar with the KELS prior to undertaking a study.

Another problem was in the follow-up contact. Nineteen patients were not living alone at 40 to 60 days after discharge from the hospital. The study did not have a method to sort out legitimate reasons for not living alone. Only the yes-no response was analyzed. With the data, it could not adequately be determined if the patient was not living alone due to the failure to perform living skills or some other valid reason. In some cases, roommates moved in, or the patient went to a residential mental health program, either of which could have had nothing to do with living skills. For many of the patients, no reason was identified. Because of the extreme limitations found in the research design, the results were disappointing. If the study were repeated, some of the problems in the research design could be eliminated.

Brown, Moore, Hemman, and Yunek published a research study that investigated whether interview and simulation methods of assessment were as effective as observation of the task in the natural environment.[24] Two items from the KELS were used—Use of Money in Purchasing Items (task) and Basic Knowledge of Transit System (interview). Twenty subjects with severe mental illness were selected by convenience sampling from a community support services program. All of the subjects were living in the community. The two KELS items were administered at the program, and interrater reliability was achieved at 100% on scoring of the two items. Immediately after completion of the KELS items, the research assistants had the participants purchase a bar of soap at a nearby store and take the local bus to a location that was new to them. Money was provided and the participants were allowed to obtain additional information or assistance from the environment, other than asking the research assistants who were accompanying them.

The findings indicated that agreement occurred in both methods of testing for the item Use of Money in Purchasing Items with chi-square equal to 5.96 and $p < .05$. For the item Basic Knowledge of Transit System, only 60% of the time did both methods of testing agree. With chi-square equal to 1.25 and $p > .05$, the hypothesis was supported that the interview KELS item would be unrelated to assessment in the natural environment. There was concern by the authors that some false positives occurred in the transit item. In their conclusions, it was suggested that the real-life experience was more complex than that portrayed by the KELS simulation and interview methods. A limitation of the study is that it only examined two of the 17 items of the KELS and did not examine the test as a whole. The KELS was not designed for the items to be used individually, although the items may indicate a need for further testing in a particular area. It is also important to note that the KELS was not intended to be the sole determinant of a person's living environment. This study does reinforce the need for occupational therapists to not rely too heavily on assessments not done in the patient's actual living environment. It is always preferable to test clients with demonstration of actual performance in the environment in which they must function. When considering time and practicality, occupational therapists must use their judgment to determine the most effective and efficient method of assessment to get the highest quality results.

SUGGESTED FURTHER RESEARCH

The research studies completed as of early 1987 all contributed to making the Third Edition of the Kohlman Evaluation of Living Skills an effective assessment tool. Studies conducted after that date will be included in future editions under the

Research section. Further research is needed to more completely establish the reliability and validity of the KELS. Larger sample sizes, broader geographical representation, and greater variety in research design is needed. Some suggestions for further research are:

1. Interrater reliability—Multiple observers score videotapes of the KELS being administered.
2. Consistency in administration—Comparison of groups learning the KELS by the manual only versus the manual and videotape instruction.
3. Predictive validity—Studies using a variety of populations and time frames to determine how accurately the KELS predicts over time, and which other factors affect success in community living.
4. Concurrent validity—Studies in a variety of settings with many populations to examine if patterns of living skills occur within specific populations and settings.

Additional studies administering the KELS, using large sample sizes and wide geographical representation while collecting demographic data about people with chronic psychiatric conditions who are living alone, would also be helpful.

These are only a few of the many possible research projects that are needed. More studies investigating the validity of the KELS are necessary but difficult to design. Isolating living skills as the only changing variable can be very challenging, particularly over an extended period of time. This is especially true when the patient populations of interest may lead very unstable lives. Even though the research designs may be difficult, the studies are needed to give occupational therapy practitioners a living skill assessment that is even more reliable and valid.

SUMMARY

The Kohlman Evaluation of Living Skills is a valuable assessment tool for occupational therapy practitioners. Research was conducted on the validity and reliability of the tool, but more studies are needed. The KELS is an effective measure in assisting occupational therapy practitioners to determine the living skills of a patient and whether a patient can live alone. With the current health care trends of shortened hospital stays and community living, an assessment of this nature is critical. The KELS is an assessment that can be used in a variety of settings with many patient populations. It can be given in a short period of time and the administration procedures can be learned easily. The Kohlman Evaluation of Living Skills is an essential assessment tool for occupational therapy practitioners and occupational therapy programs.

REFERENCES

1. Johnson TP, Vinncombe BJ, Merrill GW. The independent living skills evaluation. *OTMH.* 1980;1:5-17.
2. Black BJ, Chapple ED. Rehabilitation through productive participation: Still waiting in the wings? *Psychiatric Q.* 1981;53:85-92.
3. Fidler GS. *Overview of OT in Mental Health.* Unpublished. Rockville, Md: American Occupational Therapy Association. 1981;1-17.
4. White RW. Motivation reconsidered: The concept of competence. *Psychol Rev.* 1959;66;297-333.
5. Broekema MC, Danze, KH, Schloemer CU. Occupational therapy in a community aftercare program. *Am J Occup Ther.* 1975;29:22-27.

6. Gauger AB, Brownell WM, Russell WW, Retter RW. Evaluation of levels of subsistence. *Arch Phys Med*. 1964;45:286-292.

7. Diasio K, Moyer E. On psychosocial assessment. *OTMH*. 1980;1:1-3.

8. Casanova JS, Ferber J. Comprehensive evaluation of basic living skills. *Am J Occup Ther*. 1976;30:101-105.

9. Sarno JE, Sarno MT, Levita E. The functional life scale. *Arch Phys Med*. 1973;54: 214-220.

10. Switzky HN, Rotatori AF. Community living skills assessment inventory: An instrument to facilitate deinstitutionalization of the severely developmentally disabled. *Psych Rep*. 1978;43:1335-1342.

11. Graver H, Birnbom BA. A geriatric functional rating scale to determine the need for institutional care. *J Am Geriatr Soc*. 1975;23:472-476.

12. Pfeiffer E, Johnson TM, Chiofolio RL. Functional assessment of elderly subjects in four service settings. *J Am Geriatr Soc*. 1981;29:433-437.

13. Cairl RD, Pfeiffer E, Keller DM, Burke H, Samis HV. An evaluation of the reliability and validity of the functional assessment inventory. *J Am Geriatr Soc*. 1983;31:607-612.

14. Linn MW, Linn BS. Self-evaluation of life function (SELF) scale: A short comprehensive self-report of health for elderly adults. *J Ger*. 1984;39:603-612.

15. Donaldson SW, et. al. A unified ADL evaluation form. *Arch Phys Med*. 1973;54:175-179.

16. McGourty LK. *Kohlman Evaluation of Living Skills*. Seattle,Wash: KELS Research; 1979.

17. Morrow M. *A predictive validity study of the Kohlman evaluation of living skills*. Master's thesis. University of Washington; 1985.

18. Leonardelli C. *The Milwaukee Evaluation of Daily Living Skills (MEDLS)*. Thorofare, NJ: SLACK Incorporated; 1988.

19. Ilika J, Hoffman NG. *Reliability study of the Kohlman evaluation of living skills*. Unpublished. 1981.

20. Ilika J, Hoffman NG. *Concurrent Validity Study on the Kohlman Evaluation of Living Skills and the Global Assessment Scale*. Unpublished. 1981.

21. Kaufman L. *Concurrent Validity Study on the Kohlman Evaluation of Living Skills and the Bay Area Functional Performance Evaluation*. Master's thesis. Gainesville, Fla: University of Florida; 1982.

22. Tateichi S. *A Concurrent Validity Study of the Kohlman Evaluation of Living Skills*. Master's thesis. Seattle, Wash: University of Washington;1984.

23. McGourty LK. *Kohlman Evaluation of Living Skills — A Predictive Validity Study*. Unpublished. 1987.

24. Brown C, Moore WP, Hemman D, Yunek A. Influence of instrumental activities of daily living assessment method on judgments of independence. *Am J Occup Ther*. 1996;50:202-206.

The Milwaukee Evaluation of Daily Living Skills

Carol Leonardelli Haertlein, PhD, OT, FAOTA

The Milwaukee Evaluation of Daily Living Skills (MEDLS) was developed to provide a behavioral measure of the abilities of people with serious mental illness to do basic and complex activities of daily living. Classical methods of test development were used to develop the instrument as it was originally published.[1] Since that time, techniques of modern test theory, such as Rasch analysis, have been increasingly used in the development of functional assessments in rehabilitation. This chapter will describe the reasons for applying techniques of modern test theory to the functional assessments of people with mental illness that are used by occupational therapists and discuss revisions in the MEDLS, following application of these techniques.

ISSUES INFLUENCING ASSESSMENT OF PEOPLE WITH MENTAL ILLNESS

Occupational therapists regularly measure a wide range of markers of clinical change during treatment programs. These markers include such phenomena as strength, memory, agitation, mobility, and activities of daily living, or ADLs, including basic ADLs, such as dressing and eating, and more complex ADLs, such as using transportation and homemaking tasks. Most often, the measurement tools used are ordinal scales that provide a rank ordering of common representations of the phenomenon under review.[2] Examples include the Functional Independence Measure, Katz ADL Index, and the Barthel Index. The determination of the ranking is typically based on direct rater observation, family caregiver or other health care provider reports, or patient self-report. The use of these methods depends on the phenomenon being considered and the characteristics of the individuals being measured. For example, direct observation might be used to determine the strength of an elderly person after a cerebrovascular accident, self-report to determine the mobility status of a well elderly person, and report by family caregivers to evaluate memory deficits of a person with dementia.

Several issues that influence the evaluation of basic and complex ADLs of people with mental illness must be considered. These include: a) the method of evaluation used, ie, self-report or report by others versus direct performance evaluation; b) the measurement of specific abilities that contribute to performance of ADLs, eg, motor ability and cognitive ability versus measurement of the ADL skills themselves; c) the usefulness of norm as compared to criterion-referencing as a basis for determining skills of people being tested; and d) the importance of targeting evaluation instruments to specific disability groups.

Method of Evaluation

Assessment instruments, which are designed for direct observation of self-care skills under standardized conditions, are usually considered to provide the most useful information, although they are the most costly in time and evaluator knowledge level.[3] But since self-report of self-care levels, including questionnaires and interviews, has been identified as generally unreliable in psychiatric populations, especially schizophrenics,[4] the trade-off—higher costs in exchange for meaningful information—seems worthwhile.

The occupational therapist, faced with the need to choose between assessment modes, must consider the characteristics of the clinical population as well as other, more obvious factors, such as time constraints, personnel and space limitations, qualities of the evaluation, and so forth. There was consensus among therapists participating in the original content validation of the MEDLS that people with serious mental illness underestimate the difficulty of a skill, deny inability to perform it, or overestimate their abilities.[1]

Assessment of Skills Versus Abilities

It is most common that ADL skills are evaluated on what a person can or cannot do, eg, get dressed, take a bath, or prepare a meal; rather than on why the person can or cannot do the activity, eg, adequate strength, sufficient memory, or good balance. These two levels of function have been distinguished as *skills* and *abilities*.

Christiansen distinguishes between abilities and skills, based on the work of Fleishman and colleagues in the area of human performance analysis.[5] Fleishman "defines abilities as general traits that are a product of genetic makeup and learning, much of which occur during childhood and adolescence."[5] Some examples are written comprehension, inductive reasoning, manual dexterity, and stamina. Skill is defined by Fleishman as "the level of proficiency in a specific task. The assumption is that skill in complex tasks can be explained by the presence of various underlying general abilities."[5] Self-care activities can be characterized as groupings of skills involving many abilities. For example, dressing for rainy weather conditions involves deductive reasoning (deciding what to wear), information ordering (arranging the dressing process), spatial orientation (locating clothing), and several motor abilities (coordination, dexterity, strength, flexibility, and stamina) to don clothes. Whether or not an individual puts any of these abilities into action depends on self-concept, motivation (intrinsic and extrinsic), knowledge (conditions of situation), and judgment (sociocultural expectations). The actual performance of skills is dependent on abilities, knowledge, and internal or external forces driving the person to act. Yet the evaluation and treatment of dressing impairment of a person with mental illness does not focus on deductive reasoning and spatial orientation. Rather, the level of skill performance is addressed, for example, assisting the person to dress in an acceptable manner. If the person cannot decide which clothing is appropriate for rainy weather, a decision-making process for clothing choices is taught, with examples and cause-effect relationships. If he or she cannot locate clothing, visual or written reminders of where clothing is stored are provided.

Fisher reports that research has not shown a strong enough relationship between abilities and ADL skills to be able to make valid predictions about performance of daily life tasks based on motor, cognitive, or psychological test scores.[6] The assessment and treatment must occur at the level of skill performance, with the potential for remediation of underlying abilities occurring at the same time.

Normative Versus Criterion Standards

Four evaluations of basic and more complex ADLs, in addition to the MEDLS, that have been published in the occupational therapy literature are targeted to people with mental illness.[7-10] At least 15 to 20 such instruments for the physically impaired have been published in the rehabilitation and aging literature.[11-14] For the most part, these evaluation instruments represent a wide range of minimal to moderate standardization, and validity and reliability data. For those instruments developed by therapists in clinical settings, this may reflect clinicians' lack of sophistication in test development procedures. For the other instruments it "may, in part, reflect the recognition that 'norms' are not meaningful in the measurement of [basic and more complex] ADLs ."[6]

Performance of basic and more complex ADL skills must meet a criterion, or standard, to be acceptable. It is assumed that people with "normal" abilities will be able to perform all tasks or skills without difficulty and achieve maximum scores.[6] Although different subgroups of a disabled population, eg, institutionalized versus community-living people with mental illness, will display success or failure on different items of an evaluation, there is not an average, or mean, score, or rating for the overall disabled group. The standard for evaluation success is that people achieve maximum scores on all relevant tasks, with the criterion being the ability to perform skills without difficulty. Standardized, norm-referenced evaluations cannot accomplish this goal; criterion-referenced instruments are needed.

Targeting Evaluation Instruments to the Population

The individual for whom the MEDLS was originally designed is operationally defined as "an adult, age 18 and above, with a history of mental illness of at least 2 years duration who has been hospitalized or under care at a skilled nursing facility, community-based residential facility, halfway house or so forth for a cumulative period of at least 6 months within the past 2 years; or is receiving outpatient treatment due to a mental or emotional disorder for a minimum of 2 years."[1] This person is often described as having severe and persistent or serious mental illness, and is found in many different treatment settings.

According to traditional test theory, one of the criteria to be met in the content validation procedure of an evaluation instrument is targeting items to the population for whom it is intended (face validity). If a measurement instrument is sampling behaviors to make predictions or explanations about a set of skills, the sampled behaviors must be valid representatives of the larger set. This validation process of the MEDLS for people with serious mental illness demonstrated that the behaviors assessed in the instrument represent important ADLs for the target population.[15] This same validation process has not occurred for the MEDLS for other clinical populations.

Several ADL evaluation instruments are available for populations other than that of people with mental illness.[11,13,14] The instruments described in these sources are primarily developed for physical rehabilitation settings or for the elderly population. They could not be used appropriately for people with mental illness because they exclude relevant items, eg, selection of suitable clothing for specific situations, and include irrelevant items, eg, transfers and mobility. Although there are other important criteria to consider in selection of evaluation instruments, eg, administration time required, clarity of administration procedures, interpretation and usefulness of results, the need to select evaluations that are designed for the clinical population under consideration cannot be overlooked.

DEVELOPMENT OF ORIGINAL MEDLS

Occupational therapists have a long-standing interest in the functional status of the disabled individuals whom they serve. Several years ago leaders in the profession established assessment of function as one of its most pressing priorities.[16] For occupational therapists, functional status "relates primarily to the ability of the individual to perform the daily life tasks [occupations] that he or she wants and needs to perform…[and is most meaningfully expressed] within the context of his or her actual performance of [those] daily life tasks."[17]

Assessments of functional status provide information that can be used for at least three different purposes: a) to describe a problem or diagnosis, b) to formulate a prognosis and direct treatment, and c) to evaluate the effectiveness of intervention programs.[13,18]

The MEDLS is a functional assessment that addresses the second identified purpose, which is to be predictive and directive regarding basic and more complex ADLs of people with serious mental illness.[1] It was developed out of a desire to provide, as much as possible, a measure of the behavioral performance of basic and complex ADLs for the target population.

The MEDLS was designed using methods and techniques of traditional test theory. Its development followed a four-phase process of planning, construction, quantitative evaluation, and validation that was consistent with the process of test construction discussed by Nunnally[19] and others.[20,21] The process is described in greater detail elsewhere[15,22] and is briefly summarized here.

The planning phase consisted of stating a purpose for the MEDLS, identifying the domains of the assessment (basic and more complex ADL), and identifying the target population (people with serious mental illness). During the construction phase, items (subtests) and the testing format were established and reviewed. Subtests were revised in accordance with reviewers' suggestions.

Quantitative evaluation consisted of a pilot administration of the MEDLS to a normal population to establish minimum time criteria for subtests, and to further refine administration procedures and scoring criteria. A reliability study, with a sample from the target population, was completed. Following this study, revisions were made in some of the MEDLS subtests. Validation studies, particularly construct and predictive, were not conducted prior to its publication.

The MEDLS, as originally published, consists of 20 subtests (skill areas) of basic and more complex ADLs, which are selected to be administered based on patients' anticipated deficits and needs.[1] Subtests are scored based on the number of individual skills passed for that subtest. For example, bathing has four skills with 1 point per skill; patients receive a score in the range of 0 (failed all skills) to 4 (passed all skills). The scoring is ordinal in nature—a 1 on one subtest does not mean the same as a 1 on another subtest. Subtests are scored individually and there is no cumulative or summed total score for the MEDLS. Most skills are evaluated by having the patient perform or simulate performance of the skill. Self-report is kept to a minimum.

At the time of its publication the MEDLS represented the best effort to measure basic and complex ADLs of people with serious mental illness. It was the intent of the author that the MEDLS would meet certain criteria of sound measurement instruments. The criteria met via the development process used for the MEDLS were a) standard administration procedures (to enhance reliability), b) specific criteria to determine levels of function in skill areas (to enhance validity), c) comprehensiveness, yet individualization, based on anticipated patient need, and d) appropriateness for many types of mental health settings.[15] Content validity, interrater reliability, and standards of performance for the sample population used in the reliability studies also were determined.

AREAS TARGETED FOR IMPROVEMENT

The MEDLS has many characteristics that make it a useful assessment of the functional skills of people with long-term mental illness. It combines basic, more complex ADLs to provide a set of test items that range in difficulty. However, beyond an identified need to add more difficult items, the relative difficulty of the test items is not known. The construct validity of items included in the revised MEDLS has not been determined. An analysis of validity should include confirmation that the items measure the construct(s) assessed by the MEDLS. The flexible and individualized testing allowed by the MEDLS means patients do not have to be tested on irrelevant test items, and raters do not have to try to interpret a total test score that is not meaningful, ie, if there were a total score of 100, a score of 90 might mean deficits in bathing and dressing or in use of money and transportation. On the other hand, the lack of a total score makes it difficult to: a) measure patient change, b) compare patients to each other, or c) compare patients to another standard of performance. The ability to use the MEDLS to identify problems or evaluate change requires that a method of cumulative scoring be developed that simultaneously allows for flexible and individualized testing.

Application of the Rasch Model of Analysis

Since the publication of the MEDLS, concepts of item response theory, and specifically the Rasch measurement models, have been applied to functional assessments by other test developers.[23] For the most part, the evaluation instruments under development using Rasch, employ ordinal rating scales, as does the MEDLS, and are criterion-referenced measures. The traditional statistical procedures used in their earlier development are primarily based on interval data and are probably not valid for the purposes used. The Rasch models of analysis are especially useful because they convert ordinal rating scale data into linear measures in which item difficulties and person abilities are calibrated on the same linear scale. The Rasch models also are useful when missing data must be accommodated, which occurs when irrelevant subtests are not administered to a patient, as in the case of the

MEDLS and other functional assessments. Rasch models also provide the same advantages as other item response approaches, including: (a) person ability estimations that are independent of the particular choice and number of items in subsets of test items assuming that the domain of items is homogeneous and measures a single ability, allowing for comparison of examinees, even though they have taken different subsets of test items, which is a condition common to the MEDLS; and (b) item difficulty estimations that are invariant across sub-groups of examinees from a targeted and identified population.[24]

Another dimension of Rasch analysis is its usefulness in creating scales of test items that reflect unidimensional traits or abilities, or constructs. If items do not characterize single traits or abilities, the statistical analysis will reveal that. At the time of the development of the MEDLS, it was assumed that the ability to do basic and more complex ADLs represented one underlying trait. However, it is likely that more than one trait is being assessed by the current items. It is now hypothesized that there is a subset of items that assesses ADL knowledge/judgment, ie, the capacity to know or discern something gained through experience or association, and another group of items that assesses ADL performance, ie, the ability to carry out an action or pattern of behavior in a prescribed manner. Rasch analysis is able to determine which items, or specific skills within subtests, underlie each of these traits. Because Rasch analysis allows for missing data, it is also possible to generate total scores for traits, even though all test items have not been administered. If items can then be ordered hierarchically within traits, it will be possible to administer test items around an individual's ability level. This will facilitate the process of administering the most relevant items as part of individualized assessment based on patient need. That is to say, items obviously too easy or too hard need not be administered.

In summary, the Rasch model of analysis is able to assist in addressing existing limitations of the MEDLS. Specifically for the revised version of the MEDLS, Rasch analysis provides: a) a hierarchical ranking of the test items by difficulty level, b) validity and reliability data on the newly hypothesized constructs, and c) cumulative ability measures, or a scale of each construct, while maintaining the flexibility of the instrument.

REVISED MEDLS

Initial Analysis

The MEDLS was initially revised, using the data from the original reliability study. Only 18 of the 20 subtests were analyzed as an all-male population, and facility limitations during the original study prevented data collection on the subtests *Makeup Use* and *Hair Care*.[1] For this first analysis, each skill of each subtest was treated as an individual test item so that 72 items were analyzed, following the accepted protocol for Rasch analysis. Three subscales were conceptually hypothesized by a group of expert reviewers who determined which items defined which trait. This process yielded three scales—performance, knowledge/judgment, and social, ie, those skills that reflect the ability to form cooperative and interdependent relationships with others. Twenty-nine items defined the knowledge/judgment trait, 37 items the performance trait, and six items the social trait. The six items on the social trait were insufficient in number and range to provide a scale; therefore, the social scale was eliminated from the MEDLS, and only the knowledge/judgment and performance scales were analyzed.

A low-count item in the original study showed that few people (n = 3) in the target population wear dentures and, therefore, could be scored on the *Denture Care* subtest. In Rasch analysis, it is difficult to determine stable parameter estimates on a group smaller than 30; an item that is rarely used is considered to be of little overall value. Consequently, this subtest was eliminated from the MEDLS.

Rasch analysis was used to evaluate the remaining items for their fit to the remaining two hypothesized scales. The results of this analysis indicated that the knowledge/judgment and performance items defined single, unidimensional constructs, but that neither contained enough difficult items suitable for testing more capable patients. In response to the need for more difficult items, six more subtests anticipated to be more difficult, eg, cleaning activities, were developed for the revised MEDLS.

The revised MEDLS comprises a total of 95 items within 24 subsets. Table 16-1 lists the items by subtest. The 95 items were divided into the 64-item performance scale and the 31-item knowledge/judgment scale (see Table 16-1). Table 16-2 lists the items for the performance scale by subtests.

Study to Examine Revised MEDLS

The revised MEDLS, with six new subtests, was administered to 100 people with serious mental illness, as defined earlier in the chapter following the procedures described by Leonardelli.[1] Three raters, the author and two assistants, participated in data collection. The participants were solicited from two mental health treatment programs that serve people with mental illness via a wide range of programs, including residential care, community support, and day treatment. A heterogeneous sample group was used, representative of the range of dysfunction seen in people with serious mental illness, ie, those living in highly structured institutional settings to those living on their own with the help of a community support program. Three specific subgroups were identified.

Group 1 (n = 30) included people who needed 24-hour supervision. This was the least able group. They were characterized as lacking the skills to perform moderate to difficult functional tasks and needing assistance or supervision with basic ADL.

Group 2 (n = 41) were people living in group homes or community-based residential facilities who were engaged in outside programs on a regular basis, such as day treatment, school, or supported or regular employment. These individuals were characterized as independent in basic ADL tasks, but possibly having difficulty planning and preparing their own meals, caring for their clothing, providing their own transportation, and so forth.

Group 3 (n = 29) was the most able group and included people who live independently but receive help via a community-support program. These individuals might need assistance or supervision in monitoring their medications, following a regular budget, or handling emergencies.

There were 53 male and 47 females in the sample population. Men and women were equally divided among the three groups, with the exception of group 3 which had 30% more men. The age range for group 1 was 18 to 65 years (average 45.9), 19 to 62 years for group 2 (average 34.5), and 20 to 65 years for group 3 (average 41.2).

Table 16-1
Knowledge/Judgment Scale (n = 31) for the Milwaukee Evaluation of Daily Living Skills

Subtest	Item
Makeup	Applies Acceptable Amount*
Clothing Selection	Selects Summer Clothes Selects Winter Clothes
Health Care	Cold Symptoms/Treatment Flu Symptoms/Treatment
Community Safety	Cross Street Lock Door Uses Sidewalk Hitchhike
Home Safety	Reports Emergency Location Reports Injury Danger/Stove Danger/Wire Danger/Smoking
Medications	Knows Names Knows Purpose Knows Side-Effects Knows Amount Knows Renewal
Time	Reads Regular Clock Reads Digital Clock Aware of Schedule
Money	Counts Makes Change Plans Budget
Telephone	Finds Phone Number
Transportation	Names Bus Route Reads Bus Schedule Return From Store Going Shopping
Eyeglasses	Describes Repair

* Items deleted from Rasch analysis.

There was a statistically significant difference for ages between the groups 1 and 2.

Following administration of the revised MEDLS, the subtests were individually scored for each examinee and then transcribed to the performance scale (P Scale) and knowledge/judgment scale (K/J Scale). Items that were completed by 30 or fewer participants were eliminated from the data analysis (n = 11). Scores for the remaining 84 items on the two scales (54 on the $P >$ Scale and 30 on the K/J Scale) were evaluated, using the many-faceted Rasch analysis computer program FACETS.[25]

Results and Discussion

Construct Validity and Difficulty of Items

When applying Rasch analysis, construct validity is confirmed by goodness-of-fit statistics, specifically mean square residual values and standardized fit statistics. These statistics provide a measure of the degree to which the items, examinees, and raters fit the Rasch model—easier items are easier for all people; people with greater ability pass more difficult items; and raters rate items of different difficulty and people of different ability consistently. For the P Scale, only four items did not fit the Rasch model by the criteria set for the study. Based on further examination of the data, two items may not fit the construct—one item may need clarification in the scoring procedures, and one item may be redundant with other items on the scale. For the K/J Scale, all items fit the Rasch model.

The Rasch analysis was able to determine item difficulty estimates, including standard errors of these estimates. When considering item difficulty rankings, it is useful to consider items together, as they compose a subtest as well as individual items. On the P Scale, many of the subtests had items spread throughout the scale by difficulty. There was a logical order of difficulty for many items, eg, rinsing dishes is confirmed to be easier than dusting, which is easier than sewing on a button. Items rated as more difficult, ie, performed correctly by fewer people, were often related to socially appropriate behaviors, such as washing hands after using the bathroom or cleaning the area after doing nail care or shaving. For the K/J Scale, the logical ordering of items by difficulty also was confirmed, for example, reading a clock is easier than recognizing cold or flu symptoms, or counting money is less complex than making change and planning a budget. Many items had close item-difficulty estimates, suggesting overlap and possible redundancy among test items.

Interpretation of the item difficulty estimates must be considered tentative, because of the large standard errors of estimate found for many items and the relatively low number counts for several items (>80 examinees) on the P Scale.

Rater Consistency and Severity

Can the MEDLS be reliably scored by different raters? Do raters judge examinees' abilities with different degrees of severity? Analysis of the P Scale shows that the raters judged the examinees' abilities consistently and with the same degree of severity. For the K/J Scale, the analysis shows that the raters judge examinees with the same degree of severity. Two raters were consistent in their scoring, but one rater was not. The P Scale can be used with confidence in agreement among raters. This is less true with the K/J Scale and suggests that an examination of the scoring criteria for several items is warranted.

Item Difficulty Targeted to Sample and Ability to Differentiate Among Groups

A goal of test development is to target the difficulty of items to the potential examinees' ability to determine differing levels of ability among test takers. For the P Scale, the items are appropriately targeted to approximately the least able 25% of the sample group; for the K/J Scale, the items are appropriate for approximately the bottom 50% the sample. Thus, the P Scale items are not difficult enough for 75% of the sample group, and the K/J Scale items are not difficult enough for 50% of the group.

The revised MEDLS described here included six cleaning activities—washing dishes, taking out garbage, changing bedsheets, dusting, vacuuming, and bathroom cleaning—which were added with the intent of increasing the item difficulty. All items from these subtests are on the P Scale. This attempt was only partially successful in that only two of these subtests included items that were among the more difficult on the scale.

The assumption that people with serious mental illness who live more independently in the community will score higher on the MEDLS scales than those individuals requiring more supervision was not supported in the study described here. The differences in mean scores on the scales among the three sample groups was not significant. This suggests that people with serious mental illness who live in the community but receive considerable assistance with basic and more complex ADLs have essentially the same ability to carry out these activities as people requiring minimal assistance. Other factors besides ability, eg, confidence and motivation, are apparently influencing the implementation of ADLs by people with serious mental illness living in the community.

FUTURE PLANS

Potential directions for more research with the MEDLS include clarification of the scoring criteria for items on the K/J Scale, with a subsequent interrater agreement study; the development of more subtests with items in the more difficult end of the range; and inclusion of people with serious mental illness in sample groups who demonstrate more impairment.

SUMMARY

The many-faceted Rasch model of analysis provides comprehensive and detailed reliability and validity data for the purposes of test development and revision. The data analysis suggests interrelationships among several items on each scale. The MEDLS needs to be reevaluated for redundant items. However, most participants in the study described here fit the theoretical measurement model proposed by Rasch, thus the scales of the MEDLS are useful for people with serious mental illness.

It is inaccurate to assume that what appear to be basic ADL tasks, such as dressing and brushing teeth, are easier than what appear to be more complex ADL tasks, such as washing dishes and making the bed, for people with serious mental illness. Each task has several component skills that require different degrees of ability, and most tasks require abilities in both areas of performance and knowledge/judgment.

The training provided for raters in this study—viewing of a videotape of the administration of the MEDLS, observing one session of the MEDLS administration by the author, and a practice session on a family member/friend—is sufficient to assure reliability when using the P Scale. The criteria for determining pass/fail scores on the K/J Scale should be clarified on some items. Once accomplished, the training provided for raters to assure reliability should be sufficient for the K/J Scale as well.

The MEDLS still lacks a sufficient number of difficult items to accurately evaluate the ability of the more capable end of the spectrum of people with serious mental illness. More difficult subtests that could be developed include meal planning, meal preparation, ironing, and using a checkbook.

Table 16-2
Performance Scale (n = 64) for the Milwaukee Evaluation of Daily Living Skills

Subtest	Item	
Maintains Clothing	Washes Clothes Dries Clothes	Stores Clothes Sews Button
Hair Care	Shampoos* Combs* Cleans Area*	
Teeth	Applies Toothpaste Brushes	Rinses Cleans Sink
Makeup	Uses Makeup Correctly*	
Shaving	Prepares Skin Removes Hair	Shaves Safely Cleans Area
Bath	Puts Mat Down* Enters Exits	
Health Care	Applies Medicine Applies Bandage	
Home Safety	Makes Emergency Call	
Medications	Reports Taking*	
Time	Reports Attendance*	
Telephone	Money* Dials	
Eyeglasses	Cleans Stores	
Nails	Cuts Fingernail Cuts Toenail	Cleans Nails Cleans Area
Eating	Chews Food* Uses Utensils	Uses Cup Ingests Adequate Amount*
Vacuuming	Plugs In Vacuums Floor Removes Objects	Unplugs Stores Vacuum
Dusting	Removes Objects Dusts Disposes Dust	
Garbage	Removes Takes Bag Out Inserts New Bag	
Dishes	Gets Dishpan Fills Sink/Pan Washes Rinses	Dries Drains Sink/Pan Cleans Sink/Pan
Bedsheets	Removes Clean Sheets Dirty Sheets in Laundry	
Bathroom	Applies Cleaner Inside Toilet Flushes Toilet Wipes Tub	Rinses Tub Uses Spray Cleaner Washes Hands

* Items deleted from Rasch analysis.

Finally, the MEDLS evaluates the abilities of people with mental illness to do a wide range of activities of daily living. It does not determine whether or not the individual actually carries out these activities on a daily basis. The MEDLS is only one part of a comprehensive evaluation of the functioning of people with mental illness. Additional data must be gathered regarding motivation, self-confidence, and so forth

REFERENCES

1. Leonardelli CA. *The Milwaukee Evaluation of Daily Living Skills: Evaluation in Long-term Psychiatric Care*. Thorofare, NJ: SLACK Incorporated; 1988:40.
2. Merbitz C, Morris J, Grip JC. Ordinal scales and foundations of misinference. *Arch Phys Med Rehab*. 1989;70:308-312.
3. Christiansen C. Occupational performance assessment. In Christiansen C, Baum C. *Occupational Therapy: Overcoming Human Performance Deficits*. Thorofare, NJ: SLACK Incorporated; 1991:375-421.
4. Glazer W, Sholomskas MS, Williams D, Weissman M. Chronic schizophrenics in the community: Are they able to report their social adjustment? *Am J Orthopsychiatry*. 1982;52:166-171.
5. Christiansen C. Occupational therapy: Intervention for life performance. In Christiansen C, Baum C. *Occupational Therapy: Overcoming Human Performance Deficits*. Thorofare, NJ: SLACK Incorporated; 1991:3-43.
6. Fisher AG. *Assessment of Motor and Process Skills*, ed 5-R. Chicago, Ill: University of Illinois at Chicago; 1990:2.
7. Casanova J, Ferber J. The comprehensive evaluation of basis living skills. *Am J Occup Ther*. 1976;30:143-147.
8. Clark EN, Peters M. *The Scorable Self-Care Evaluation*. Thorofare, NJ: SLACK Incorporated: 1976.
9. Johnson TP, Vinnicombe BJ, Merrill GW. The independent living skills evaluation. *OTMH*. 1980;1:5-18.
10. Thomson LM. *The Kohlman Evaluation of Living Skills*. Rockville, Md: American Occupational Therapy Association; 1993.
11. Eakin P. Assessments of activities of daily living: A critical review. *British Journal of Occupational Therapy*. 1989;52:11-15.
12. Guralnik JM, Branch LG, Cummings SR, Curb JD. Physical performance measures in aging research. *Journal of Gerontology*. 1989;44:141-146.
13. Law M, Letts L. A critical review of scales of activities of daily living. *Am J Occup Ther*. 1989;43:522-528.
14. Ottenbacher KJ, Christiansen C. Occupational performance assessment. In Christiansen C, Baum C. *Occupational Therapy: Enabling Function and Well-Being* (2nd ed). Thorofare, NJ: SLACK Incorporated; 1997:104-135
15. Leonardelli CA. The process of developing a quantifiable evaluation of daily living skills in psychiatry. *OTMH*. Winter,1986;6:17-26.
16. Yerxa EJ. Research priorities. *Am J Occup Ther*. 1983;37:699.
17. Fisher AG. Functional measures, part 1: What is function, what should we measure, and how should we measure it? *Am J Occup Ther*. 1992;46:183-185.
18. Fisher AG. Functional measures, part 2: Selecting the right test, minimizing the limitations. *Am J Occup Ther*. 1992;46:278-281.
19. Nunnally JC. *Psychometric Theory*, 2nd ed. New York, NY: McGraw-Hill; 1978.
20. Allen MJ, Yen WM. *Introduction to Measurement Theory*. Monterey, Calif: Brooks/Cole Publishing Co; 1979.

21. Crocker L, Algina J. *Introduction to Classical and Modern Test Theory.* New York, NY: Holt, Rinehart and Winston; 1986.

22. Leonardelli CA. The Milwaukee evaluation of daily living skills. In Hemphill BJ. *Mental Health Assessment in Occupational Therapy: An Integrative Approach to the Evaluative Process.* Thorofare, NJ: SLACK Incorporated; 1988:151-162.

23. Teresi JA, Cross PS, Golden RR. Some applications of latent trait analysis to the measurement of ADL. *Journal of Gerontol.* 1989;44:196-204.

24. Hambleton RK, Cook LL. Latent trait models and their use in the analysis of educational test data. *Journal of Educational Measurement.* 1977;14:75-96.

25. Linacre JM. *FACETS Computer Program for Many-Faceted Rasch Measurement.* Chicago, Ill: MESA; 1988.

17

The Comprehensive Occupational Therapy Evaluation

Karen R. Kunz, OTR
Sara J. Brayman, PhD, OTR/L, FAOTA

The comprehensive occupational therapy evaluations (COTE and KidCOTE) are behavioral rating scales for use in psychiatric programs. The impetus guiding the development of the original COTE was the need to delineate occupational therapy's unique role in comprehensive adult mental health programs, and to provide a standard and objective means of reporting patient behaviors observed by occupational therapists. The KidCOTE was developed nearly 20 years later to address the similar needs of therapists working with children and young adolescents. Each of the scales enable the therapists to report a large volume of diverse and pertinent information quickly in a consistent format, using defined terminology. Each of these instruments, the COTE and the KidCOTE are fully described in this chapter. The descriptions include a listing of the behaviors addressed in each scale and the procedure for scoring them. A brief case study is included to illustrate the application of each instrument.

COTE

The COTE was developed in 1975 by the occupational therapists, a psychiatrist, and a psychologist practicing at the Greenville Hospital System in Greenville, South Carolina. The instrument was designed to address four objectives. The first objective concerned the focus of the instrument—to identify the behaviors that occurred in and were particularly pertinent to the practice of occupational therapy. The behaviors included in the COTE Scale reflect the profession's traditional emphasis on occupational performance. Occupational therapy often provides the only opportunity for patients to practice behaviors necessary to interact with objects in the environment and perform daily life tasks.[1] Daily life requires that individuals interact with others and master the tasks necessary to function in their occupational environment. Occupational therapists use activities to teach these skills and to shape the adaptive behaviors that individuals need to resume their roles and responsibilities.[2] Many of the behaviors included in the COTE were identified in 1954 by Ayres as being important factors in successful participation and production in a work setting.[3] These behaviors, which include punctuality, organization, initiative, responsibility, dependability, attention to detail, neatness, interest, and concentration, serve as the basis of this instrument.

The second objective guiding the development of the COTE was to define the behaviors in a manner that would allow the observations of different occupational therapists to correspond. Each of the behaviors included on the COTE was defined and subdivided into five levels of performance. These definitions, complete with the description of each level of performance, are printed on the instrument. This immediate reference decreases misinterpretation by both the reader and the therapist, and eliminates the use of vague descriptions.

The third objective related to finding an efficient and effective tool to communicate a great deal of information to the physician and other members of the treatment team. Therapists were overwhelmed by the amount of documentation required by the facility and the payors, and by the excessive time needed to complete the paperwork. This resulted in documentation that contained little useful information about patient performance. Narrative notes often reflected single events occurring during therapy, rather than ongoing patient behaviors. The physicians valued occupational therapy and wanted more information about how their patients performed during OT. The COTE imposes a structure for reporting observations made during the occupational therapy process.

The fourth objective guiding the development of the scale was to provide an efficient means of retrieving data needed for treatment planning and evaluating treatment results. Since the COTE uses numbers to rate behaviors, progress or change in behaviors can be easily noted and measured.

Readers familiar with the COTE will note few changes since its introduction in 1975. The format of the document has evolved to reflect the shorter lengths-of-stay. The definitions and descriptions are now printed on the back of the form for easy reference. Some of the behaviors have been redefined to reflect current terminology, and some behavioral parameters have been tightened to aid in interrater reliability. One item, conceptualization, which addresses the ability to abstract, has been added to the list of behaviors. Punctuality was replaced by attendance. When the COTE was developed, patients were housed on open units and were able to attend therapy independently. In the current health care environment, patients are often on closed units and must depend on others to escort them to and from therapy sessions.

Behaviors Assessed by the COTE Scale

Twenty-six behaviors are included in the COTE. These are divided into three areas: 1) General Behaviors, 2) Interpersonal Behaviors, and 3) Task Behaviors. All behaviors are rated on a 5-point scale. The eight behaviors included in part one of the scale provide information about the patient's general functioning. These behaviors are not uniquely observable in occupational therapy, but are included to provide some general information about the patient's overall performance.

The six behaviors listed in part two involve interpersonal skills, which are also observed by other members of the treatment team. These behaviors are included because the occupational therapy environment provides opportunities for the patient to interact with others during structured and non-structured activities. Patients may behave differently during occupational therapy than they do during group therapy or while on the ward. Part three of the COTE Scale consists of 12 behaviors that relate to task performance, an area central to occupational therapy. The COTE's emphasis on task behaviors emphasizes the importance of occupation.

Rationale for Scoring

Part One Behaviors

Behaviors in part one provide for an evaluation of the patient's general level of functioning. While these behaviors are also reported by other professionals, occurrence during the occupational therapy process provides additional perspective in the patient's overall behavior. The scoring parameters for each of the six behaviors appear in the Appendix (Appendices A & B).

Behavior 1A. *Appearance* tells how the patient is caring for himself or herself. The six factors were selected because they are within the control of the patient in the hospital. Appearance is rated according to the number of factors involved.

Behavior 1B. *Non-Productive Behavior* includes such behaviors as rocking, playing with hands, and talking to oneself. They prevent the patient from becoming involved in day-to-day experiences. Excessive socialization is also considered non-productive. When these behaviors interfere with activity participation or relationship building, they are considered to be non-productive and are recorded on the COTE Scale by the amount of treatment time involved.

Behavior 1C. *Activity Level* may be two-directional. A normal level of activity is balanced between hyperactivity and hypoactivity. The level of activity is problematic when it is so high or low as to attract the attention of others, disrupt performance, or prevent participation. Activity level is rated according to its effect on participation.

Behavior 1D. *Expression* includes the many elements that can provide indications of a patient's feelings. Some of these elements are body language, volume and tone of voice, facial expression, posture and bearing, and the degree of animation displayed. Expression is rated according to its appropriateness to the situation.

Behavior 1E. *Responsibility* is a measure of the patient's accountability for his or her actions. This behavior is reflected by attendance patterns, adherence to known rules, care of equipment and supplies, and adherence to behavioral contracts. Responsibility is measured according to the degree it is assumed.

Behavior 1F. *Attendance* is a behavior that reflects a patient's commitment and motivation to participate in therapy. The amount of encouragement needed for attendance is the basis for rating attendance.

Behavior 1G. *Reality Orientation* addresses the patient's awareness of person, time, place, and situation. The behavior rating is based on the number of factors of which the patient is unaware.

Behavior 1H. *Conceptualization* represents the patient's level of learning and response to situations. It is rated on a continuum that reflects responses that range from concrete to abstract.

Part Two Behaviors

Interpersonal relationships affect performance in all social activities. Effective performance of tasks in daily living often depends upon effective social interaction. Occupational therapy provides both structured and non-structured opportunities for these interactions to occur.

Behavior 2A. *Independence* shows how independently the patient can function in occupational therapy. While occupational therapy may include structured activity, opportunities exist in each session for a patient to be independent.

Behavior 2B. *Cooperation* indicates how well the patient cooperates with the program. Indicators used for rating this behavior are compliance and opposition to the program and therapist.

Behavior 2C. *Self-Assertion* is divided like behavior 1C, *activity level*. Normal assertion lies midway between passive, compliant behavior and dominating behavior. Assertion is rated according to the time the patient's behavior is passive, compliant, or dominant.

Behavior 2D. *Sociability* describes how well the patient socializes with the staff and other patients during the therapy session. This behavior is rated by whether or not the patient can participate, initiate, or respond to social interaction.

Behavior 2E. *Attention-Getting Behavior* reflects the amount of time that the patient spends seeking attention. Examples include repeated questions, frequent requests for assistance, overt requests for approval, or doing nothing in order to get attention.

Behavior 2F. *Negative Response From Others* is an indicator of the patient's effect on the therapists and other patients. Examples of this behavior include asking or demanding special privileges or interactions with fellow patients that result in negative responses. This behavior is rated according to the number of negative responses evoked from other people during the session.

Part Three Behaviors

Behaviors in part three of the COTE (Appendix A) reflect occupational therapy's emphasis on task performance. Occupational therapy often provides a unique opportunity to observe a patient's behavior during activities that reflect the challenges of daily life. The occupational therapist can select numerous types of activities that involve task performance. Various activities are included as examples to clarify these 12 task behaviors and to illustrate how these behaviors are rated on the COTE. It is possible to evaluate most behaviors by using most treatment activities.

Behavior 3A. *Engagement* reflects motivation toward work or activity. Because no task can be completed unless it is initiated, this task behavior is significant. The patient's willingness to participate in a magazine collage activity can illustrate the degree of engagement displayed and would be scored as follows:

0—After receiving directions, the patient chooses a magazine, gathers scissors and glue, and selects items for the collage. The items selected are cut out, arranged, and glued as directed.

1—The patient performs as above but requires gentle encouragement to begin.

2—The patient participates in the activity but needs to be encouraged, by name, to begin and then further encouraged to continue.

3—The patient needs frequent support and encouragement at each step of the activity.

4—The patient is unable to participate in the activity.

Behavior 3B. *Concentration/Attention Span* is an important factor in the ability to perform life tasks and is measured by the amount of time spent attending to the activity. When participating in a copper tooling activity, the patient's performance would be rated as follows:

0—The patient is able to attend to the activity, work throughout the session, and resume after interruptions.

1—The patient has difficulty resuming the activity after interruption, exhibiting some non-productive behaviors.

2—The patient is able to participate in the task for only half of the session and is unable to resume the activity after interruption without therapist intervention.

3—The patient is easily distracted and is able to concentrate on the tooling activity less than one-quarter of the session, requiring therapist's reminders to resume.

4—The patient loses concentration in less than 1 minute and lapses into non-productive behaviors.

Behavior 3C. *Coordination* is an indicator of how well the body and brain function together. Coordination can serve as a measurable monitor of the patient's response to medication or other treatments. Glazing a ceramic stein is an activity in which coordination can easily be noted.

0—The patient applies underglaze or stain, and can conform to the fine detailed features of the bisque ware.

1—The patient can stay within the lines, except in very precise areas.

2—The patient has some difficulty, but can glaze neatly in large areas.

3—The patient can manage a one-color overglaze only because of unsteady hands.

4—The patient is unable to manipulate the brush.

Behavior 3D. *Following Directions* is an important aspect of many daily life skills. The occupational therapist may use games, such as charades, to assess the patient's ability to follow directions. This behavior would be scored as follows:

0—The patient actively plays charades and once learned, responds to and uses standard game symbols without reinforcement.

1—The patient remembers most of the rules, but may forget some of the common symbols of the game.

2—The patient needs assistance and reinforcement regarding the procedure; reminders about rules or symbols may be needed each time the patient takes a turn.

3—The patient requires guidance from the therapist at each step of the activity.

4—The patient is unable to participate in the activity.

Behavior 3E (a-b). *Activity Neatness or Attention to Detail* are listed as opposites on the COTE scale, and only one or the other is rated. The behaviors relate to how well a patient can accomplish a task and to the quality of his work. Either of them can be readily observed while the patient is engaged in a tile trivet activity. These behaviors are scored as follows:

a) *Activity Neatness*

0—Given directions, a large box of assorted tile, a trivet, and glue, the patient creates a pleasing design, selects, places, and glues the tiles neatly in place within a 30-minute session.

1—The design is disorderly or excessive glue is dribbled on the surface of the tiles. However, the activity is completed within the allotted time.

2—The design may be haphazard and the surface of the tiles may be spotted with glue.

3—The patient's work is sloppy; glue may be spilled onto hands and work surfaces, and the tiles may be scattered and glued on the wrong surface.

4—The therapist has to intervene during this activity, as the patient requires close supervision and is apt to streamline the task by pouring large quantities of glue onto the trivet before dumping the tiles into it.

b) *Attention to Detail*

0—Given directions, a large box of assorted tile, a trivet, and glue, the patient creates a pleasing design; and selects, places, and glues the tiles neatly in place within a 30-minute session.

1—Tiles are selected carefully and placed on the trivet with precision. A full 60 minutes is used to accomplish the task.

2—Excessive time is used to create the design or select the tiles. However, once these steps are accomplished, the remainder of the task is completed in the allotted time.

3—Two sessions are required to complete the activity. Each tile is painstakingly placed, and the patient may even use the tools to assure proper alignment of the tiles.

4—The patient takes many sessions to complete the task, if it is completed at all. The tiniest tiles available are selected. Calipers may be used to set and space the tiles on the trivet.

Behavior 3F. *Problem Solving* occurs in many different situations. A group puzzle activity provides the opportunity to observe this behavior. The patients are each given a package containing all but one piece of a simple jigsaw puzzle, plus one odd piece belonging to another puzzle. Each patient is directed to bargain with other patients and trade puzzle pieces, so that each person's puzzle can be assembled. Problem-solving behavior is scored as follows:

0—Given instructions, the patient quickly recognizes the odd puzzle piece and approaches others to trade the odd puzzle piece, secure the missing piece, and complete the puzzle.

1—The patient systematically assembles the puzzle, notes the missing piece and the extra piece, and seeks advice from the therapist. The patient attempts to locate the missing puzzle piece by going from person to person, trying all odd pieces until the puzzle is completed.

2—The puzzle is assembled by trial and error. After discovering that a puzzle piece is missing, the patient goes from person to person, trying all odd pieces until a match is found.

3—The patient is able to put together the puzzle with effort. Repeated attempts are made to fit the odd piece into the puzzle. The patient does not recognize that the odd puzzle piece does not belong to the puzzle.

4—The patient is unable to assemble the puzzle.

Behavior 3G. *Complexity and Organization of Tasks* can be rated using multilevel activities, such as leather lacing. Each style of lacing carries its own degree of complexity. Lacing with a double buttonhole stitch requires more organization and is far more complex than lacing with the whip stitch.

0—Given instructions, the patient is able to accomplish the double buttonhole stitch and can begin, end, and splice the lacing without difficulty.

1—The patient can do the lacing but cannot figure out how to splice, begin, or end it, even with detailed instructions.

2—The patient can do the lacing, but has difficulty keeping the twist out of the lace. The lacing is accomplished one stitch at a time, and requires cueing from the therapist.

3—The patient can only do simple stitching, such as the running stitch or the whip stitch, and needs reinforcement from the therapist.

4—The patient cannot manage the task.

Behavior 3H. *Initial Learning* is evaluated when the patient is performing an activity that is unfamiliar and requires instruction. Assembling a leather link belt can provide an excellent opportunity in which to observe this behavior.

0—The patient follows all written or verbal instructions, and begins assembly of the belt without assistance from the therapist.

1—The patient requires additional instruction and assistance from the therapist before beginning to assemble the belt. After the therapist inserts the first two links, the patient is able to continue independently.

2—The patient is unable to do double wide-links but can accomplish a single-wide variety with minimal assistance from the therapist. However, as above, the therapist must begin the belt.

3—The patient is unable to assemble the link belt without occasional assistance from the therapist throughout the activity.

4—The patient does not participate and is unwilling to be a spectator.

Behavior 3I. *Interest in Activity* illustrates the patient's willingness to try new or different activities. This behavior can be observed, using the parachute, during a gross motor activity and is scored as follows:

0—The patient participates with enthusiasm.

1—The patient is willing and does participate, though somewhat guarded at first. After 10 or 15 minutes, participation is enthusiastic.

2—The patient participates only by being present, otherwise demonstrating no interest or commitment to the activity.

3—The patient may join in the activity for the first 5 minutes, but then stands or sits outside the circle and watches the others participate.

4—The patient does not participate and is unwilling to be a spectator.

Behavior 3J. *Interest in an Accomplishment* indicates whether the patient can set goals and work toward them by taking the necessary steps. Craft activities, such as decoupage, require many separate steps and a commitment to complete it. This behavior is scored below.

0—The patient carefully selects his or her design or article to be decoupaged, prepares the wooden surface appropriately, and sands between coats. An effort is made to assure that everything is done correctly and that the completed project will be pleasing.

1—The patient wants to do the activity and initially makes the investment, although interest wanes before the project is completed. The first steps of the activity are done with care, but the last steps are hastily finished.

2—The patient expresses interest in the activity, but seems to want to get finished as quickly as possible. No substantial investment in the activity is demonstrated, although desire to complete the task is expressed.

3—The patient does the activity only with substantial therapist encouragement. No investment or commitment to complete the activity is exhibited.

4—The patient demonstrates no interest or pleasure in the activity and does not complete it. The project may be discarded or abandoned when the patient prepares to leave the session.

Behavior 3K. *Decision Making* is an integral part of daily living and may depend on the number and kinds of choices and degree of support available. The process of selecting an activity during occupational therapy can illustrate this behavior.

0—After discussion with the therapist regarding the goals for treatment, the patient chooses an activity from those available and proceeds independently.

1—After discussion with the therapist regarding the goals for treatment, the patient selects an appropriate activity, occasionally seeking the therapist's approval.

2—The patient makes decisions about the activity, but often seeks reassurance from the therapist.

3—The patient selects an activity from two alternatives.

4—The patient cannot or refuses to make any decision.

Behavior 3L. *Frustration Tolerance* can be an indicator of the patient's ability to persevere in activities when each phase does not come easily. This behavior can be seen when patients are asked to assemble wooden kits.

0—The patient assembles the wooden pieces of a tool rack, carefully planning each step of the assembly. The project is completed even with minor difficulties, such as lost nails or dry stain.

1—The patient becomes frustrated with tasks requiring several steps but is able to accomplish the tasks.

2—The patient often becomes frustrated with any task requiring more than one step, but is able to accomplish the task.

3—The patient becomes frustrated by all aspects of assembly, but attempts to continue the activity.

4—The patient is unable to complete the task.

Case Example: COTE

The format of the COTE is helpful in developing a treatment plan. The COTE graphically displays areas of strengths and weakness, and can help the therapist to determine treatment priorities. For example, the behaviors of a 49-year-old female patient with a diagnosis of depressive neurosis were evaluated using the COTE scale. This patient was escorted to occupational therapy by the therapist. She sat quietly at the table, seemingly unaware of the activities around her. She responded only when approached and answered direct inquiries, but did not volunteer information or initiate conversation. The therapist directed her to sit in a chair at a table with two other women and introduced them to each other. To assess task behavior, the therapist selected a tile trivet activity. The patient was directed to select tiles of any three colors, place a small amount of glue on each tile and glue it to the trivet in any pattern or design she selected.

The patient needed to be encouraged three times to begin selecting tiles. She was unable to determine a design or pattern for the tile and began gluing only after the therapist had suggested a design. She manipulated the tiles and the glue bottle, and placed the tiles face side up on the trivet. However, some tiles were placed and glued somewhat haphazardly. She was unable to complete the task and demonstrated no interest in the activity or in the activities around her.

While recording this patient's performance on the COTE scale, the therapist was identifying the patient's problem areas. The patient's major difficulties were found to be in the areas of independence, self-assertion, sociability, and concentration. Based on her history and her performance in occupational therapy, the therapist discussed the patient's performance with her. The therapist and the patient collaborated in the development of treatment goals to increase independence, socialization, self-assertion, and self-esteem.

KidCOTE

The KidCOTE was developed in 1995 by an occupational therapist at the University of Texas Medical Branch at Galveston to provide the psychiatrist with more comprehensive information about the child's behavior and developmental performance. The creation of the KidCOTE was initiated to address needs similar to those guiding the development of the COTE 20 years earlier. The KidCOTE is also a performance-based instrument, formatted as a behavioral grid.

Behaviors Assessed by KidCOTE

The KidCOTE includes 27 behaviors that are divided into four specific areas—general behaviors, sensory motor performance, cognitive behaviors, and psychosocial behaviors. As in the COTE, the behaviors included in the general behavior section are also addressed in other settings and may be evaluated by other members of the treatment team. When noted during the occupational therapy session, perspective and dimension are added to the composite assessment of the patient. Behaviors included in this section are activities of daily living, expression, responsibility, reality orientation, and attendance/punctuality. Behaviors are rated on a 4-point scale, according to their intensity and frequency of occurrence. (See Appendix C.)

Rationale for Scoring

General Behaviors

Activities of Daily Living (ADL) addresses how well the child performs basic self-care. ADLs include dressing, eating, grooming, oral hygiene, bathing, and showering. Functional performance is rated according to the child's chronological and developmental ages. For example, a 5-year-old child might be expected to select clothing and dress without assistance, while an 11-year-old might take more care in appearance and be concerned about oral hygiene and hairstyle.

Responsibility reflects how the child accepts accountability for his or her actions. Responsibility is demonstrated by following unit or school rules and by modifying behavior in response to feedback. Although young children may blame others when confronted, as a child matures, the level of responsibility is shown by the assumption of accountability for behavior.

Reality Orientation illustrates the child's level of awareness of self, place, time, and situation. A child's age, both chronological and developmental, determines awareness of his reality. However, even young children may recognize a daily routine and activity schedule, expecting their OT after lunch and therapeutic recreation after school.

Attendance/Punctuality reflects commitment and motivation to attend and participate in scheduled treatment sessions. The behavior reflects the child's readiness to participate and is demonstrated by being ready for therapy, having his or her shoes on, gathering his or her belongings, following the rules, and avoiding timeouts. In the facility where the KidCOTE was developed, children move from the nursing unit to the classroom and to therapy during the day. Transition from one activity to another requires that the child adapt to changing situations and authority figures. Transition between activities or therapies is often unstructured, providing occasion for acting out that may result in tardiness. Frequency of tardiness is the basis for measuring this behavior.

Cognitive Behaviors

Cognitive Behaviors reflect occupational therapy's unique emphasis on task performance. Behaviors included in this section describe how the child approaches and completes tasks, and organizes thoughts and actions. The occupational therapist may assess behaviors, using any activity that is appropriate to the developmental or educational level of the child.

Attention Span/Concentration reflects the degree of distractibility exhibited by the child. This behavior is graded by the relationship of the child's performance, as it corresponds to his or her developmental and chronological ages. The actions of a 7-year-old boy with depression who is doing a copper tooling activity may be rated as follows:

0—Concentration on the activity for more than 30 minutes in a group setting without requiring redirection from the therapist.

1—Concentration of 15 to 30 minutes in a group setting, requiring redirection once or twice during that period.

2—Concentration on the activity 10 to 15 minutes in a group setting, requiring redirection three to five times, or concentration for at least 15 minutes when removed from the distractions of the group.

3—Inability to concentrate in either an individual or group setting without constant redirection.

Memory reflects the degree to which a child applies previously learned skills. In this sense, it involves short-term learning. The memory demonstrated by a 5- year-old boy engineering a Lego™ community may be demonstrated as follows:

0—Independently retrieves the Lego™ bucket from the cabinet and announces to the therapist his plans to finish building his city.

1—In response to the therapist's inquiry about what he was doing the day before in occupational therapy, he runs to get the Legos™ and resumes his activity, requiring no further prompting from the therapist.

2—The child needs reminders about the previous day's activity and plan, and may also need assistance in retrieving the Legos™.

3—The child is unable to recall the previous day's activity or the plan for the day. When told, he needs help to locate and retrieve the Legos™.

Sequencing and Categorization can easily be demonstrated by a young boy playing Duck Duck Goose. The child must take turns, proceed around the circle, pat each child on the head in turn, while chanting "duck-duck-duck." When reaching the child that he chose to be named "goose," he pats the child's head and shouts "goose," and then must circle the group and return to his space.

0—The child participates, completing all facets of the game without cueing or redirection from the therapist.

1—Mild—The child completes all facets of the game, but can only complete his turn after some prompting from the therapist.

2—The child completes the game with staff prompting at each step.

3—Staff accompaniment is needed for the child to participate in the activity.

Concept Formation involves the ability to abstract to develop a plan. Twelve-year-old boys engaged in playing the Ungame™ may demonstrate varying degrees of this skill. Participants in this activity are required to respond to and formulate questions. The queries may pose superficial or substantive challenges.

0—The child is able to respond to each question, using abstract thinking. For example, in response to a question as to what he would do if he found a thousand dollars, he is able to elaborate on how he would spend the money, report his find, ask for advice, etc.

1—The child initially responds concretely, but is able to expand on his answer with encouragement.

2—The child's responses are concrete and limited.

3—The child does not appear to comprehend the questions.

Problem Solving/Judgment reflects how well the child appears to assess situations. A 12-year-old girl participating in a trust walk must determine a course of action to direct her partner safely to a specified location. The child is given general directions and guidance to assure safety.

0—The child understands the activity, and safely and successfully navigates her partner to the target destination without further help or direction from the therapist.

1—The child occasionally seeks further clarification and assurance from the therapist regarding the activity.

2—The child needs prompts and reassurance at each obstacle on the course.

3—The child is unable determine an appropriate or safe course for the activity.

Following Directions reflects the ability to respond to predetermined guidelines necessary for participation in an activity. A 9-year-old girl creating a sand art poster is given both oral and written directions for completing the activity. The written directions include diagrams and illustrations of patterns and techniques.

0—The child participates in the activity according to the guidelines given.

1—Further explanation or demonstration is sought prior to starting the activity.

2—Further explanation of the directions and demonstration are required during the activity.

3—The child completes the task only with repeated demonstration at each step.

Organization includes recognizing and completing the steps needed to begin activities, such as gathering all the supplies, preparing the work surface, and finding the appropriate tools. Making brownies from a mix provides an opportunity to observe an 11-year-old girl's ability to organize.

0—After reading the directions on the box, she washes her hands, prepares a work space, gathers the ingredients and the implements, and preheats the oven prior to beginning the activity.

1—The child completes the necessary preparations with occasional cueing from the therapist.

2—The child is able to complete the activity only when a structure is provided that identifies the necessary steps.

3—External structure and demonstration are required at each step of the preparations.

Decision Making is the ability to make choices and to follow through on those choices. Options of activity, color, partner, or place may be offered when appropriate. The child may be asked to choose between two similar alternatives or to choose from many different alternatives.

0—When given a choice between similar or different options, the child is able to quickly determine a course of action.

1—The child can make a selection when options are fully explained.

2—The child makes a selection only after seeking direction from the therapist or direction from peers.

3—The child cannot make a choice in any situation.

Initial Learning. Children face many new experiences as they mature. This behavior was included because it represents how well the child performs new activities or skills when given the instructions and the opportunity. An 8-year-old boy who is inexperienced with computers may respond as follows when introduced to an action game.

0—The child explores the computer, handles the mouse and the keyboard, and recognizes that the action on the screen depends on the movement of the keyboard or mouse. The game is played with minimal instruction from the therapist.

1—Some direction and encouragement is required from the therapist before the child comfortably handles the computer and begins the game.

2—Frequent direction, encouragement, and some hands-on assistance from the therapist is required before the child is able to begin the activity.

3—The child cannot participate in this activity without the therapist's guiding the child's hands on the mouse throughout each step of the game.

Interest in Activity illustrates the child's enthusiasm about the activities in which he is engaged. A group of 6-year-old boys planting marigolds provides an opportunity to see various degrees of interest.

0—The child remains at the table, retrieves supplies eagerly, makes frequent eye contact with the therapist and peers, asks pertinent questions, and manipulates the soil as directed.

1—The child seems uncertain whether he wants to participate, but is able to complete the activity. Enthusiasm is limited or sporadic.

2—The child has difficulty staying engaged; his behaviors may reflect resistance or even disgust with the activity.

3—The child refuses to participate. He may remain with the group, but does not engage in the activity.

Interest in Accomplishment demonstrates the degree of meaning an activity has for a child. A 12-year-old girl engaged in building a birdhouse may demonstrate interest in accomplishment as follows:

0—The child tells the therapist why she wants to build the birdhouse. She follows the directions in the kit and maintains interest at each step of the activity. She demonstrates pride in the finished product.

1—The child initially invests in the activity, but loses interest when the steps become tedious or challenging.

2— The child initially invests in the activity, but quickly loses interest when completion of the project is delayed.

3—The child is not interested in the activity and does not seem to take any pleasure from it. She participates only with steady encouragement from the therapist and peers.

Psychosocial Behaviors

This section of the KidCOTE includes those behaviors that represent the child's values, social behaviors, self-management skills, and insight. Self-concept, social conduct, self-expression, coping skills, and time management reflect the AOTA's *Uniform Terminology* (1994).[4] Insight is also included here to address the child's degree of awareness or understanding of his or her situation. The observation of psychosocial behaviors is not unique to occupational therapy, but is included here because children often respond differently to the demands present in various treatment environments. The child's behavior in OT, where he or she participates in an activity with other children, may differ greatly from behavior in a "talk therapy" session with a physician or social worker.

Occupational therapy provides an opportunity for the child to explore the self. This exploration can be demonstrated by the following components:

1. Self-concept reflects the child's perception of his or her needs and abilities as they relate to feelings, conflicts, and satisfaction.
2. Social conduct reflects the quality of the child's interaction with others. The use of manners, personal space, eye contact, gestures, active listening, and self-expression are indicators of social conduct.
3. Self-expression involves how the child reveals thoughts, feelings, and needs, including elements that may indicate a child's feelings. Factors included in self-expression are body language, facial expression, volume and tone of voice, and other styles of self-expression appropriate to the situation.
4. Coping reflects how the child identifies and responds to day-to-day stressors.
5. Time management includes the ability to plan and participate in a lifestyle balanced between school, play, rest, and self-care.
6. Insight describes the child's awareness of the gravity and consequences of his or her circumstance, and the knowledge of how he or she is perceived by others.

Sensory Motor Performance

Sensorimotor Performance provides the therapist with the opportunity to examine the child's developmental status. Performance is examined by observing sensory awareness and processing, neuromuscular skills, and fine and gross motor skills during activities. The therapist also screens for problems in posture, gait, coordination, balance, reaction response and tone, vision, perceptual motor skills, and audition and speech. When difficulties are noted in any area, further testing may be indicated.

Case Example: KidCOTE

A 7-year-old boy with a diagnosis of bipolar disorder was admitted to the hospital because of aggressive behavior, opposition, poor social relations, and hyperactivity. He was escorted to occupational therapy by the nurse. He was well groomed and neatly dressed, but did require some assistance tying his shoes. Although occasionally oppositional, he was in a pleasant mood and cooperated with the therapist during the evaluation process. At times he seemed to be preoccupied but was highly distractible by background noises. He confided to the therapist that he "was not feeling happy" about being in the hospital.

The patient was given a copper tooling activity to assess his performance. He was able to select a template and the mounting plaque, and choose the paint. He worked on his project for 15 minutes before redirection from the therapist was required. The therapist provided him with directions and demonstration at each step of this activity. He had difficulty arranging his tools and organizing his work space and the items needed for the activity. He had some difficulty manipulating the modeling tools. He twice sought reassurance from the therapist about his performance. He appeared to enjoy the activity and told the therapist that he planned to do "five more." However, motivation waned and he rushed through the last steps of activity.

The therapist noted problem areas in sensory motor performance, psychosocial behaviors, and cognitive behaviors. The treatment plan included further sensory motor testing, with treatment focusing on improving independence, problem solving, following directions, organization, and concept formation.

Reliability and Validity

Interrater reliability of the initial COTE was determined by computing percentage agreement between the ratings of two therapists, with five different therapists involved. Ratings within 1 degree of each other were considered acceptable and the percent agreements for 55 patients ranged from 76% to 100% and averaged 95%. Percentage agreements for exact agreements ranged from 36% to 84 % and averaged 63%.

Subsequent Review of Interrater Reliability

Initial interrater reliability on the KidCOTE demonstrated 100% agreement within one degree. No child's KidCOTE scores reflected total agreement. Disagreement among raters occurred most often on the behavior *expression*. An examination of the criteria for rating this behavior is necessary in order to clarify its interpretation.

In personal correspondence from the director of occupational therapy of a large general hospital with a 13-bed psychiatric unit, reliability data were reported on seven patients. Percentage agreements for ratings within one degree of each other ranged from 96% to 100% and averaged 98%. Thus, reliability data from three different settings were very comparable.

Validity was determined by randomly selecting the charts of five discharged patients from a group of 400. Total scores for the first and last days in occupational therapy were compared. The scores averaged 31 and 17, respectively, and the drop in the score agreed with the observation of other professionals in the acute hospital setting. In a similar review, comparing initial and discharge scores, showed average admission scores of 33.5, with a discharge score of 22.25 and an average variance of 10.8.

In a study conducted by an occupational therapy student in the psychiatric unit of a medical university hospital, it was observed that a patient's total scores decreased from the first to the last day in occupational therapy. To insure validity of each day's ratings, the student scored the patients on a new scale each day to avoid the influence of the score from the previous day. The average score for the first day of occupational therapy was 20 with a range of 0 to 28. The average decrease in scores was 11 points, with a range of 0 to 57. Again, similar results in a different setting support the validity of the instrument.

FORMAT

Both the COTE and the KidCOTE are designed as checklists with grids to display numerical scores for each behavior. The COTE originally provided a means for daily documentation of patient performance over the span of the hospital stay. The grid format was used to display daily profiles, which were helpful in identifying changes in patient performance during the course of treatment. Sixteen spaces were allocated to record ratings of each behavior on each day of the patient's hospital stay.

This document was used by the team and the patient to review progress, plan further intervention, or to process performance.

The marked decrease in lengths-of-stay no longer affords the opportunity to examine and respond to a sequelae of changes in behavioral profiles. Hospital stays now average less than four days, barely enough time for medication regimens to be established or for the members of the treatment team to gain rapport with the patient. However, the grid format does afford the opportunity to easily compare and contrast patient admission and discharge behaviors, thus providing information about functional outcomes.

The actual COTE document has been designed so that the parameters of each behavior are printed on the back of the document. This was done in response to physicians' requests for clarification of the reports. This was not done on the KidCOTE, as the parameters, normal, mild, moderate, and severe reflect the milieu of the facility's behavior programs.

The COTE and KidCOTE each includes opportunities for the clinician to record short-term treatment goals, test results, pertinent demographic information, and a statement of the patient's expectations. This information is on a supplemental sheet that is tailored to meet the specific demands of each clinical team. This information is supplemental to the patient's scores and assures compliance with the documentation requirements of the facility and the payors.

APPLICATION

The COTE and the KidCOTE create structures for organizing and recording diverse patient behaviors that may be addressed in therapy. Because the listing of behaviors is expansive and includes more than one performance area, the rater is compelled to consider many components of patient performance and can contribute more comprehensive information to the treatment planning process. The grid simplifies comparison of variances in patient behaviors, and is especially helpful when reviewing the effects of a new medication or a change in treatment intervention or milieu. The numerical scores can be easily monitored and provide hard data that is useful in documenting patient outcomes for quality improvement.

Quality management/improvement initiatives are data-driven, and the comparison between admission and discharge behaviors offers measurable performance outcome data. The emphasis of COTE and KidCOTE on function is compatible with accreditation standards and patient-focused care. For example, since entries on the COTE are numerical, outcome criteria can be expressed numerically. For example, discharge criteria for patient with a diagnosis of depressive neurosis may be: 1) able to socialize with more than one person at a time, 2) follow three-step directions, and 3) function independently in occupational therapy. The retriever would be directed to look for scores of 0 to 1 in behaviors 2A (independence), 2D (sociability), and 3D (following directions), entered on the last day of hospitalization. If the scores are higher, then the treatment objectives of occupational therapy were not met.

Another focus of quality management is to improve the efficiency of service delivery. With rapid patient turnover, increasing productivity standards, and greater demands for records, documentation must be made more effective and efficient. It takes less than 3 minutes to complete a COTE or KidCOTE, far less time than it takes to write a meaningful narrative note. The structure of these instruments guides the therapists' reports so that the patient's functional performance is documented.

The COTE and KidCOTE provide a strong foundation for discussion of patient goals and treatment priorities. During the peer review process, colleagues examine patient records to determine the appropriateness of treatment provided to the patient. Because the behavioral assessment is straightforward and the parameters guiding the assessment are evident, therapists can make judgments based on similar information. Discussions regarding differences in goals, treatment approaches, and expected outcomes can be based on performance data.

The COTE and KidCOTE also provide a mechanism for teaching students and new therapists how to observe and document patient behaviors in occupational therapy. Because many different behaviors are addressed on each instrument, the supervising therapist can identify learning needs through concurrent evaluations with the student or therapist.

A peer review of patient records allows therapists to discuss goals and treatment priorities. A comparison of the COTE or KidCOTE with treatment plans can also be useful in assessing whether patient goals and treatment plans appropriately reflect patient performance.

The COTE and the KidCOTE can assist the therapist in defining occupational therapy services in psychiatry. The listing of behaviors is straightforward and relates directly to functional performance. Discussing the COTE score with the patient allows the therapist to explain how the patient's behaviors affect his or her performance. Using the profile outlined on the COTE, the patient and the therapist can collaborate on the appropriate treatment plan. Discussing a child's score on the KidCOTE with parents can provide them with greater insight about their child's behaviors and how those behaviors impact the ability to attend school, play with other children, and function satisfactorily in the family.

SUMMARY

The COTE and the KidCOTE provide a structure to clinical observation by occupational therapists. Their formats guide the therapist's attention to diverse behaviors. These instruments can be successfully utilized with most activities and in most psychiatric settings The instruments serve only to evaluate observed behaviors and to communicate those observations. The behaviors included on both scales are directly related to functional performance. The evaluation is recorded numerically so changes in behavior can be easily measured, compared, and retrieved for study. The COTE and the KidCOTE are effective and efficient instruments for use in the evaluative process in psychiatric occupational therapy.

REFERENCES

1.   Ayres AJ. A form used to evaluate the work behavior of patients. *Am J Occup Ther.* 1954;8(2):73-74.
2.   Brayman SJ, Kirby TF, Meisenheimer AM, Short MJ. The comprehensive occupational therapy evaluation scale. *Am J Occup Ther.* 1976;30(2):94-100.
3.   Brayman SJ, Kirby TF. The comprehensive occupational therapy evaluation. In Hemphill BJ, ed. *The Evaluative Process in Psychiatric Occupational Therapy.* Thorofare, NJ: SLACK Incorporated; 1982.
4.   American Occupational Therapy Association. Uniform terminology for occupational therapy, 3rd ed. *Am J Occup Ther.* 1994;48(11):1047-1059.

PART VII:
ASSESSMENT BASED ON A BIOLOGICAL THEORY

18

The Cognitive Adaptive Skills Evaluation

Gladys N. Masagatani, MEd, OTR/L, FAOTA

The Cognitive Adaptive Skills Evaluation (CASE) was developed by Gladys N. Masagatani, MEd, OTR/L, FAOTA, Catherine S. Nielson, OTR/L, and Elizabeth R. Ranslow, OTR/L, between 1979 and 1981. It was developed to provide the practicing therapist with a tool to evaluate cognitive skills. As occupational therapists, the authors were frustrated by the lack of assessment tools that were designed to evaluate cognitive skills in adults independent of other performance components and that did not focus on determining an intelligence quotient. Many of the evaluation tools on the market had a tendency to evaluate several performance components (psychosocial, sensorimotor, and cognitive skills) within a single assessment tool, and not in much depth. Few tests focused on performance-based cognitive skills exclusively. After a review of occupational therapy and psychological literature and retail markets, the authors decided to develop the CASE. This chapter describes the development, use, and administration of the CASE, including research studies, scoring, and analysis of results.

HISTORY OF DEVELOPMENT AND THEORETICAL BASE

The CASE was developed to identify thought processes used by an individual while engaged in the performance of a task and responding to questions related to the task. The CASE is a skills inventory utilizing data collection methods of observation and interview. During the evaluation, the examinee is asked to perform a task and to respond to interview questions related to the task. The examinee is then asked to repeat the task and respond to a second set of interview questions. By observing how the examinee selects and uses the available materials and listening to the way in which he or she describes what is done with the materials, the examiner forms hypotheses about the examinee's thought processes. These hypotheses relate to the examinee's ability to organize perceptions, respond appropriately to the task, and perceive objects, events, and their relationships.

The tool provides the therapist with a uniform system for gathering data, analyzing that data, and reporting the findings, according to a theoretical base. The objective of the tool is to facilitate a more efficient and consistent method for collecting information about a person's cognitive skills during an initial evaluation or reevaluation session. The CASE examines the following cognitive behaviors:

- The ability to engage in imitation and circular reactions
- The ability to develop and use object permanence, time concepts, language, images, classifications, and relational and number skills
- The ability to use judgment and engage in moral behavior.

These behavior categories are matched with subskills of cognitive development as outlined by Mosey,[1] Ginsburg and Opper,[2] Singer and Reveson,[3] and Allen.[4] The classification levels of cognitive development are: Movement (level 2), Egocentric Causality (level 3), Establishing a Goal (level 4), Trial and Error Problem Solving (level 5), Beginnings of Thought (level 6), Pre-Operational Thinking (levels 7 and 8), Concrete Operational Thinking (level 9), and Formal Operations (level 10).

The performance task selected for the structured observation portion of the evaluation is the "Making of a Calendar for One Week," a single or multidimensional product representing a 7-day week. This task was selected because it is a task that uses a limited number of novel or potentially unfamiliar equipment and tools, the end product is relatively familiar and non-threatening to most individuals, the process of making a calendar lends itself to the observation of several categories of behavior, and the calendar may be used by the therapist to develop a patient program schedule. Additionally, the materials needed to complete the evaluation are economical and easily replaced. The performance tasks, interview questions, directions, categories of behavior, and levels of cognitive development are printed on evaluation forms called Protocol Sheets. (See Appendix D for CASE Protocol Sheets.)

The Protocol Sheets are structured to direct the examiner to watch and listen for the demonstration of cognitive behaviors. The Protocol Sheets are hierarchically structured to permit the review of cognitive behaviors in a developmental and categorical sequence. The levels of cognitive development are listed horizontally and in hierarchical sequence, and the categories of behavior are listed as vertical column headings. Each cognitive skill listed on the Protocol Sheet is followed by a number to indicate the order of that subskill. It does not imply a quantitative value for that level, or that the qualitative value from one level to another is the same between each and every level. As a skills inventory, the CASE is intended to identify the presence or absence of cognitive processing skills relative to a specific task and specific interview questions. The CASE is not intended for use as a predictor of diagnoses. The CASE provides the therapist with a systematic way to collect and categorize data and to establish a baseline from which to develop a treatment program.

The CASE may be used with any individual experiencing a cognitive skills problem. It was initially developed for use with adult patients diagnosed with psychiatric conditions; however, since its development, it has been used with children (ages 6 and above), and adult individuals diagnosed as mentally retarded or having neurological problems, eg, adults who have experienced cerebral vascular accidents or traumatic brain injuries.

The CASE was developed on the premise that to help individuals experiencing cognitive disorders, it is necessary to first identify the nature and quality of the cognitive skills used by the individual. Once the nature of the individual's thinking has been identified, it is possible to apply Mosey's[1] Theory of Recapitulation of Ontogenesis to develop a treatment program to help the individual to achieve whatever degree of adaptation possible to fulfill life roles. The CASE is based on a developmental frame of reference, specifically the adaptation and cognitive theories of

Mosey[1] and Piaget. The clinical research method used by Piaget to study the development of cognition was used to establish the structure of the CASE. This method includes the observation of an individual's interaction with the environment, conversation with the individual concerning this interaction, and the development of conclusions about the individual's thought process.

The Protocol Sheets were developed through a series of structured analyses. The draft protocol was compiled by doing an activity analysis of the task of "Making a Calendar" and the listing of cognitive behaviors that corresponded to the process. Behaviors reflecting cognitive processing identified by Mosey,[1] Ginsburg and Opper,[2] and Singer and Reveson[3] were related to each step in the process of making the calendar. A psychologist was consulted for input on the structure of the evaluation as a skills inventory. The resultant draft evaluation was administered to two practicing therapists for further content analysis. The draft evaluation was also administered to two groups of five non-patient/non-therapist individuals on separate occasions. This process validated the content by demonstrating that a relationship between the task performance and the variables being measured did exist. Individuals being tested reported on cognitive behaviors identical to those listed on the Protocol Sheet. Specific cognitive processes were used while engaged in designated steps of the task, and these relationships were identical to those identified by the developers of the CASE in their content analysis process. Following structural and grammatical refinements of the initial protocol sheets, the revised evaluation was administered to a group of 10 volunteer occupational therapists. These therapists reported that the cognitive behaviors listed on the protocol sheets were used during the performance of the task.

Further testing for content validity was conducted, using the expert opinion method of analysis. Five experts were selected on the basis of their a) knowledge of the theory base, b) years of practice in the area of mental health, and c) recognized leadership in occupational therapy. Three of the five experts responded with an analysis, and they unanimously indicated that the battery did appear to be measuring the construct (cognitive processing) it was intended to measure.

Two interrater reliability studies were conducted on the CASE. The first was a pilot study conducted by the developers. They videotaped three non-patient individuals taking the test and independently analyzed their performance. Rater reliability was demonstrated by the evaluators on all three tapes. The tapes were then shown to a group of four therapists with instructions to rate the examinee's performance. Again, the degree of agreement among raters was high. The assessment of behaviors by the raters was consistent on all three tapes. A second interrater reliability study was conducted by Catherine Lees.[5]

In the Lees study, 30 volunteer staff members were administered the CASE in the standard manner by an evaluator and the study investigator. Each evaluator simultaneously and independently scored each subject's performance on the CASE. Interrater reliability between the investigator and each evaluator was determined using a Spearman rho ranking method. Since the two correlation coefficients were in excess of 0.98, both evaluators' subjects were grouped to maximize sample size (n = 30). The level of significance was held at 0.05 for all comparisons in this study. Pearson product-moment correlation coefficients were generated between the subjects' demographic characteristics, the investigator's ratings, and the evaluators' ratings on the CASE. Intrarater and interrater product-moment correlation coefficients were generated to determine the linking phenomena in the CASE model. Comparisons of these correlations were done to demonstrate the consistency between the theoretical base and the CASE Protocol Sheets, thereby substantiating the construct validity of the instrument. The Lees study found that an exceptionally high interrater reliability was established for the CASE, using a normal population, and that construct validity of the CASE was supported by the results. The empirical model of the tool appears to exhibit a developmental nature similar to Piaget's theory of cognitive development. For this reason, it is strongly recommended that potential users of the CASE familiarize themselves with the cognitive theories of Piaget and Mosey.

ADMINISTRATION OF THE EVALUATION

All materials, directions, and general introductions are listed on the cover page of the Protocol Sheets, along with spaces to record patient demographic information. Evaluation materials include:

1. A 12-inch ruler with numbers
2. One sheet each of 8 1/2- by 11-inch paper (yellow, blue, pink, and white)
3. A No. 2 pencil with an eraser
4. Three pens (1 blue, 1 red, 1 black)
5. A box of 8 assorted wax crayons
6. A sample calendar
7. Beginning directions typed on an index card.

All materials, with the exception of the sample calendar, listed under evaluation materials are to be laid out directly in front of the examinee. Writing tools and crayons are to be placed in the same general area in a group. All sheets of paper are to be in a loose pile, with each sheet being visible to some degree.

Before beginning the evaluation, the examiner presents a general introduction of the evaluation process to acquaint the examinee with what is to take place. Questions of a general nature may be answered at this time. Specific questions related to actual performance should be deferred until after the evaluation is complete. (See Appendix D for specific instructions.) The Protocol Sheets are structured with the instructions listed in the far left column. The entire evaluation is designed to allow for different functioning ability, from the patient who is able to read the initial instructions and is able to act on these instructions, to the patient who requires step-by-step verbal directions and a sample finished product. The entire performance task is broken down into steps with directions to the examiner about how to modify the evaluation to facilitate a response from the patient.

As the evaluation begins and behaviors are demonstrated and observed, or reported by the examinee, the examiner checks the appropriate box on the Protocol Sheet that corresponds to the behavior. This recording is to be done while the examinee is engaged in the task or responding to interview questions. A check mark is a "yes" response, indicating that yes, the behavior was observed or reported. Additional observations and interview responses are noted in the Comments Column of the Protocol Sheets. At the completion of the evaluation, the examiner may review any notes in the Comments Column and, if necessary or appropriate, check additional behaviors listed on the Protocol Sheets. At the conclusion of the evaluation, all individual check marks are transferred from the body of the Protocol Sheets to the Evaluation Summary Sheet found at the back of the Protocol Sheets. Each check mark is recorded in the corresponding category and classification , eg, a behavior with a numerical 8 after it should be recorded in the Level 8 row under the appropriate category; images, and relations column.

SCORING AND ANALYSIS OF RESULTS

The check marks recorded on the Evaluation Summary Sheet should be reviewed and analyzed according to the following criteria:
a) Repetition of skills or behaviors demonstrated
b) Clustering of behaviors demonstrated
c) The scattering of behaviors
d) The categories of behaviors demonstrated.

Repetition of skills or behaviors refers to the frequency with which the same behavior is demonstrated by the examinee. It may be assumed that if a behavior is demonstrated with repeated frequency, the examinee has either integrated the skill, or he or she is functioning through the use of that particular skill. For example, if the examinee repeatedly demonstrated that "words have personal meaning" to him or her, he or she uses reasoning based on past experiences; his or her reasoning may be presumed to be personalized and concrete in nature for the task at hand.

The clustering of behaviors refers to the number of behaviors demonstrated by the individual within specific classification levels of cognitive development. The clustering of behaviors demonstrated or reported within a particular level may imply that the individual is functioning at that level of cognitive skills development, or that he or she is using cognitive processes characteristic of a particular level of development. For instance, repeated check marks at Level 3 across several categories of behavior indicates that the individual is either functioning at the Egocentric Causality Level of cognitive development, or that during the evaluation the individual utilized egocentric causative thought processes.

A scattered profile, behaviors randomly scattered throughout several levels of cognitive development, should be carefully analyzed to determine if there is a relationship between the category of behavior and the level of processing used by the individual. Isolated behaviors may be viewed as chance occurrences or the indication of the potential for development of a specific skill, and cannot be assumed to be evidence of integrated development.

A review of the categories of behavior will enable the examiner to identify the nature or quality of the cognitive processes being used. The quality of specific cognitive skills, such as decision making, use of language, and having and using images may be delineated by the examiner. Based on this analysis procedure, the examiner then compiles a list of cognitive assets or strengths and weaknesses or problems. An asset is viewed as the ability to engage in a cognitive process as evidenced by the demonstration of a behavior or the verbal reporting of the process. A weakness or problem is viewed as the inability or limited ability to demonstrate or report a behavior given the age of the individual. These findings are then discussed with the examinee, along with any comments or additional observations noted by the examiner. This process serves as a validation of the examiner's observational analysis. Revisions or disagreements are noted and modifications are made as necessary.

These items may require additional evaluations or become items for careful observation during the treatment process.

The examiner and examinee will then cooperatively develop appropriate treatment goals. Learning approaches or treatment methods are suggested, based on a review of categories of behavior. Learning approaches may be motoric, visual, verbal, kinesthetic, or social, or any combination of these methods of interacting with the environment. Patient interests and levels of functioning are considered in a final determination.

The Protocol Sheet, including the Evaluation Summary Form, is not intended to be used as a report writing form. Notes may be taken from the Protocol and Summary sheets to prepare a formal written report. No specific reporting format has been developed for the evaluation. It is recommended that institutional or departmental procedures be considered in the selection of a specific format. It is, however, recommended that behaviors be reported in the same terms as used on the Protocol Sheets. This use of the language will reinforce the application of the frame of reference used in the development of the evaluation. It will also increase the probability of providing reliable information from one administration of the evaluation to the next, and from one examiner to another. This process will also increase the reliability and validity of the tool.

SUGGESTIONS FOR FURTHER CASE RESEARCH

Further studies of reliability and validity of the tool are warranted. In addition, studies that examine the predictive potential of the tool would add greatly to the value of the instrument.

REFERENCES

1.   Mosey AC. *Three Frames of Reference for Mental Health*. Thorofare, NJ: SLACK Incorporated; 1970.
2.   Ginsburg H. and Opper S. *Piaget's Theory of Intellectual Development*. NJ: Prentice-Hall; 1969.
3.   Singer D, Reveson, TR. *A Piaget Primer, How a Child Thinks*. New York, NY: New American Library; 1978.
4.   Allen C. *Thought Process and Activity Analysis Charts*. Unpublished; 1972.
5.   Lees C. *An Interrater Reliability Study of The Cognitive Adaptive Skills Evaluation*. Unpublished thesis; 1983.

BIBLIOGRAPHY

Aiken LR. *Psychological Testing and Assessment*. Boston, Mass: Allyn and Bacon, Inc; 1979.
Allen C. *Thought Process and Activity Analysis Charts*. Unpublished; 1972.
Arieti S. *The Intrapsychic Self*. New York, NY: Basic Books; 1967.
Davitz JR, Davitz LL. *Evaluating Research Proposals in Behavioral Sciences: A Guide*, enlarged 2nd ed. New York, NY: Teachers College Press; 1977.
Ginsburg H, Opper S. *Piaget's Theory of Intellectual Development*. New Jersey: Prentice-Hall; 1969.
Line J. Case Method as a Scientific Form of Clinical Thinking. *Am J Occup Ther*. July-August 1969;23:308-313.
Mosey AC. Recapitulation of Ontogenesis, A Theory for Practice of Occupational Therapy. *Am J Occup Ther*. September-October 1968;22:426-432.
Mosey AC. *Three Frames of Reference for Mental Health*. Thorofare, NJ: SLACK Incorporated; 1970.

PART VIII:
COMPUTERIZED ASSESSMENTS USED IN MENTAL HEALTH

19

OT FACT Applications in Mental Health

Roger O. Smith, PhD, OT, FAOTA

The conceptualization of OT FACT and its initial development stages began in 1985 with a small seed grant from the American Occupational Therapy Foundation (AOTF).[1] Since that time, that initial work—not only the OT FACT instrument, but the test and measurement theory from which the OT FACT data collection process is grounded—has matured. OT FACT differs from most traditional assessments. Like several newer assessments, OT FACT is based on modern test and measurement theory, derived from the decision sciences and health outcomes assessment, rather than on traditional psychological and educational testing. Consequently, a significant portion of this chapter describes the theoretical basis and structure of OT FACT. To appropriately apply OT FACT, the user should have a solid understanding of both traditional and newer measurement theories.

The instrument itself is a functional assessment approach that is designed into software. The assessment has three aspects, each of which will be discussed separately. The first is the taxonomy of questions and the theory in which it is framed. Second, the software uses a questioning methodology called "Trichotomous Tailored Sub-Branching Scoring," or TTSS. The TTSS method is made feasible through its computer presentation. (OT FACT data collection is not practical using traditional paper and pencil administration.) Third, the OT FACT software includes a number of features to assist in data collection for patient-progress documentation, program evaluation, and outcomes research.

These three aspects introduce OT FACT. Following that introduction, this chapter describes psychometric aspects of OT FACT, including its theoretical foundation, reliability, and validity.

THE OT FACT TAXONOMIC ORGANIZATION: HUMAN OCCUPATIONAL PERFORMANCE PRACTICE INTEGRATION THEORY (HOPPIT)

Overview of HOPPIT

OT FACT is structured around a human performance theory that is based on occupational therapy practice. This theory describes the relationships between dif-

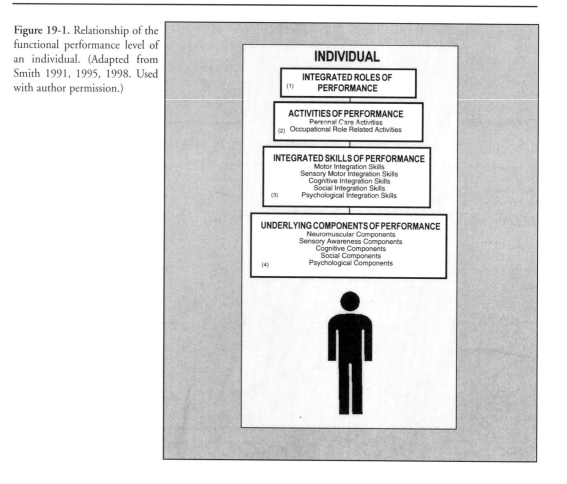

Figure 19-1. Relationship of the functional performance level of an individual. (Adapted from Smith 1991, 1995, 1998. Used with author permission.)

ferent functional areas, provides the foundation, and explains how OT FACT tallies the scores and how results are interpreted.

The HOPPIT model is organized as a hierarchy of four levels that depict the individual's functional areas (Figure 19-1). Integrated Roles of Performance, which includes such items as role balance, continuity of roles across time, and meeting role expectations of others, are at the top of the hierarchy. Successful role performance, however, is dependent upon performance in these activities. Activities of Performance is the second level, underneath the integrated roles. Personal maintenance areas of activity as well as occupational role-related activities fall into this level of function. Categories within the personal maintenance area address basic self-care skills, such as toileting, eating, and other traditional activities of daily living. Included in the occupational-role-related activities are areas typically described in the gerontological literature as IADLs, or instrumental activities of daily living, such as meal preparation, household safety, and community mobility. Additionally, categories, such as educational, vocational, caregiving, and religious activities, are encompassed in role-related activities.

How well individuals perform these activities depends on yet a third level called Integrated Skills of Performance. This third level includes such items as problem solving, hand function, and management of maladaptive behavior. The lowest level

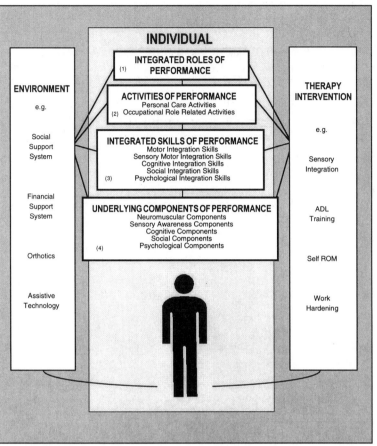

Figure 19-2. Three HOPPIT domains. (Adapted from Smith 1991, 1995, 1998. Used with author permission.)

on this hierarchy is Components of Performance, which is the most fundamental and which enable the Integrated Skills of Performance. The component level includes such items as memory, ability to initiate a task, ability to terminate a task, endurance, and pain.

These four levels are arranged in a dependency hierarchy, as each is believed to contribute to the functions above it. HOPPIT, however, acknowledges that individual function is dependent on outside influences (Figure 19-2). Therefore, on the perimeter of the individual's function, beyond these four hierarchical levels, lie the Environment and Therapeutic Interventions. The domain of the Environment is physical and social-cultural areas. The domain of Therapeutic Interventions includes all potential therapeutic methods. Both the Environment and the Therapeutic Interventions can target any of the four levels of individual performance. For example, in the environment an individual in a wheelchair may encounter an inaccessible bathroom, which would directly impact the Activities of Performance. Or a lack of social support systems in the Environment could directly impact several levels of the person's functional performance. Likewise, Therapeutic Interventions can address the specific areas of functional performance. For example, a list of steps that could be used for someone with difficulty in sequencing tasks could be created as an assistive technology intervention. This could help with several of the categories within the Components of Performance domain. As another example, social interaction strategies that impact social functional performance in the Integrated Skills of Performance domain could be taught to individuals.

One additional important domain lies over the Activities of Performance level, resulting in a three-dimensional HOPPIT model. This functional-activity domain is the Co-Variates of Performance, which includes two major types. The first is the skill/component type, representing every category on the Integrated Skills of Performance and the Components of Performance levels of the HOPPIT model. For example, whether an individual is functional in self-care activities might be dependent on the component of pain. The importance of the co-variate domain to the HOPPIT model is that functional performance can be scored by OT FACT for any given co-variate. A specific component, such as an individual's delusional or hallucinatory processes can be viewed as a skill/component co-variate. The result of this co-variate scoring is the percent contribution of a thought process impairment to functional performance deficits.

The second type of co-variate is the Task Attribute. Task Attributes include factors that contribute to functional performance, such as the quality of performing an activity, the speed in completing an activity, or the safety in which an activity is completed. Figure 19-3 highlights how these two types of co-variates overlay each of the Activities of Performance categories. OT FACT integrates this HOPPIT model and makes each of these co-variates scorable assessments in themselves.

HOPPIT Development

The HOPPIT was initially developed the mid-1980s with many revisions through the 1990s. The hierarchical relationships of the four functional performance levels were developed through extensive discussion and review from occupational therapy practice. The development of the taxonomy was initiated with the first edition of AOTA's Uniform Terminology,[2] and further developed in conjunction with the revisions included in Uniform Terminology II.[3] The AOTA Uniform Terminology III[4] added the context domain that includes environmental and temporal types of considerations already framed into the HOPPIT model.

The importance of viewing the HOPPIT in this way is to identify an individual's functional capacities and the relationships of these capacities across levels. It also clearly recognizes the two domains outside intrinsic performance and how they interact with a person's functional performance outcome.

The development of AOTA's Uniform Terminology versions and the development of the OT FACT taxonomy also have run parallel to other major efforts. The National Center for Medical Rehabilitation Research's Taxonomy[5] and the Institute of Medicine Taxonomy[6] have modeled human performance as well. All of these taxonomies have many commonalities. The HOPPIT model retains the gestalt scope, yet incorporates functional performance detail. This model provides the foundation for the current version of OT FACT.

The Number of Categories in the OT FACT Taxonomy

The approximately 1,000 categories in version 2.03 of OT FACT create the potential questions for occupational therapy practitioners to use. The large number of cat-

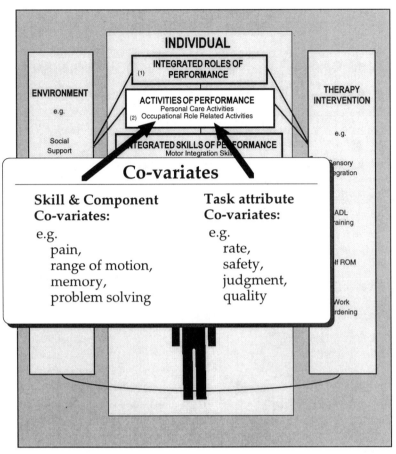

Figure 19-3. Co-variate HOP-PIT domain as it interacts with activities of performance. (Adapted from Smith 1991, 1995, 1998. Used with author permission.)

egories is designed to accommodate the prominent areas of occupational therapy practice—physical disabilities, pediatrics, and mental health practice. Any given practice setting however, may want to skim over the detail of many OT FACT categories that are specific to other specialty areas of practice. For example, practitioners working in mental health may want to avoid the depth required in range of motion, sensory testing, or strength, which are desirable in physical disability settings. Therefore, while OT FACT includes 1,000 categories, the software provides a mechanism to customize the depth of questioning so as to de-emphasize the detail of practice areas less relevant to a given population or setting. In this way OT FACT is packaged for a comprehensive occupational therapy program assessment across disability types, diagnoses, and practice settings, while its customization of questions allows the detail required for specialty areas of practice.

Mental Health Categories Within the OT FACT Taxonomy

While the philosophy of OT FACT and the HOPPIT model support the concept that all occupational therapists assess the same generic categories of human functioning, primary areas of practice do have focuses. Thus, while occupational therapists working in mental health must acknowledge a cursory review of neuromuscular, skeletal, and sensory functioning, they do not need to delve into detail. On the other hand, more detailed categories specific to mental health issues fall within various levels and domains. Excerpts of categories from OT FACT relating to mental health are included as Appendix E.

TTSS: THE SOFTWARE QUESTION METHODOLOGY OF OT FACT

OT FACT uses a trichotomous scale. All the questions throughout the instrument follow the same format. A score of 2 is given if an individual has met all of the criteria in the category, basically having no deficit in that area. A score of 0 is given to a person in the category if none of the criteria are met for that particular question, and indicates that an individual has a total deficit in that area. A score of 1, partial deficit, is given for all situations where an individual has some function in a given area, but the function is neither complete nor totally dysfunctional.

The scoring of TTSS is tailored by tallying "non-applicable" for a category of function. Many questions in other tests and assessments are dependent on gender, age, vocation, culture, or other individual characteristics that might render a given question inappropriate for the particular person being assessed. The TTSS approach allows a category to be omitted from the total scoring process when it is irrelevant. The result of this customization of questions is that the total scores obtained using the TTSS approach are comprised only of questions relevant to individuals in their particular contexts. Therefore, 100% performance of people using a TTSS strategy is 100% performance of these individuals for their particular needs in their particular situations. The implications of this are profound. The question set for any individual may differ from that of other individuals, as the question set is no longer standard across every person. This also has implications for the validity of the question set to an individual's needs. The questions, uniquely gathered to those of other types of tests and measures, are specifically selected because they are deemed valid to an individual's functional areas of concern.

Sub-branching is the characteristic of scoring that moves the questioning process from one category to the next, depending on how the previous question was answered. The use of a computer for TTSS allows this quick and efficient presentation of questions. Generally, the algorithm used by TTSS is simple. If an individual scores a 2 or a 0, then the TTSS process goes on to the next category in the same level of questioning. If a score of 1 is obtained, and a person is identified as having some deficit in an area, then TTSS branches into further detailed categories to follow this line of questioning. In this way, every question is a screening question. If there is no deficit or a total deficit in the area, then no further questioning is required. However, if some deficit has been identified, then the TTSS requires, "Tell me more about this deficit." Figures 19-4 a-c highlight this branching process, using medication routine as the category of focus.

The result of this sub-branching process is to make the questioning procedure more efficient. Indeed, the TTSS methodology used in the OT FACT taxonomy of questions can result in a practitioner scoring less than 100 questions or as many as 1,000. The detail prompted by the software is totally dependent on an individual's particular needs, which must be assessed, as determined by the scope of their deficits.

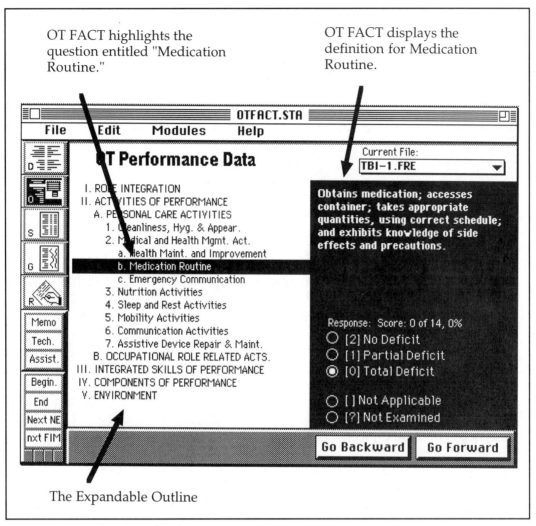

Figure 19-4a. TTSS branching of medication routine.

OT FACT SOFTWARE FEATURES

Data Entry and Data Use

All of the data that are entered into OT FACT are available for merging into reports. Various types of reports can be printed, saved to disk, or compiled into databases. The standard reports include data summaries or prose. Any data of any type entered into OT FACT can be included in a report. Once the performance data have been collected, OT FACT allows viewing the information in summary tables or graphs. Up to three given administrations of OT FACT can be compared side-by-side. For example, data collected for an initial evaluation, a progress note, and a discharge summary can be placed side by side. Figure 19-5 highlights one window of data as an illustration of the summary (the window can be scrolled to see additional categories). Figure 19-6 shows other questions depicted in graph form. Both the table summaries and graphs can be printed or incorporated into prose reports.

If a question is scored a [2] or [0], then OT FACT branches to the next logical question on the same level.   In this case, the category Medication Routine had been scored a [0], Total Deficit. OT FACT interpreted that there was no need for additional questioning since the deficit was total. Therefore, it branched to the next question called "Emergency Communication."

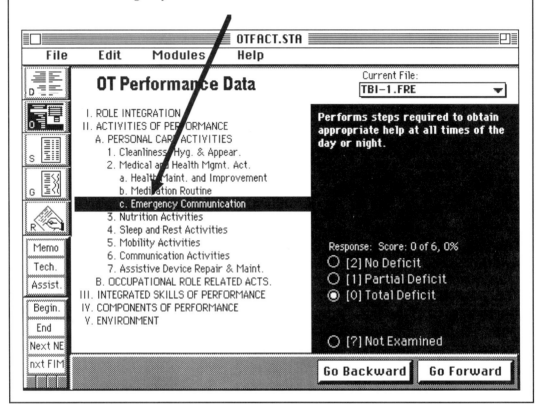

Figure 19-4b. TTSS question progression if no deficit or total deficit.

Many different types of comparisons can be made. The previous example of initial progress and discharge assessments is a method of comparing across time. Comparisons also can be made between perspectives. For example, an individual's perspective of his or her performance, a practitioner's perspective of performance, and a family member's perspective of performance can be compared. Comparisons can be made across interventions. For example, a person's performance in self-care skills when at home alone can be compared to his or her self-care skills when at home with a supportive family member. These two could be examined side by side to view the impact of family support. OT FACT will also calculate the differences between any two data sets.

Demographics

OT FACT has three types of demographic data that allow a practitioner to collect administrative information, such as dates of assessments, dates of admissions,

If the response was [1], Partial Deficit, OT FACT would pursue the line of questioning within Medication Routine to obtain more detail. In this case, a Medication Routine sub-category called "Schedule" is the next question.

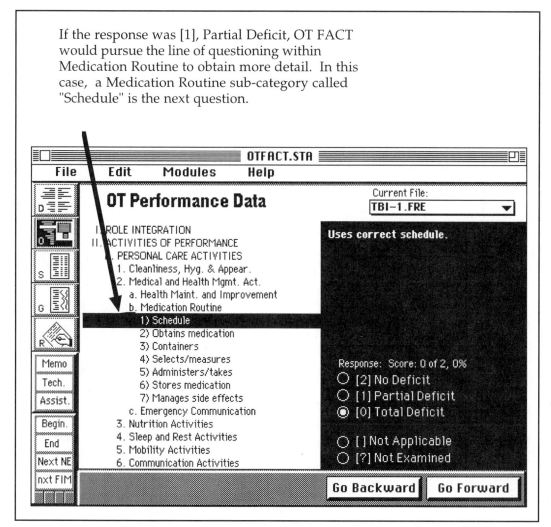

Figure 19-4c. TTSS question progression if partial deficit.

and frequency of OT sessions; and patient information, such as name, diagnoses, and prior living status; and extended demographics, such as other disciplines involved in intervention, sources of payment, primary language, socioeconomic status, and education completed. None of the demographic fields are required, but all are available.

File Types

OT FACT data have many uses. Figure 19-7 highlights the File Type screen of OT FACT. As can be seen, OT FACT data can be collected for a number of purposes and using various frames of reference. Purposes can include initial assessments, progress assessments, discharge assessments, goal setting, or other data collection. If other data collection purposes are identified, the practitioner can enter a specific description. There are also several scoring types that can be selected in OT FACT. These include environment-free, indicating a person's performance without any support systems; environment-adjusted, indicating that some accommodations are

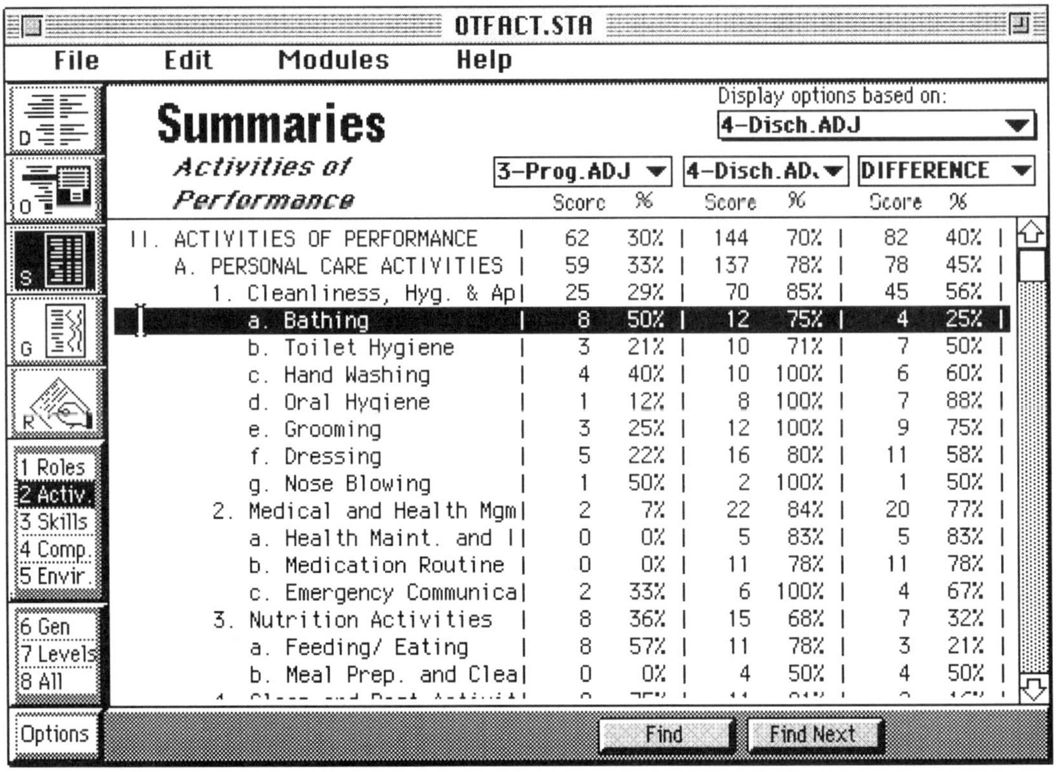

Figure 19-5. OT FACT summary window comparing progress and discharge notes.

made in the environment; environment-assisted, indicating that personal assistance is provided; self-satisfaction, portraying how an individual feels about his or her performance; co-variate scoring, specific co-variates to be described, such as safety and judgment; or other types of scoring, as delineated by the software user.

Report Writing

OT FACT includes a report generation module. This module includes features that help the practitioner write a report. One mechanism is using a form-merging feature. OT FACT allows a practitioner to develop a form, including codes that incorporate OT FACT demographic and performance data into the prose text in the report. Thus, once a form a has been developed, the practitioner saves time by selecting the form and simply pressing a button that states, "Fill in data." This process merges the data from the OT FACT assessments and drops the information into the report, using the previously designed format. These reports can be printed as paper copy or saved as an electronic text file. Refer to Appendix H for an example of a case study and reporting data.

Pick Lists, Memos, and Templates: Additional Data Collection and Report Strategies

Pick lists are simply lists of text items that can be selected and "pasted" into a report. These may be lists of such commonly used goals as interventions and interpretations.

This bar graph displays three sets of scores for comparison. Here, we see performance from an Initial assessment compared to a Progress reassessment and a third assessment repeated at Discharge.

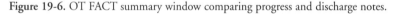

```
▤▢▬▬▬▬▬▬▬▬▬▬▬▬▬▬ OTFACT.STA ▬▬▬▬▬▬▬▬▬▬▬▬▬▬ ▢▤
   File      Edit      Modules     Help

▦  ▤        Graphs             • TBI-1.FRE      ▼
D▤▤                            * TBI-2.ADJ      ▼   Display options based on:
  ▤          Activities of     + TBI-3.ADJ      ▼   TBI-1.FRE              ▼
0▤▤         Performance        0%          50%            100%

   ▤      II. ACTIVITIES OF PERFORMANCE                                    ⇧
 S ▤                TBI-1.FRE  ●●●●●●●●●●27%
                    TBI-2.ADJ  ********************27%****63%
   ▤                TBI-3.ADJ  ++++++++++++++++++++++++++++++++88%
 G ▤          A. PERSONAL CARE ACTIVITIES
                    TBI-1.FRE  ●●●●●●●●●●●●33%
 R ▤                TBI-2.ADJ  *****************************70%
 ▤▤                 TBI-3.ADJ  ++++++++++++++++++++++++++++++++++92%
 1 Roles        1. Cleanliness, Hyg. & Ap
 2 Activ.           TBI-1.FRE  ●●●●●●●●●●●●33%
 3 Skills           TBI-2.ADJ  ***************************73%
 4 Comp.            TBI-3.ADJ  ++++++++++++++++++++++++++++++++++91%
 5 Envir.        a. Bathing
                    TBI-1.FRE  ●●●●●●●●●●●29%
 6 Gen              TBI-2.ADJ  ****************************74%
 7 Levels           TBI-3.ADJ  ++++++++++++++++++++++++++++++++++++100%
 8 All           b. Toilet Hygiene
                    TBI-1.FRE  ●●●●●●●●●●●33%                              ⇩

 Options  ▓▓▓▓▓▓▓▓▓▓▓▓▓▓▓▓▓▓▓▓▓▓     Find      Find Next
```

Figure 19-6. OT FACT summary window comparing progress and discharge notes.

OT FACT also makes available areas in which practitioners can attach memoranda information to any question or category being assessed. For example, if an individual has extreme difficulty organizing time, and the chosen intervention being tried is an electronic scheduler, the details of this scheduler could be described in the assessment itself, using a memo category. All memos can automatically be merged into the report.

Templates are simply pre-written parts of the data collection process. For example, if another assessment is commonly used in an intake assessment, this form can be built directly into the OT FACT data collection process by placing the intake data collection categories into OT FACT memo areas. It is essential to recognize, however, that many of these extended features of OT FACT, like any significant software package, demand time to learn and customize.

Program Evaluation and Outcomes Research

OT FACT includes a mechanism for compiling large data sets so that information can be placed into a spreadsheet or a statistic package for an examination of group data. While OT FACT generates no specific program evaluation or outcomes report, it does have a "plug-in" available that allows the data to be compiled for additional investigative research studies.

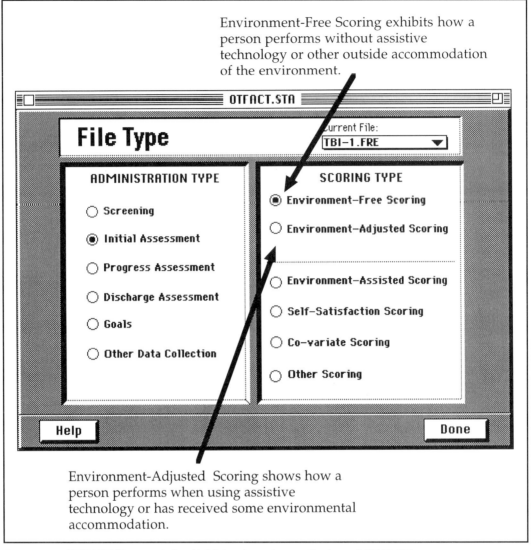

Figure 19-7. OT FACT file type window highlights the various applications of OT FACT.

PSYCHOMETRIC ASPECTS OF OT FACT

Criterion-Referenced

OT FACT is a criterion-referenced assessment. Many occupational therapy assessments are based on normal distributions and compare individual scores to a mathematical mean by examining standard deviations or standard scores. OT FACT does not subscribe to the concept of normal functional performance. Moreover, OT FACT does not even suppose that there are normal functional areas that must be assessed to determine whether an individual is functional. OT FACT is criterion-referenced and founded on the concept that individuals can range from being able to perform 100% of the specific tasks and life activities they need to perform, to being totally unable to perform any of the specific tasks and life activities. Thus, the score represents a person's function in the tasks, not a comparison to any normative group.

Nomothetic Versus Idiographic Approach

Additional to the OT FACT criterion-referenced orientation, the tasks and activities assessed specifically target the needs of the individual. Again, this sets OT FACT apart from most assessments used in occupational therapy practice. The items in the OT FACT assessment may differ from one person to the next as previously described in the tailoring aspect of the TTSS approach. Traditional test and measurement instruments, even criterion-referenced tests, tend to use a standard set of questions enabling a nomothetic application. OT FACT individualizes the questioning process to better match the concept of an idiographic assessment approach.[7] The construct that OT FACT targets is the functional performance of individuals in their own environmental, physical, social, cultural, and developmental contexts.

Data-Based Theory Versus Decision-Based Theory

The measurement theory closest to OT FACT methodology is called decision-based theory, as opposed to data-based theory. Data-based theory collects data and obtains distributions of data to which an individual's score is compared. Typically in classical test and measurement theory, the assumed distribution is a bell-shaped curve, which sets the backdrop for comparing an individual's score to the normal distribution.

Recognizing non-bell-shaped distributions, however, has become more popular in recent years. For example, the types of assessments that use item-response theory can assume non-normal distributions which have been obtained from prior data sets.[8] Item response theory applications, including Rasch Scale Measurement,[9] use item difficulty to ascertain distributions. These distributions are often not normal, but are consistent with assessments created from data-based theory, as they require previously collected group data for proper interpretation. Data-based theory can also drive the selection of items within a given assessment. For example, Rasch Scaling Analysis Methods allow the omission of a test question because previously collected data has documented the item difficulty of each question. Rasch Scaling allows the interpretation of the meaning of an individual's score by simply adjusting the "difficulty" ruler.[10]

OT FACT is one assessment used in mental health and occupational therapy whose use and interpretations do not depend on prior data, thus reflecting a decision-based theoretical perspective. In OT FACT, questions are included in the assessment and scores interpreted specific to the individual. Additionally, OT FACT, like other decision-based assessments, relies heavily on subjective information, subjective weighting of question items, and adaptive interrogation. Question selection is dependent on the individual and answers to prior questions. Many mental health assessments that collect data using the interview technique are similarly based on this type of theoretical perspective.

Validity and Reliability Design Implications of TTSS

Inherent in the fundamental structure and design of the TTSS approach is an attempt to optimize reliability and validity. For example, the branching component of TTSS theoretically increases the reliability of response. In most assessments, when an individual response is being elicited and the individual administering the assessment does not know the answer because of a poor understanding of the question or an ambiguity in the definition, the practitioner must respond by either guessing or leaving missing data. In the case of the TTSS data collection methodology, if an individual does not understand a given question or how an individual should be scored in that category, the proper scoring response is "1." What the TTSS software proceeds to do in these situations is to expand the question into more detail, breaking down the particular construct of the question category. The more detailed questions explain the question construct with more concrete behaviors and make it easier to provide an accurate response. In this way the TTSS methodology allows the data collector to clarify questions for consistency of response.

Additionally, the TTSS design attempts to increase reliability throughout its trichotomous scale. The trichotomous scale provides only three options, allowing the data collector to quickly and confidently tally a score. The more common assessments, which have a 5-point or 7-point scale require more data collection deliberation, as there are more intermediate points on the scale. Often these types of assessments require special training sessions for data collectors.

A third characteristic of the TTSS approach that helps optimize reliability is its number of questions. The trichotomous and sub-branching aspect of TTSS permits rapid data collector response. Thus, the data collector can efficiently answer many more questions in a similar amount of time as would be used with a complicated scaling system. The Spearman-Brown formula statistically proves that increasing the number of questions on a test increases its reliability.

The TTSS methodology also attempts to maximize the validity of functional performance assessment in three ways. First, the TTSS structure enables a prompting system. The comprehensive nature of the OT FACT taxonomy presents functional performance categories to the data collector for consideration of each area. While a given question may not be applicable, the range of questions offered allows appropriate questions to be completed for an individual's assessment of functional performance. Thus, fewer questions are left out due to inadvertent omissions or an assessment's attempts to standardize questions across the population (many assessments lose richness of detail as the questions move toward the lowest common denominator).

Validity also is addressed with the non-applicable questions. Not only does the OT FACT taxonomy prompt a comprehensive performance review, but the ability to omit questions as non-applicable individualizes the question set. The resulting process performs a mini-validation of each question to match the needs and diversity of people with disabilities.

In addition, the validity of the TTSS methodology is forwarded by the methods in which the OT FACT taxonomy was generated. The taxonomy of questions was developed from field research and multiple iterations of feedback from occupational therapy practice from more than 30 feedback sessions. Two national field tests supplemented early taxonomies that were based on practice from AOTA's Uniform Terminology.

A number of small reliability and validity studies have been performed during the development of OT FACT. Some of these studies were performed early to identify whether the TTSS process was going to be sufficiently robust, other studies are confirmation. Table 19-1 charts the overall results of these studies. While these studies are just beginning to identify the usefulness of OT FACT, these are viewed as indicators of the potential of software data collection.

Contemporary Reliability and Validity

In the early 1990s, it became apparent that the TTSS process was developing innovative types of dynamic scaling that traditional reliability research methods were only partially able to address. TTSS is not an instrument for which we can confirm or reject reliability. It is a scaling approach. Unfortunately, traditional test and measurement methodology is attuned to examining instruments, not approaches. Therefore, to investigate the reliability of TTSS, which is a decision-based theory method, one study used a decision-theory technique. The TTSS approach was examined by sensitivity analysis, comparing it to the traditional 7-point scale.[11] The results of this study showed that the TTSS method was more stable than a 7-point scale method. The study examined how rater error affected the true score. The results showed that when a rater was within 30% of the true score, the TTSS method was extremely stable compared to the 7-point scale method. When rater error exceeded 30% of the true score, however, the TTSS scale became volatile, resulting in an exaggerated amount of error. In contrast, under the scenario of high rater error, the traditional 7-point scale method was more stable. Given the features of the TTSS design to improve the inherent reliability of data collectors, highlighted earlier, and the high correlations of preliminary interrater reliability studies,[1] it seems quite plausible that occupational therapy raters would remain within the 30% tolerance. Therefore, the TTSS scaling structure could very well be viewed as more likely to score the true functional abilities of an individual than the traditional 7-point scale method. Obviously, additional studies are required, but these initial steps to validate the method seem promising.

USE OF OT FACT TO TEACH HOLISTIC PHYSICAL AND MENTAL HEALTH PERSPECTIVES IN OCCUPATIONAL THERAPY

Since the HOPPIT taxonomy is comprehensive, it allows a unique way for professionals entering occupational therapy to view disability and individual functional performance of people with disabilities. Several university and college programs training occupational therapy students have used the OT FACT software to help students review and document functional performance across all domains relevant to occupational therapy. While specialization in occupational therapy fragments functional assessment into areas of practice, it becomes important for occupational therapy students to view practice from a much wider perspective. OT FACT allows students to consider all aspects of human dysfunction and human performance abilities in one data collection scheme to frame a mental model that encapsulates all of occupational therapy.

Use of the HOPPIT model can frame curricular content to ensure appropriate coverage and help students identify where the different areas of course work apply to overall human performance. The OT FACT software has assisted students in Level I and Level II fieldwork placements, as the prompting of categories helps teach practitioners in training to avoid inadvertent omission of important assessment and intervention areas.

Table 19-1

OT FACT Reliability and Validity Development

Type of Reliability or Validity Activity	N	Procedure	Statistical Outcome	Interpretation	Reference
Content Validity Development		Began with AOTA Uniform Terminology; design team worked with AOTA Uniform Terminology II in parallel development		OT FACT taxonomy of questions based on practice accepted uniform terminology.	Smith, 1992
Rater Reliability Development		Up front deliberate design		Scoring procedure designed to minimize rater error.	Smith, unpublished
Construct Validity Development	41 surveys from workshops	Likert style survey on paper and pencil version	Wide range depending on question	Predominantly positive about the conceptualization of the instrument. Skepticism about paper and pencil version being the right tool for their particular area of practice. Specific question asking about whether the tool should be computerized resulted in overwhelming agreement that it should.	
Content Validity Development	>30 regional workshops and group feedback sessions	Informal focus group discussion		Seven major versions were generated. Two major versions of taxonomy in software.	Smith, 1990; Smith, 1998
Construct Validity Development		Development of theory as foundation		The HOPPIT model was developed and is discussed in the chapter in more detail.	Various
Content Validity Development		National field-test computer version 1.0		Comments on taxonomy and procedures. Resulted in new versions.	
Alternate Form	National field data of n=127	Pearson and Spearman correlations	All $r > .97$	Short-form and long-form virtually identical.	Smith & Rust, 1992
Content Validity	National field data of n=127	The above analysis also subjects the test to interval scaling analysis	As above	The score of 1 average to be equidistant between 2 and 0.	Smith & Rust, 1992
Content Validity	25 patients with mulitple sclerosis	Krippendorff coefficients and rater agreement	0.89 five 5 OT raters; agreement between OT raters and patients 94%; 86% agreement with patients 10 days later	OT FACT categories highly correlated with activity configurations used in practice.	Bhasin & Goodman, 1992

Table 19-1 (continued)
OT FACT Reliability and Validity Development

Type of Reliability or Validity Activity	N	Procedure	Statistical Outcome	Interpretation	Reference
Interrater Validity	13 pairs of diversly trained therapists	Pearson correlations, Spearman correlations, item agreement	15 of 24 of the correlations resulted in p values of <.005. 9 of 24 r values >.9, 8 additional >.7, percent exact agreement of summed categories ranged from 62 to 92%	Strong indications that the TTSS/OT FACT approach demonstrated a high degree of interrater reliability.	Smith, 1998
Rater Reliability	Two sets of true data were used for this analysis. For 7 point scaling there were 3456 primary data cells (24 questions*144 tests) and for TTSS there were 13,064 (21 branches and 21 bottom level leaves totaling 92 questions*142 tests)	Sensitivity analysis	Almost zero resulting error below 30% forced rater error, over 30% forced rater error explodes resulting error substantially	Assuming that OT FACT raters produce less than the 30% error tolerance, rater reliability is excellent. Traditional 7-point scale was not stable at error levels below 30% tolerate error as well.	Smith, 1993b

Bhasin CA, Goodman GD. The use of OT FACT categories to analyze activity configurations of individuals with multiple sclerosis. *Occupational Therapy Journal of Research.* 1992;12(2):67-82.
Smith RO. *OT FACT,* versions 1.0 and 1.1 (computer software and manual). Rockville, Md: American Occupational Therapy Association Inc; 1990, 1998.
Smith RO. *Impact of Computer Technology on Functional Assessment.* Paper presented at the American Occupational Therapy Foundation Symposium on Measurement and Assessment: Directions for Research in Occupational Therapy. Chicago, Ill: 1991.
Smith RO. *Comparative Reliability of Dynamic Trichotomous Tailored Sub-Branching Scoring (TTSS) and Static Functional Assessment Methods.* Paper presented at the American Congress of Rehabilitation Medicine. San Francisco, Calif; 1992.
Smith RO. Rust KL. *Construct and Content Validity of Dynamic Tailored Questions Sets Used in Functional Assessment.* Paper presented at the American Congress of Rehabilitation Medicine. San Francisco, Calif; 1992.
Smith RO. *Sensitivity Analysis of Trichotomous Tailored Sub-Branch Scoring (TTSS) and Traditional Scales.* Unpublished PhD dissertation. Madison, Wis: University of Wisconsin-Madison; 1993b.
Smith RO. *OT FACT,* version 2.0, version 2.03. [Computer software and manual]. Rockville, Md: American Occupational Therapy Association Inc; 1998.

PAST, PRESENT, AND FUTURE

Contribution of Occupational Therapy to Measurement

The development of OT FACT, over its more than a decade of maturation, has provided a concerted effort to optimize reliability and validity in every step of the design process. This is attempted through careful attention in design to unique methods of scaling, its comprehensive approach, and its theory-grounded approach to the construct of function. One might ask why, when measurement of people's disabilities has been around for decades, this type of approach has been suggested only recently. Interestingly enough, this answer has two major reasons. One is that occupational therapists have only become interested in measurement in recent decades. As a profession of occupational therapy and a discipline of occupational science, the profession is relatively new and has not been ready to propose new ways of looking at measuring human performance and function of people with disabilities. The literature and chapters in this text highlight much of the interest in assessment and measurement in occupational therapy, as it has risen in recent decades. Only recently have the occupational therapy profession and the occupational sciences discipline been ready to offer and contribute functional assessment and holistic approaches to disability. Second, the technology and instrumentation potential used in OT FACT was not ready for computerized implementation until the 1990s. Computer power and computer costs have only recently become practical for daily practice in occupational therapy. Complex assessment schemes offered by the TTSS method and the OT FACT taxonomy have only become possible in the past decade.

Future Use of OT FACT

Computer technology's sufficient availability to occupational therapists in recent years made OT FACT possible. Computer portability with laptops and accessibility because of the decreasing cost of powerful computers has finally made computerized assessment realistic in occupational therapy practice. OT FACT, with customization potential to tune its use across many applications, is a comprehensive tool available to occupational therapists. While it is able to customize to specific specialized areas in occupational therapy practice, the unique contribution of OT FACT is its ability to view patients from a comprehensive and holistic perspective, based on a practice theory generated from the field. The software provides a consistent method for collecting data and merging the data into various types of reports.

Although the OT FACT software is available for use through the AOTA, it is the theoretical foundation and new measurement methods that deserve the most serious examination and comparison to other assessment approaches. OT FACT offers a new model. Other applications of OT FACT are also being explored. For example, the OT FACT structure is being viewed as a possible mechanism for "teasing out" the specific impact of assistive technology and its contribution to overall functional performance.[12-15]

While the OT FACT's innovativeness continues to require intensive research efforts to validate specific applications within areas of occupational therapy practice, it remains a versatile measurement, documentation, and reporting tool for occupational therapy practitioners and an innovative tool for the profession.

Occupational therapy practice is comprehensive in scope. It spans diagnostic populations and stretches across a full spectrum of practice settings. This extremely wide scope of practice is unique to occupational therapy and provides a rich basis for organizing a scheme to assess the degree and outcome of disability. This extraordinary perspective of the occupational therapy profession is the foundation of OT FACT. Through the use of computerized data collection, this scheme has become feasible to apply. OT FACT brings together a practice theory model of human performance, modern test theory, and technology.

SUMMARY

This chapter provides an overview of the OT FACT data collection software, the theory undergirding its scoring methodology, and its use. The scaling approach, Trichotomous Sub-Branching Scoring is described as a data collection method that has only become feasible with the use of computer technology in the practice setting. The chapter also summarizes the psychometric characteristics of the instrument. Excerpts of OT FACT psychosocial categories and definitions, as well as an OT FACT profile, have been included in Appendices E and F.

REFERENCES

1. Smith RO. *OT FACT,* version 2.0, version 2.03. [Computer software and manual]. Rockville, Md: American Occupational Therapy Association Inc; 1998.
2. American Occupational Therapy Association, ed. *Occupational Therapy Product Output Reporting System and Uniform Terminology for Reporting Occupational Therapy Services.* Rockville, Md: Author; 1979.
3. American Occupational Therapy Association Uniform Terminology for Occupational Therapy, 2nd ed. *Am J Occup Ther.* 1989;43:808-815.
4. American Occupational Therapy Association Uniform Terminology for Occupational Therapy, 3rd ed. *Am J Occup Ther.* 1994;48(11):1047-1054.
5. National Center for Medical Rehabilitation Research. *Research Plan for the National Center for Medical Rehabilitation Research.* Washington, DC: US Dept of Health and Human Services, Publication No. 93-3509; 1993.
6. Institute of Medicine. Models of Disability and Rehabilitation. In Brandt J, Edward N, Pope AM, eds. *Enabling America: Assessing the Role of Rehabilitation Science and Engineering.* Washington, DC: National Academy Press; 1997.
7. Silva F. *Psychometric Foundations and Behavioral Assessment.* Newbury Park, Calif: Sage Publications Inc; 1993.
8. Hambleton RK, Swamihathan H, Rogers HJ. *Fundamentals of Item Response Theory.* Newbury Park, Calif: Sage Publications Inc; 1991.
9. Wright BD, Masters GN. *Rating Scale Analysis.* Chicago, Ill: Mesa Press; 1982.
10. Fisher W. Scale-free measurement revisited. *Rasch Measurement Transactions.* 1993;7(1):272-273.
11. Smith RO. *Sensitivity Analysis of Trichotomous Tailored Sub-Branch Scoring (TTSS) and Traditional Scales.* Unpublished PhD dissertation. Madison, Wis: University of Wisconsin-Madison; 1993b.
12. Smith RO. *Using the Occupational Therapy Comprehensive Functional Assessment (OTCFA) to Evaluate the Efficacy of Technological Intervention in Rehabilitation.* Paper presented at the RESNA '87. Washington, DC; 1987.
13. Smith RO. *Assessing the Impact of Assistive Technology Using OT FACT Version 2.0.* Paper presented at the RESNA '93. Arlington, Va; 1993a.
14. Davel N, Smith RO. *Functional Impact of Assistive Technology on People With Hemiplegia From Stroke.* Paper presented at the RESNA '96 Conference. Salt Lake City, Utah; 1996.
15. Bhasin CA. Review of OT FACT. In Vitaliti LU, ed. *RESNA Resource Guide for Assistive Technology Outcomes: Assessment Instruments, Tools, and Checklists From the Field.* Arlington, Va: RESNA; 1998, vol 2, pp 22-31.

20

Adolescent Risk-Taking Behaviors: Computer-Assisted Questionnaire

Maureen M. Black, PhD, OTR
Jeanne Gordon, MA
John Santelli, MD, MPH

Adolescence is a period of transitions as children undergo biological, social, emotional, and psychological changes from childhood into adulthood. During this period experimentation with risk-taking behaviors is common, even expected, as youths try out behaviors that signify adult status, such as smoking. In most cases experimentation is transient and does not lead to a chronic pattern of risk-taking behavior.[1-3] However, the possibility of negative consequences increases when risk-taking behaviors are initiated early in adolescence[4,5] and when multiple risk-taking behaviors co-occur.[6] In the current social context, risk-taking behaviors, such as violence, substance use, and early sexuality, can lead to life-threatening consequences. Indeed, the highest rates of human immunodeficiency virus (HIV) infection occur among young adults, most of whom probably acquired the infection during their teen years.[7] This chapter proposes criteria to be considered in the development of a protocol for interviewing youths about risk-taking behavior, with attention focused on methodological, psychometric, developmental, and ethical issues.

RISK-TAKING BEHAVIORS

Risk-taking behaviors are often divided into four domains.[8] The first domain is early sexuality, which can lead to pregnancy or sexually transmitted diseases (STDs).[9-11] Issues such as number of partners and methods of protection against pregnancy and STDs are included in this domain. The second domain addresses substance use and trafficking, and includes youth involvement with cigarettes, liquor, marijuana, and cocaine. Early use of substances that are legal for adults, such as alcohol or cigarettes, increases the likelihood of progression to illegal substances, including marijuana, cocaine, and crack.[4] School failure is the third domain and includes performance below expectations, truancy, and school dropout. The lack of a high school degree limits opportunities for stable employment and increases the likelihood of either dependence on public assistance or criminality.[12] The final domain, delinquency, includes stealing, lying, vandalism, aggression, and other forms of criminal behavior that may result in involvement with the juvenile justice system. Youth violence is a particular concern, because it has reached endemic proportions and is a major public health problem.[13-15]

Theories of Risk-Taking Behavior

In many adolescent subcultures the primary risk-taking behaviors co-occur,[16-19] resulting in a general pattern of deviance or problem behaviors. Problem Behavior Theory (PBT) is a widely recognized developmental theory that provides one possible explanation to early risk-taking.[6,20] Briefly, the theory implies that risk-taking behaviors occur when youths reject social norms and regard risk-taking behavior as beneficial and normative.

Explanations for risk-taking behavior are often based on risk and protective factors. Risk factors increase the likelihood of youths engaging in risk-taking behavior, and protective factors reduce the likelihood or buffer the youths from engaging in risk-taking behavior, even when risk factors are present.[21] Risk and protective factors are not necessarily opposite ends of the same dimension, although they are often negatively correlated.

Jessor and colleagues[20] have outlined six risk factors related to risk-taking behavior. First, expectation for success includes the anticipated positive outcomes in aspects of life, including family, friends, and employment. Low success expectancy is a risk, because without hope for success, youths are more likely to use maladaptive means to achieve goals. Second, low self-esteem is a risk because youths lacking self-confidence may also lack the skills to resist temptations to engage in risk-taking behavior, or may engage in risk-taking behavior to compensate for low self-esteem. Depression, which includes feelings of hopelessness and social alienation, is the third risk factor. A fourth risk factor involves the degree of risk-taking behavior among friends. Adolescents are influenced by perceptions of their friends' behavior.[22] Having friends who engage in high-risk behavior makes the behavior enticing, and provides adolescents with an opportunity to learn how to engage in the behavior and where to obtain the necessary materials. Fifth, a preference for friends, as opposed to parents, is a risk factor because parents often control deviant behavior and model more conventional behavior. The final risk factor is low grade-point average. Poor academic performance can lead to detachment from school, and have a negative impact on achievement expectations and self-esteem.

Jessor and colleagues[20] also outlined seven protective factors that may reduce the likelihood that an adolescent will engage in risky behavior. First, a positive orientation toward school is a protective factor, because it reflects an acceptance of a traditional institution as a primary socializing agent for youths. The second protective factor, a positive orientation toward health, reflects a personal commitment to refrain from behaviors that may jeopardize health and well-being. An intolerance of deviance is the third protective factor, because it signifies a recognition of conventional behavior and an objection to norm violations. The fourth includes positive relations with adults, which indicates that the youth uses adults as socializing agents and imitates conventional behavior modeled by adults. A fifth protective factor is perceived regulatory controls. A youth's perception of his or her parents (or other adults) as being concerned reduces the likelihood of his or her engaging in risk-taking behavior and increases the youth's awareness of the distinction between acceptable and unacceptable behavior. Sixth, having friends who model conventional behavior serves as a protective factor, because it indicates that the adolescent interacts with conventional peers who engage in norm-appropriate behaviors. The final buffer is pro-social activities. When youths engage in pro-social activities, eg, sports, they are building social networks that are congruent with a conventional lifestyle.

Questionnaires About Adolescent Health and Risk-Taking Behavior

Information about risk and protective factors is essential, because it aids clinicians in planning preventive services for adolescents who are not engaging in risk-taking behaviors or in planning intervention services for youth who are engaging in risk-taking behaviors.[23] Thus, prevention and intervention programs for adolescents often begin with questions designed to collect information about the individual adolescent's current health status, risk-taking behavior, and risk and protective factors. The primary method of gathering this information is through questionnaires, either completed by the adolescent individually or used by clinicians as interview guides.

Individually administered questionnaires rely on adolescents' reading skills and ability to sustain attention on a questionnaire. Interview guides require interviewer time and rely on the skills of the interviewer in eliciting truthful responses from adolescents. Concerns have been raised about adolescents' level of comfort with the sensitive questions necessary to collect information about risk-taking behavior, eg, sexuality, and about their willingness to give truthful responses.[24,25]

An alternative to questionnaires is to use computers programmed to administer questions, using the same rules that would be used by a live interviewer. With the technical advancement of "talking" computers and the "mouse," questions can be presented through two modalities concurrently—aurally through headphones and visually through the screen. Adolescents select their desired response through touch screens or clicking the mouse. Decisions as to whether to ask highly sensitive questions are based on responses to less sensitive questions. For example, adolescents may be asked if they ever experienced a particular type of event. Those who respond in the affirmative would then be asked more questions about the event. In contrast, those who denied prior experience would not receive the follow-up questions. Computer-administered interviews have been used with youths as young as 9 to 15 years of age to ask very sensitive questions about sexual and drug behavior.[26-28]

COMPUTER-ADMINISTERED QUESTIONNAIRES

Computer-administered questionnaires have been used successfully in clinical settings with children.[29] In examining responses as a function of mode of administration, no differences have been reported on computer-administered versus written tests of attitudes or personality variables among adults[30,31] or of routine health behaviors among adolescents.[32] However, adolescents attending health care clinics were more likely to report frequent alcohol or marijuana use, and more likely to respond to sensitive questions about family problems, emotional issues, and requests for information on contraceptives, when questions were administered through a computer rather than through a written questionnaire.[33] Similarly, adolescent girls were more likely to report sexual experience when questions were administered on a computer, rather than through a face-to-face interview,[34] and adolescent and young adult patients in a sexually transmitted disease clinic were more likely to report highly sensitive HIV risk-taking behaviors, eg, unprotected anal intercourse, in a self-administered audio interview (portable cassette player) than in a written or face-to-face interview.[35] Although audio interviews administered through cassette players may facilitate accurate responding to sensitive questions, they are limited by their inability to alter presentation of questions based on prior responses, ie, skip patterns. In a recent national survey of adolescent males, rates of high-risk and illegal behaviors were three times higher with computer-administered, rather than self-administered questionnaires.[36]

There are several other potential benefits to computer-administered questionnaires. First, software is available to store a high-quality digitized recording of an interviewer's voice. Thus, the adolescent may hear a culturally familiar voice asking the questions. Second, computer-administered interviews afford privacy. Respondents select their choices and do not have to worry about others "hearing" their answers. Third, because adolescents do not have to consider reactions from the interviewer, they should be more likely to endorse sensitive behavior when it has occurred and less likely to provide socially desirable responses. Paperny and colleagues reported that 89% of the youths in their study preferred answering sensitive questions on the computer, often because they found it "easier to talk more honestly with a computer than with a person."[33] Fourth, the multimodal input enables youths with limited reading or computer skills to participate in computer-administered questionnaires. They hear and see the questions simultaneously and have the option of repeating questions if they desire. Fifth, questions are presented in a systematic manner without subtle individual differences introduced by different interviewers. Sixth, the computer can be programmed to scan responses and alert the interviewer if the adolescent gives answers that demand immediate attention. For example, the computer could be programmed to inform the interviewer if the youth makes a logical error, answers in an apparent response set, or indicates an immediate or severe problem. Seventh, the data are recorded and saved in electronic format. Not only is there less probability of data errors because responses are fixed, but the risk of errors during data entry and the associated costs are eliminated. Eighth, the process is novel and interactive, thus reducing the possibility of boredom and distractibility. Using a color monitor and interspersing popular icons in the interview protocol should enhance attention and enjoyment. Ninth, computers are portable, enabling interviews to be conducted in any location that is convenient for the youth and the interviewer. Finally, depending on the availability of computers, multiple interviews can be conducted concurrently by one interviewer, making the procedure very cost effective.

Despite these benefits, there are several potential limitations to computer-administered questionnaires that should be considered. First, the personal rapport that is often established in interviews is eliminated. A skilled interviewer can pick up on subtle verbal and non-verbal cues, and know when and how to probe. In a computer-administered interview, the branching of questions is dependent upon prior responses, and non-verbal signs are missed. Second, respondents who are "computer-phobic" may be uncomfortable interacting with a machine. However, because computers are widely available in most school systems and commercial establishments, many youths have been exposed to computers and are in fact very enthusiastic about using them.[33] Finally, technical problems may interfere with the recording and storing of responses. Investigators working with 9- to 15-year-old youths residing in public housing projects report that the interview was completed successfully by 98% of the children who agreed to participate.[37] Youths learned to use the computer with a few minutes of instruction, appeared to enjoy interacting with the computers, displayed little fatigue or lack of interest, and asked when there would be subsequent opportunities to use the computers.

CONSTRUCTION OF THE COMPUTER-ASSISTED QUESTIONNAIRE ON ADOLESCENT RISK-TAKING

Questionnaire construction regarding adolescent risk-taking behavior is a complex process because it requires careful attention to reliability, validity, adolescent development, and ethical issues.

Reliability

Reliability is a critical consideration in questionnaire construction because it refers to the consistency of scores if the same individual were to answer the questions on two occasions.[38] There are four types of reliability. *Test-retest* is the most well known type of reliability and consists of administering a questionnaire twice over a brief time period. The time period depends on the reactivity of the questionnaire, but rarely exceeds 6 months. A reliability coefficient is calculated by correlating the responses from the two sets of scores. One potential drawback to this type of reliability is in recall that occurs when respondents are asked to answer the same questions over a brief period.

Alternate-form is another type of reliability. In this case the interviewer uses two different forms of the test, which presumably are similar. The respondent answers one form during the first administration and the other form (counter-balanced across respondents) at the second administration. Again, correlation analysis is used to calculate a reliability coefficient.

A third type of reliability is *split-half*. The respondent answers questions on only one occasion, but the questionnaire is divided into two halves and scored separately. Not all questionnaires lend themselves to this type of reliability. It must be possible to ensure that the two halves are similar. Correlation is used to calculate a reliability coefficient.

Internal consistency is another type of reliability used to ensure that items on a questionnaire are consistent. For example, a questionnaire may include six questions that address depression. The interviewer may want to sum the responses to create a construct that represents depression. However, before summing the responses, the interviewer should ensure that respondents gave consistent responses to the six items by calculating their internal consistency. Coefficient alpha and Kuder-Richardson reliability are two statistical procedures used to calculate internal consistency.

Validity

Validity is a critical issue in the development of an interview protocol because it refers to what the interview measures and how well. There are several types of validity that are relevant to the development of an interview protocol—content, criterion (including concurrent and predictive), construct, convergent, and discriminant.[38]

Content validity determines if the questions represent youths' perspectives on risk-taking behavior. One way to enhance content validity is to incorporate qualitative procedures into the development of the interview to ensure that the questions on the interview are culturally and developmentally appropriate.[39]

Criterion validity refers to the effectiveness of the interview protocol to predict individual performance and is often divided into concurrent and predictive validity. *Concurrent validity* determines if the interview protocol differentiates individuals as would be expected from theory. For example, do youths who engage in risk-taking behavior report different risk and protective factors from youths who do not engage in risk-taking behavior? *Predictive validity* is used to predict what will happen in the future. For example, on the basis of their responses, is it possible to predict which youths are likely to engage in risk-taking behaviors?

Construct validity examines whether the interview protocol measures a specific theoretical construct. Developing interview protocols based on theoretical and empirical information about risk-taking behavior provides some protection against the threat of violating construct validity. Statistical procedures, such as structural equation modeling, may also be used to examine the relationship between youths' perspectives on risk behaviors and their social adaptation.

Convergent validity indicates that the interview should correlate with other measures of the same construct. This objective is often met by comparing the responses from the youths' questionnaires with those from their parents and other informants.[40] Using agreement between parent and adolescent perceptions also has shortcomings. Because parents and adolescents do not necessarily share the same memory, perspective, or knowledge, their agreement may be only low to moderate,[41,42] even if both reports are "correct."[43]

Discriminant validity indicates that the interview should not correlate with variables that assess different constructs. Discriminant validity is difficult to assess because risk-taking behavior has been associated with many other aspects of behavior and development. Care should be taken to ensure that interviews about risk-taking behavior are guided by theories of risk-taking behavior.

Social desirability or lie scales are often included to assess the veracity of youths' responses. Lie scales typically include frequent responses to ideal behavior, such as always being kind to others. When youth have elevated scores it may be unclear whether they are intentionally faking well or whether they have an inflated view of themselves. In either case, youths with elevated scores represent those with a high need for social desirability[44] and their responses to the risk-taking questionnaire should be viewed with skepticism.

The lie scale from the Children's Revised Manifest Anxiety Scale[44] has been developed for youths between ages 6 and 19. This scale consists of nine items, eg, "I like everyone I know," which could be interspersed through the interview. There are ethnic, age, and gender-specific norms for 4,972 youths in the national standardization sample.

For a detailed discussion of reliability and validity, refer to Chapter 22.

Adolescent Development

Both the structure and content of the questions in the interview protocol should be oriented to the cultural background and developmental level of the youths. Assessments of reading level and word frequency may be used to assess language structure.[45] To ensure clarity, questions should be context-based, which may be provided by vignettes[46] or introductory screeners.[47] For example, Finkelhor and Dziuba-Leatherman used an introductory screener to ask about family assault: "Sometimes kids get pushed around, hit, or beaten up by members of their own family, like an older brother or sister or parent. Has anyone in your family ever pushed you around, hit you, or tried to beat you up?" "Has anyone in your family gotten so mad or out of control you thought they were going to hurt you badly?"

Adolescence provides a unique opportunity for health promotion, because behaviors that are associated with mortality and morbidity during adulthood often begin in adolescence, eg, smoking.[48] Adolescents are at a healthy phase of life and most of their health-related problems are explained by negative consequences of risk-taking behavior (injuries, homicide, and suicide account for 75% of the morbidity).[23,49]

The American Medical Association (AMA) has developed the Guidelines for Adolescent Preventive Services (GAPS) to assist clinicians and policy makers in identifying and providing the services needed by adolescents.[50] GAPS emphasizes the importance of ensuring that services are developmentally and culturally appropriate for each adolescent and are provided within an atmosphere of confidentiality.

Ethical Concerns

Interviewing youths about their risk-taking behavior raises ethical concerns. If youths reveal that their safety is in danger or that they have been harmed, eg, sexually abused, it may be necessary to contact the state's protective service agency. Interviewers must also be prepared to deal with youths' reports of illegal behavior. If the interviews are conducted in the context of research, developmentally appropriate consent forms should be prepared for both parents and youths, indicating that sensitive questions are included. Respondents must be told that they may refuse to answer any questions or to participate altogether, even after the interview has begun.

It may also be useful to institute a debriefing procedure at the end of every interview to assess possible trauma from the interview.[51] Youths are debriefed by an experienced interviewer who acknowledges the sensitivity of the questions and informs the youths how to obtain consultation immediately or in the future. If the youths express concern or the interviewer has concerns about them, a clinician should be contacted immediately.

Existing Questionnaires of Adolescent Risk-Taking Behavior

There are several excellent recent examples of questionnaires regarding adolescent risk-taking behavior that have been published and have undergone careful scrutiny of their psychometric properties. Much can be learned from these questionnaires that can be incorporated into a computer-assisted questionnaire for adolescent risk-taking behavior.

The Safe Times Questionnaire consists of 45 items and covers a comprehensive set of risk domains, including sexuality, substance abuse, affect, education and employment, family life, immunizations, medical exams, mineral intake, and safety.[52] Adequate validity and reliability have been established with African-American youths, and the authors are currently examining validity and reliability in other populations. The clinical utility of this self-report measure as a screening instrument has also been established. The physicians who used the information gathered in the Safe Times Questionnaire to guide the interview portion of the office visit completed the interview in a less time than the physicians who did not have access to the screening information. In addition, physicians who used the Safe Times Questionnaire had a higher level of agreement with a psychologist, when identifying youths at risk for family problems and depression. In short, the Safe Times Questionnaire improved physician efficiency and accuracy in identifying at-risk youths.

The Adolescent Child Health and Illness Profile (CHIP) is a recently developed questionnaire that includes 107 items and 46 questions regarding specific injuries or diseases.[53] The CHIP can be self-administered in approximately 30 minutes. It consists of six domains, including discomfort, disorders, satisfaction with health, achievement, risks, and resilience. Adequate reliability and validity have been established for African-American and white middle school and high school students in both urban and rural settings. This questionnaire is particularly useful when describing the health behaviors of groups of adolescents.

A third health assessment is the Youth Risk Behavior Surveillance System (YRBS), developed by the Centers for Disease Control and Prevention. The YRBS is a 75-item questionnaire that assesses six domains, including unintentional/intentional injuries, tobacco use, alcohol and drug use, sexual activity, dietary behaviors, and physical activity.[54] It takes approximately 35 minutes to self-administer this survey. The reliability of many items on the questionnaire has been established for white, Hispanic, and African-American high school students in rural and urban environments.

SUMMARY

Computer-administered technology offers a promising information-gathering strategy when care is taken to satisfy the methodological, psychometric, developmental, and ethical criteria necessary for interviewing youths about risk-taking behavior. Interactive computer technology offers an innovative opportunity for intervention, demonstrated by the computer games that have been used to promote health-related knowledge and attitudes among children with asthma,[55] and information and attitudes regarding parenting, child rearing, and contraceptive use among high school students.[56] Logical extensions are to use the information gathered from interviews with youths about health, risk-taking behavior, risk factors, and protective factors to develop and evaluate interactive computer games to prevent risk-taking behavior and to promote adaptive behavior among youths.

REFERENCES

1.   Newcomb MD, Bentler PM. *Consequences of Adolescent Drug Use*. Newbury Park, Calif: Sage; 1988.
2.   Newcomb MD, Bentler PM. Substance use and abuse among children and teenagers. *American Psychologist*. 1989;44:242-248.
3.   Shedler J, Block J. Adolescent drug use and psychological health: a longitudinal inquiry. *American Psychologist*. 1990;45:612-630.
4.   Kandel D, Yamagucki K. From beer to crack: Developmental patterns of drug involvement. *Am J Public Health*. 1993; 83:851-855.
5.   Tonkin RS. Adolescent risk-taking behavior. *Journal of Adolescent Health Care*. 1987;8:213-220.
6.   Jessor R, Jessor SL. *Problem Behavior and Psychosocial Development: A Longitudinal Study of Youth*. New York, NY: Academic Press;1977.

7.   Hein K. Adolescents at risk for HIV infection. In DiClemente RJ. *Adolescents and AIDS: A Generation in Jeopardy*. Newbury Park, Calif: Sage Publications; 1992:3-16.

8.   Dryfoos JG. *Adolescents at Risk: Prevalence and Prevention*. New York, NY: Oxford University Press; 1990.

9.   Forrest J, Singh S. The sexual and reproductive behavior of American women,1982-1988. *Family Planning Perspectives*. 1990;22:206-214.

10.   Rosenthal SL, Biro FM, Succop PA, Cohen SS, Stanberry LR. Age of first intercourse and risk of sexually transmitted disease. *Adolescent and Pediatric Gynecology*. 1994;7:210-213.

11.   Ehrhardt AA, Wasserheit JN. Age, gender, and sexual risk behaviors for sexually transmitted diseases in the United States. In Wasserheit JN, Aral SO, Holmes KK. *Research Issues in Human Behavior and Sexually Transmitted Diseases in the AIDS Era*. Washington, DC: American Society for Microbiology; 1991:97-121.

12.   Hamburg DA. *Today's Children: Creating a Future for a Generation in Crisis*. New York, NY: Times Books; 1992.

13.   Koop CE, Lundberg GD. Violence in America: a public health emergency. *JAMA*. 1992;267:3076-3077.

14.   Novello AC, Shaskey J, Froehike R. A medical response to violence. *JAMA*. 1992;267:3007.

15.   Rosenberg ML, O'Carroll PW, Powell KE. Let's be clear: violence is a public health problem. *JAMA*. 1992;267:3071-3072.

16.   Donovan JE, Jessor R. Structure of problem behaviors in adolescence and young adulthood. *Journal of Consulting and Clinical Psychology*. 1985;53:890-904.

17.   Elliott DS, Huizinga D, Menard S. *Multiple Problem Youth: Delinquency, Substance Use and Mental Health Problems*. New York, NY: Springer-Verlag; 1989.

18.   Osgood DW, Johnston LD, O'Malley PM, Bachman JG. The generality of deviance in late adolescence and early adulthood. *American Sociological Review*. 1988;5:81-93.

19.   Zabin LS, Hardy JB, Smith EA, Hirsch MB. Substance use and its relation to sexual activity among inner-city adolescents. *Journal of Adolescent Health Care*. 1986;7:320-331.

20.   Jessor R, Van Der Bos J, Vanderryn J, Costa FM, Turbin MS. Protective factors in adolescent problem behavior: Moderator effects and developmental change. *Developmental Psychology*. 1995;31:923-933.

21.   Rutter M. Psychosocial resilience and protective factors. *Am J Orthopsychiatry*. 1987;57:316-331.

22.   Brown BB. Peer groups and peer culture. In Feldman SS, Elliott GR. *At the Threshold: The Developing Adolescent*. Cambridge, Mass: Harvard University Press; 1990:171-196.

23.   Irwin CE, Jr. The adolescent, health, and society: From the perspective of the physician. In Millstein SG, Petersen AC, Nightengale EO. *Promoting the Health of Adolescents*. New York, NY: Oxford University Press; 1993:146-150.

24.   Costa FM, Jessor RM, Donovan JE, Fortenberry JD. Early initiation of sexual intercourse: The influence of psychosocial unconventionality. *Journal of Research on Adolescence*. 1995;5:93-121.

25.   Rowe DC, Rodgers JL. An "epidemic" model of adolescent sexual intercourse: Applications of national survey data. *Journal of Biosocial Science*. 1991;23:162-167.

26.   Black M, Ricardo I. Drug-use, drug-trafficking, and weapon-carrying among low income, urban African-American early adolescent males. *Pediatrics*. 1994;93:1065-1072.

27.   Romer D, Black M, Ricardo I, Feigelman S, Kaljee L, Galbraith J, et al. Social influences on the sexual behavior of youth at risk for HIV exposure. *Am J Public Health*. 1994;84:977-985.

28.   Stanton B, Romer D, Ricardo I, et al. Early initiation of sex and its lack of association with risk behaviors among adolescent African-Americans. *Pediatrics*. 1993;92;13-19.

29.   Sawyer MG, Sarris A, Baghurst P. The use of interview to administer the Child Behavior Checklist in a child psychiatry service. *J Am Acad Child Adolesc Psychiatry*. 1991;30:674-681.

30.   Hart RR, Goldstein MA. Psychological assessment. *Computers in Human Behavior*. 1985;1:69-75.

31.   Wilson FR, Genco KT, Yager GG. Assessing the equivalence of paper-and-pencil versus computerized tests. *Computers in Human Behavior*. 1985;1:3-4.

32. Millstein SG. Acceptability and reliability of sensitive information collected via computer interview. *Education and Psychological Measurement*. 1987;47:523-533.

33. Paperny DM, Aono JY, Lehman RM, Hammas SL, Risser J. Computer-assisted detection and intervention in adolescent high-risk health behaviors. *J Pediatrics*. 1990;116:456-462.

34. Millstein SG, Irwin CE. Acceptability of computer-acquired sexual histories in adolescent girls. *J Pediatrics*. 1983;103:815-819.

35. Boekeloo BO, Schiavo L, Rabin DL, Conlon RT, Jordan CS, Mundt DJ. Self-reports of HIV risk factors by patients at a sexually transmitted disease clinic: Audio vs. written questionnaires. *Am J Public Health*. 1994;84:754-760.

36. Turner CF, Ku L, Rogers, SM, Lindberg LD, Peck JH, Sonenstein FL. Adolescent sexual behavior, drug use, and violence: increased reporting with computer survey technology. *Science*. 1998; 280:867-873.

37. Romer D, Hornik R, Stanton B, Black M, Li X, Ricardo I, Feigelman S. "Talking" computers: An efficient and private method to conduct interviews on sensitive health topics. *Journal of Sexual Research*. 1997;34:3-9.

38. Anastasi A. *Psychological Testing*. New York, NY: Macmillan Publishers; 1988.

39. Steckler A. Integrating qualitative and quantitative methods: An introduction. *Health Education Quarterly*. 1992;19:1-8.

40. Kaufman J, Jones B, Stieglitz E, Vitulano L, Mannarino AP. The use of multiple informants to assess children's maltreatment experiences. *Journal of Family Violence*. 1994;9:227-248.

41. Achenbach T, McConaughy S, Howell C. Child/adolescent behavioral and emotional problems: Implications of cross-informant correlations for situational specificity. *Psychological Bulletin*. 1987;101:213-232.

42. McGee RA, Wolfe DA, Yuen S. *The measurement of maltreatment: A comparison of approaches*. Paper presented at the biennial meeting of the Society for Research in Child Development. Seattle, Wash; 1991.

43. Edelbrock C, Costello AJ, Dulcan MK, Conover NC, Kalas R. Parent-child agreement on child psychiatric symptoms assessed via structured interview. *Journal of Child Psychology and Psychiatry*. 1986; 27:181-190.

44. Reynolds CR, Richmond BO. *Revised Children's Manifest Anxiety Scale Manual*. Los Angeles, Calif: Western Psychological Services; 1985.

45. Fry EA. A readability formula that saves time. *Journal of Reading*. 1968;11:575-578.

46. Weithorn LA, Campbell SB. The competency of children and adolescents to make informed decisions. *Child Development*. 1982;53:1589-1598.

47. Finkelhor D, Dziuba-Leatherman J. Children as victims of violence: A national survey. *Pediatrics*. 1994;94:413-420.

48. Millstein SG, Petersen AC, Nightengale EO. Adolescent health promotion: Rationale, goals, and objectives. In Millstein SG, Petersen AC, Nightengale EO. *Promoting the Health of Adolescents*. New York, NY: Oxford University Press; 1993:3-12.

49. Gans JE, Blyth DA, Elster AB. *America's Adolescents: How Healthy Are They?* American Medical Association, Profiles of Adolescent Health Series. Chicago, Ill: American Medical Association; 1990.

50. Elster A, Kuznets N. *Guidelines for Adolescent Preventive Services (GAPS)*. Baltimore, Md: Williams & Wilkins; 1994.

51. Gurman EB. Debriefing for all concerned: Ethical treatment of human subjects. *Psychological Science*. 1994;5:139.

52. Schubiner H, Tzelepis A, Wright K, Podany E. The clinical utility of the safe times questionnaire. *J Adoles Health*. 1994;15:374-382.

53. Starfield A, Riley AW, Green BF, Ensminger ME, Ryan SA, Kelleher K, et al. The adolescent child health and illness profile: a population-based measure of health. *Medical Care*. 1995;33;553-566.

54. Brenner ND, Collins JL, Kann L, Warren CW, Williams BI. Reliability of the youth risk behavior survey questionnaire. *Am J Epidemiol.* 1995;141:575-580.

55. Rubin DH, Leventhal JM, Sadock RT. Educational intervention by computer in childhood asthma: A randomized clinical trial testing the use of a new teaching intervention in childhood asthma. *Pediatrics.* 1986;77:1-10.

56. Paperny DM, Starn JR. Adolescent pregnancy prevention by health education computer games: Instruction of knowledge and attitudes. *Pediatrics.* 1989;83:742-752.

21

Computerized Assessment: The Stress Management Questionnaire

Franklin Stein, PhD, OTR/L, FAOTA
Daniel E. Bentley, MA
Michael Natz, MS, BFA, OTR/L

The Stress Management Questionnaire (SMQ) is a self-administered paper and pencil test that was developed in 1986 by Franklin Stein at the University of Wisconsin-Milwaukee. The SMQ consists of 158 questions. The questionnaire uses a forced-choice format for each item listed, and a section for ranking the top 10 symptoms, stressors, or copers covered in each section.

The major purposes of the SMQ are to identify the:
1. Symptoms and problems precipitated by stress
2. Stressors in the individual's life that cause a stress response
3. Coping activities that the individual currently uses to manage or alleviate stress.

The SMQ can be used clinically to help the therapist and patient develop an individualized stress management program, and as a qualitative outcome measure to evaluate the patient's improvement in managing stress.

CONCEPTUAL DEFINITION OF STRESS

Stress is defined in the SMQ as the personal responses or symptoms that are the results of daily situations or thoughts that make life difficult or create discomfort. The intensity of the stress reaction will depend upon the individual's perceived ability to cope and his or her available resources (copers). Symptoms result from the individual's inability to deal successfully with the stressors. Within the individual's life space, stressors are defined as external, while stressors that are generated by an individual, such as anticipatory anxiety, are internal. In this context stress is depicted as an effect or consequence. On a healthy level, mild or moderate degrees of stress, such as meeting time demands and public performances, can be a motivating force in the individual. This is called "eustress."[1]

THE COMPONENTS OF THE SMQ

The questionnaire has three sections, listing symptoms, stressors, and coping activities. The Questionnaire usually takes about 20 minutes to complete. Individuals completing the questionnaire are asked to check yes or no to a list of symptoms and problems resulting from stress, everyday stressors that precipitate the stress response, and the coping activities that manage or reduce stress. They are then asked to list and rank in order each symptom, stressor, and coper that they have identified. The SMQ consists of 73 items describing symptoms, 37 describing stressors, and 48 describing copers. There is also space for individuals to list other items in each of the three categories.

The symptoms and problems resulting from stress were generated from four factors:
• Physiological, such as headaches, tremors, neck/low back pain
• Cognitive, such as difficulty concentrating, remembering, decision making
• Emotional, such as feeling angry, hopeless, tense
• Behavioral, such as difficulty sleeping, eating, speaking.

Everyday stressors precipitating stress reactions were grouped under nine factors:
• Interpersonal, such as arguments with family members
• Intrapersonal, such as low self-esteem
• Time demands, such as meeting a deadline at work
• Mechanical breakdown, such as dealing with a broken household appliance
• Performance, such as taking a test
• Financial pressures, such as loss of income
• Illness, such as having the flu
• Environmental disturbance, such as excessive noise
• Complex situations, such as raising a child alone.

Everyday activities that manage or reduce stress (copers) were organized into nine factors:
• Creative, such as writing a poem
• Construction, such as knitting a sweater
• Exercise, such as walking
• Appreciation, such as listening to music
• Self-care, such as taking a bath
• Social, such as talking to friends
• Plant and animal care, such as having a pet
• Performance, such as singing in a choir
• Sports, such as swimming.

A final section of the questionnaire asks for demographic information, and also poses questions about the experience of completing the questionnaire itself.

CONCEPTUAL DEVELOPMENT OF THE SMQ

In the development of the SMQ, Stein conducted two descriptive studies, collecting data from 113 subjects in the first pilot study and from 639 subjects in the second study.[2] The results from the studies are described in Tables 21-1 to 21-5. Demographics are described in Tables 21-1 and 21-2. Tables 21-3, 21-4, and 21-5 compare results from the two studies on the individual rankings for symptoms, stressors, and copers. Table 21-6 describes the concurrence of agreement in a test-retest reliability study of 34 normal subjects. As demonstrated, the reliability ranges from .85 to .89. The instrument was later applied in three clinical research studies.[3-5] In the studies the SMQ was used to establish the extent and nature of improved stress responses and lowered stress levels following relaxation and biofeedback therapy. In general the SMQ provides a personal stress profile that helps the individual identify stressors and reduces resultant symptoms by incorporating individual copers into his or her everyday life. It is envisaged that the SMQ has wide potential for self-

Table 21-1

Frequency Distribution of Age

Study 1, Stress Management Questionnaire

Age Group	Frequency	Percentage
18-22	42	37%
23-27	25	22%
28-32	8	7%
33-37	7	6%
38-42	6	5%
43-47	3	3%
48-52	2	2%
53	3	3%
No age listed	17	15%
Totals	113	100%

n = 113
Males = 32
Females = 77

Table 21-2

Frequency Distribution of Age

Study 2, Stress Management Questionnaire

Age Group	Frequency	Percentage
20-25	263	41%
26-31	132	21%
32-37	86	13%
38-43	49	8%
44-49	39	6%
50-55	30	5%
56-61	17	3%
62-67	18	3%
68-77	5	.7%
Totals	639	100%

n = 639
Males = 210
Females = 429

monitoring symptoms, stressors, and copers as a part of holistic stress-management programs. It can serve as a comprehensive interactive measuring instrument for guided self-understanding and healthy lifestyle planning, such as in health promotion and disease prevention programs in school and work environments.

The instrument takes account of response-based, stimulus-based, and interactional-stress theories. Response-based theories describe bodily and psychological patterns of response to causes of stress—in terms of symptomatology, emotions, and personal difficulties. Examples of such theories are Cannon's fight or flight syn-

Table 21-3

Comparison of Two Descriptive Studies of Normal Subjects on Stress Management Questionnaire

	Symptoms	
Rank	Study 1 (n=113)	Study 2 (n=639)
1	Headaches	Concentrating
2	Muscle tension	Anxious
3	Concentrating	Irritable
4	Nervous*	Tense
5	Sleeping*	Headaches
6	Irritable (1)	Muscle tension
7	Fatigue	Fatigue
8	Impatient*	Sleeping
9	Moody*	Eating
10	Rapid heartbeat	Low tolerance to others
11	Low tolerance to others	Moody
12	Restless	Nervous

(1) Irritable was not listed in second study
* Tied ranks

Table 21-4

Comparison of Two Descriptive Studies of Normal Subjects on Stress Management Questionnaire

	Stressors	
Rank	Study 1 (n=113)	Study 2 (n=639)
1	Having too many things to do	Feeling too much pressure
2	Feeling too much pressure	Having too many things to do
3	Being unprepared	Arguments with
4	Arguments with	Having problems with relationships
5	Financial situations*	Being unprepared
6	Gaining or losing weight*	Having no control over situation
7	Having problems with relationships**	Financial situations
8	Meeting deadlines**	Being evaluated for performance
9	Having no control over situation	Speaking in front of groups
10	Not having any free time for oneself	Not having any free time for oneself
11	Speaking in front of groups	Failure to meet goals
12	Lack of confidence in oneself	Being late for an appointment

*, ** Tied ranks

drome,[6] and Hans Selye's general adaptation syndrome.[7] Stimulus theories are concerned with identifying stressors—the situational causes of the effects described in response theories. Familiar examples of these include life events as a cause of stress[8] or the accumulated irritations of daily life encapsulated in such measures as the daily hassles approach.[9] This approach is reflected in the SMQ's section enumerating stressful situations (stressors). Interactional theories, such as that of Lazarus and Folkman,[10] emphasize the mediating role of coping and adaptive mechanisms in

Table 21-5
Comparison of Two Descriptive Studies of Normal Subjects on
Stress Management Questionnaire

	Copers	
Rank	Study 1 (n=113)	Study 2 (n=639)
1	Talk to a friend	Talk to a friend
2	Analyze situation	Analyze situation
3	Listen to music	Listen to music
4	Relax (lie down)	Relax (lie down)
5	Crying	Hot shower/bath
6	Hot shower/bath	Being by myself
7	Exercising*	Exercising
8	Sleeping*	Meditate or pray
9	Walking	Sleeping
10	Visit friends	Crying
11	Meditate or pray	Being busy
12	Read for pleasure	Walking

* Tied ranks

Table 21-6
Percentage of Concurrence on Stress Management Questionnaire on
Test-Retest Reliability Study

Major areas	Percentage of Agreement on Rank-Ordered Items
Symptoms and problems resulting from stress	88%
Everyday stressors precipitating the stress response	85%
Everyday coping activities that manage stress	89%

n = 34
Mean age = 27
Females = 21
Males = 13

determining overall levels of stress. This approach is reflected in the SMQ section listing coping responses.

SCALING OF ITEMS

In analyzing the SMQ, individual items were combined into scales that represent the cumulative significance for the respondent of symptoms, feelings, difficulties, problems, stressful situations, and coping behavior. Justification for these scales is presented in the discussion of reliability.

VALIDITY AND RELIABILITY

To establish the viability of the SMQ, the validity and reliability were measured, and an item analysis was done to establish generalizability beyond the sample of subjects in the previous studies.[2]

Validity means that the SMQ must measure stress (as it claims to do). This could be shown by the concordance of SMQ scores with other stress measures on the same individuals, and by the success of the questionnaire in differentiating groups of people who might already be thought to differ in stress levels.

Reliability means that the questionnaire should have internal consistency, where each part (or scale, as it is called) should be measuring one thing (stress symptoms, problems, stressful situations, and coping behavior). Reliability also requires that when it is reasonable to assume that stress levels are the same on more than one occasion, this would be reflected in similar scores on the SMQ. For example, the closer repeated questionnaire scores are in time, the more similar the results should be (test-retest reliability).

The question of appropriateness for a general population can be addressed by considering the contribution made by each individual item to overall indices of validity and reliability, by specific feedback from respondents, and by considering the contribution of stress management programs to changes in SMQ scores recorded before and after treatment.

Much of this work has been accomplished with preliminary samples, and some is ongoing, but there remains a need for further research. In particular, reference norms with homogeneous groups need to be established. This will also permit the construction of scoring procedures that identify users' levels of stress, predicting the effectiveness of different coping responses, and determining the efficacy of treatment programs to reduce the level of stress in vulnerable and clinical populations.

A methodological study of validity and reliability was carried out by Bentley and Stein in 1994. The study included 70 normal subjects from a wide variety of backgrounds and occupations. The data from this study was compared with previous results from the clinical subsample of 27 subjects in Stein and Nikolic,[4] Stein and Smith,[5] and Stein.[2] The sample of 70 subjects included 44% men and 55% women who were between 21 and 70 years of age. Both normal and clinical groups had the opportunity to complete the SMQ on two occasions over a period of approximately 1 month. A subset of the normal sample (n=41) also completed the Health-Promoting Lifestyle Profile (HPLP), a measure of positive health-promoting behavior and coping style,[12] and the Survey of Recent Life Experiences (SRLE),[13] an adjusted version of the Hassles Scale.[9] The SRLE is an index of the salience of stressors and the experience of stress in daily living.

Validity

The first test of validity of the SMQ involved comparing scores with those of other instruments whose relationship with stress, though based on different underlying dimensions, were already published. The HPLP and SRLE, described above, were used for this purpose.

The HPLP has six subscales reflecting different aspects of health-promoting behavior that are related to stress management. The subscales are:
1. Self-Actualization
2. Health Responsibility
3. Exercise
4. Nutrition

5. Interpersonal Support
6. Stress Management.
   Examples of these are:
1. Enthusiastic/optimistic, feel happy/content, set realistic goals
2. Check cholesterol level, observe body for changes, question physician/get second opinion
3. Recreational activities, vigorous exercise three times a week, do stretching exercise
4. Eat three meals daily, read labels, add fiber to diet
5. Spend time with close friends, express concern/love, maintain meaningful interpersonal relationships
6. Daily relaxation time, pleasant bedtime thoughts, relax muscles before sleep.

Respondents are asked to rate themselves according to how frequently or routinely they engage in these activities or hold certain attitudes toward health. The SRLE also has six subscales:

1. Social and Cultural Difficulties
2. Work
3. Time Pressure
4. Finances
5. Social Acceptability
6. Social Victimization.
   Examples of these are:
1. Being let down or disappointed by friends, conflicts with family members
2. Dissatisfaction with work, lower evaluation of your work than you hoped for
3. Too many things to do at once, a lot of responsibilities
4. Cash-flow difficulties, failing to get money you expected
5. Social rejection, dissatisfaction with your physical appearance
6. Being taken advantage of, being cheated in the purchase of goods.

Respondents are asked to rate the degree to which such occurrences or concerns are a part of their everyday life. Although there is likely to be a clear relationship between these items and a stress response, it also seems evident that there may be variation in the connection with stress, depending on the respondent's individual concerns and personal resources available to alleviate stress.

Correlations between SMQ scores and SRLE and HPLP ratings and their subscales are presented in Table 21-7.[11]

There are significant correlations between the SRLE and cumulative stress scores relating to symptoms, feelings, problems, and situations, but not with coping behavior or stress-related difficulties. For the HPLP, the only significant correlations are with difficulties and coping behavior. The degree to which a health-promoting lifestyle is adopted, then, appears to be related only to coping responses and in parallel, perhaps, to obstacles in the way of coping. It bears no relationship with the symptomatology and causes of stress, as these are measured in the SMQ. If we examine the subscales of both the comparison measures, we find that stress symptomatology is related to social difficulties, to social acceptance, and to the extent to which the respondent feels victimized but not to other "hassles" nor to a health-promoting lifestyle. Stress-related difficulties are related to concern over one's health ("health responsibility"), to the extent of social support, and to social acceptability.

Table 21-7
Intercorrelations Between Comparison Scales

Comparison Measures	Symptoms	Difficulties	Feelings	Problems	Situations	Copers
SRLE	.41		.48	.51	.59	
SCD	.37		.31	.32	.46	
W			.31	.32	.46	
TP				.28		
F				.37	.40	
SA	.54	.33	.59	.63	.70	
SV	.42		.51	.57	.35	
HPLP		.27				.37
SACT			-.42		-.34	
HR		.37	.47	.30	.45	.34
EX						
NU						.32
IS		.39	.30			
SM						.34

Note: Correlations between Scales of the SMQ and global and sub-scale scores of comparison measures: the Survey of Recent Life Experiences (SRLE) and the Health Promotion Lifestyle Profile (HPLP).

n = 41. Only correlations significant at the the .05 level or better are reported.

Key to abbreviations of the SRLE and HPLP sub-scales:
SRLE sub-scales: SCD—Social and Cultural Difficulties, W—Work Attitudes, TP—Time Pressure, F—Financial Concerns, SA—Social Acceptability, SV—Social Victimization
HPLP sub-scales: SACT—Self-Actualization, HR—Health Responsibility, EX—Exercise, NU—Nutrition, IS—Interpersonal Support, SM—Stress Management

Stress-related feelings are inversely related to self-actualization, directly correlated with active concern over one's health, and to four of the six SRLE subscales.

Problems accompanying stress are related to health concern and also to four of the six SRLE subscales. Stress-inducing situations are inversely related to self-actualization but directly (positively) correlated with five of the SRLE subscales. The strength of coping behavior, however, was directly related to health concern, nutrition, and to stress management, but among the SRLE subscales, only to social acceptability.

It is evident that the SMQ, in its present form, matches stressors, stress experiences, and coping behavior, as identified in other lifestyle measures, but that there are also important differences, reflecting the stress-inducing characteristics of particular individual concerns.

A second test of validity involved comparing the scores on the different subscales of the SMQ between normal and clinical samples of respondents. For this purpose, t-test based comparisons were made between these two groups on all the cumulative stress-related dimensions of the SMQ. These data are presented in Table 21-8.[11]

Reliability

Four of the six SMQ scales successfully differentiated between normal respondents and those hypothesized to be at higher levels of stress. For symptoms, feelings, problems, and stressful situations, the clinical sample recorded significantly

Table 21-8

Comparison Between Normal and Clinical Groups

n = 69 in Normal Group, n = 27 in Clinical Group

Subscale	Population	Mean	Standard Deviation	Standard Error of Mean
Symptoms	Normal	6.9855	4.114	.495
	Clinical	9.0370	6.248	1.202

Mean difference = -2.0515
Levene's Test for Equality of Variance: F = 10.296 $P < .002$

Difficulties	Normal	3.7971	2.627	.316
	Clinical	4.0370	2.441	.470

Mean difference = -.2399
Levene's Test for Equality of Variance: F = .071   NS

Feelings	Normal	9.4638	4.192	.505
	Clinical	9.5926	5.563	1.071

Mean difference = -.1288
Levene's Test for Equality of Variance: F = 4.193 $P < .043$

Problems	Normal	5.4348	3.215	.387
	Clinical	7.8519	4.990	.960

Mean difference = -2.4171
Levene's Test for Equality of Variance: F = 8.088 $P < .005$

Situations	Normal	16.8841	6.921	.833
	Clinical	19.9259	9.389	.807

Mean difference = -3.0519
Levene's Test for Equality of Variance: F = 5.903 $P < .017$

Coping behavior	Normal	17.3478	7.491	.902
	Clinical	22.2593	9.151	1.761

Mean difference = -4.911
Levene's Test for Equality of Variance: F = 1.37   NS

NS = non-significant statistical results

higher average stress-expressing scores. The difficulties scale proved the weakest, and there appeared to be no significant difference between normal respondents and those in therapy on the number of coping responses. The SMQ as it stands seems to indicate stress levels in a number of areas, but if the kinds of difficulties measured in the instrument are related to underlying stress, then this must be a form of stress shared by normal and clinical groups. It appears that the number of coping responses identified by individuals are not sufficient to cope effectively with stress. The key is to incorporate coping responses into one's activities of daily living.

Reliability was measured by examining the internal consistency of the SMQ subscales and also by comparing scores over two administrations of the questionnaire, separated by approximately 1 month. These data are presented in Tables 21-9 and 21-10.[11]

Alpha (reliability) coefficients presented in Table 21-9 lie within acceptable ranges for all but the problems scale, which has a moderate correlation of $r = .63$.

Correlations between first and repeat administrations of the SMQ, displayed in Table 21-10, are high, except for stress-related feelings. It may be that this dimension represents the least stable and most situation-reactive component of the stress response.

Another issue is the degree of concordance between rankings of the personal importance of the most significant symptoms, stressors, and coping activities between the two administrations of the SMQ. There is some indication of agreement on identifying the symptoms, stressors, and coping activities; however, there is little evidence of stability in the relative rankings of the SMQ components over time. It appears that individuals can identify the major symptoms that occur from stress and the coping activities that are most helpful. However, the relative importance of each item seems to vary from day to day. In other words an individual may have a headache because of time demands one day and on another day may feel anxious after an argument. The day-to-day transactions may influence how individuals rank a particular item on the SMQ.

Generalizability

The term generalizability is used as a rubric of the general applicability of the SMQ. Feedback from respondents, as reflected in their questionnaire responses, indicated that 79% found the length of the SMQ satisfactory; 94% found it clear; 82% found it interesting; 76% felt that the range of items reflected their feelings concerning stress; 55% thought the SMQ raised their awareness of everyday stressors; 33% felt that they had learned new ways to manage stress from the SMQ alone; and 52% thought they might benefit from a stress-management program, of which the SMQ might be a part.

Further research is needed to establish general norms and to determine concurrent and discriminative validity. Another area of investigation is to relate particular score levels, especially of coping, with levels of success in managing stress.

SUMMARY OF ISSUES

The SMQ is a reliable and valid instrument, as evidenced by test-retest data ($r = .63$ to $.87$) and by the statistically significant positive correlations with the HPLP and the SRLE. In general the SMQ is able to distinguish between individuals in treatment (clinical group) and those who are healthy. The SMQ is an appropriate tool for occupational therapists to use with patients.

ADAPTATION OF THE SMQ TO COMPUTER FORMAT

Natz compared results obtained from the SMQ given in a paper and pencil form and results from a newly devised computerized version of the SMQ.[4] Results indicated that the computerized form is equivalent to the paper and pencil form.

Application of Microcomputers in Occupational Therapy

From the time of its first introduction in 1973, the microcomputer has become a common place item in more than one-third of homes and businesses in the United States. This trend is changing the manner in which people engage in work, play, and leisure. Given the unique nature of occupational therapy, the emergence of a tech-

Table 21-9

Reliability Data for the Stress Management Questionnaire
Split-Half Reliability (Alpha) Coefficients

Subscale:	*Symptoms*	
	Spearman-Brown	.8662
	Guttman Split-Half	.8646
Subscale:	*Difficulties*	
	Spearman-Brown	.7512
	Guttman Split-Half	.7491
Subscale:	*Feelings*	
	Spearman-Brown	.8709
	Guttman Split-Half	.8685
Subscale:	*Problems*	
	Spearman-Brown	.6360
	Guttman Split-Half	.6316
Subscale:	*Stressful situations*	
	Spearman-Brown	.8514
	Guttman Split-Half	.8280
Subscale:	*Coping behavior*	
	Spearman-Brown	.8494
	Guttman Split-Half	.8484

Table 21-10

Test-Retest Reliability of the Stress Management Questionnaire
Correlations Between First and Second Administrations of the Stress Management
Questionnaire, at 1 Month Apart (n = 45)

Subscale	Correlation	Significance
Symptoms	.6518	$P < .0009$
Difficulties	.6520	$P < .0009$
Feelings	.4716	$P < .001$
Problems	.7695	$P < .0009$
Situations	.8188	$P < .0009$
Coping	.7400	$P < .0009$

nology with such significant impact on activity should make computer technology an area of significant interest to all therapists.[15-19] Microcomputers are being used as essential equipment in treatment, such as cognitive rehabilitation, hand strengthening, quality assurance, test scoring, and documentation of patient progress.[20-26]

An analysis of occupational therapy literature by Angelo and Smith, covering the period 1978 to 1988, found that of 174 articles identified as specific to computer use in occupational therapy, few were found to be of an experimental or quasi-experimental type.[26] Two recent studies that would seem to meet the criteria of an experimental or quasi-experimental were found. One by King, measuring the use of the computer in therapy for hand strengthening.[23] Another by Ross studied the use of computers in occupational therapy for visual-scanning training.[27] Some additional benefits of the use of computers in occupational therapy is patient self-regulation and reduced administrative time in documenting patient progress. Computer usage in conjunction with telemedicine can expand therapist availability and coverage, including in rural and underserved areas.

Computerized Versions of Standardized Tests

A 1990 study showed that 19% of psychologists used computers clinically for test administration. Matarazzo stated, "I predict that the requisite validation research will be published during the next several decades to make such computerized psychological assessment both practical and socially responsive."[28] Lukin proposed that computerized testing techniques could provide comparable results to traditional assessments.[29] He found, based on post-test assessment, that subjects preferred using the computer for testing. Kennedy, Wilkes, Dunlap, and Kuntz found no differences by administration mode.[30] Kobak, Reynolds, Rosenfeld, and Greist found a high correlation between the two forms for all groups.[31] Booth-Kewley, Edwards, and Rosenfeld found that computer and paper and pencil modes of administration yielded similar results and that subjects found the computer version more interesting.[32] Sanitioso and Reynolds, in a computerized administration of the EPI (extroversion and neuroticism), did not show significant difference between the computer form and the paper and pencil test.[33] However, George, found statistically significant differences between computer and paper and pencil forms for the Beck and State Anxiety inventories.[34] The Depression and State Anxiety scores obtained were significantly greater for the computer condition than for the paper and pencil condition. George suggested that computer anxiety may artificially inflate negative-effect scores during computer administration. Sanitioso and Reynolds reported statistically significant differences in scores for Lie and Impulsivity scales.[27]

Assessment is a promising area for the use of the computer by occupational therapists. Computers could improve client care by providing more accuracy and reliability in evaluations and assessments. There is the potential for new assessment paradigms for understanding human performance. Greater test reliability might also be obtained due to more accurate control of stimulus material. Standardized presentation may lead to improved comparability of tests' results. Computers may provide more intrinsically motivating tests and improve privacy of testing. Computers can eliminate some (evaluator) tester bias.[20,30,33,35-37] Along with benefits there are possible concerns. Computer testing may not be equivalent to currently used standardized paper and pencil tests.[10] The reliability and validity of data for a traditional version of a test may not be equivalent to a computerized version. Some studies have found traditional psychological tests and computer versions equivalent, others have been shown to elicit different responses.[38]

Comparison of Paper Test to Computerized Version of SMQ

Natz developed a computerized version of the SMQ with printed reports of the test results and a stored database of scores obtained.[14] Once the software was written, the investigator compared the results of the SMQ in a paper and pencil form with a computerized version of the SMQ. The study was conducted over a 3-week period. Following screening, each subject was given a written form of the SMQ in the first test session. Eight students at the University of South Dakota participated in the study. One week later the computerized version of the questionnaire was given. A second paper and pencil version of the questionnaire was given to each subject at least 1 week after the computer version. In all cases the re-test was taken at least 1 week after the previous test.

There were four screening criteria for the sample group:

1. Subject ages were between 18 and 22.
2. Subjects had a Computer Anxiety Index (CAIN)[39,41] score of 116 or less. The CAIN was administered to control for computer anxiety to be certain that measurements reflect real differences in computerized forms versus printed tests and not a measurement of the computer anxiety of the study group. The CAIN is an attitude index measured on a 6-point Likert scale. Scoring was made in the forward and reverse order method common for this type of scale.
3. The subjects were available for all three test dates.
4. The subjects had not taken the SMQ prior to the study.

RESEARCH DESIGN

The computer version of the SMQ was administered on IBM PS/2 model 30s, with color displays, a keyboard, and a mouse that was used for input. Each mouse click was recorded with a date and time stamp. This allowed for the analysis of time spent per question and total time per test. Individual appointments were made with the subjects, and following instructions on the use of the computer, subjects were allowed to work independently in the Occupational Therapy Department at the university.

The primary approach to analyzing data in this study was to find the percentage match for paired dependent samples. This measured the concordance between the answers given on paper forms of the SMQ and the computer form. Paper-to-paper results were compared, and participants' evaluations of the SMQ were reported.

On the computer screen the SMQ provided subjects with a list of symptoms, stressors, or coping activities, and asked the subjects to indicate whether items in the list applied (selection items). Upon completion of each of these sections, the subject was asked to choose and rank items from 1 to 10. If an item was selected or ranked in the first paper session and was selected again when a subject completed the computerized form, this was counted as a match. This procedure was used for all session data. The SMQ paper forms and computer-administered forms were compared in two ways. All selection items (SI) on the questionnaire were compared and frequency counts taken. Subject ranked items (SRI) were then matched and frequency counts taken. The data from the three sessions were labeled as paper-to-computer (PC), computer-to-paper (CP) and paper-to-paper forms (PP). Subject-ranked data (SRD) were labeled in the same manner—paper to computer-ranked (PCR), computer to paper-ranked (CPR), and paper to paper (PPR).

A comparison with data available from two studies of the SMQ by Stein,[2] and Bentley and Stein[11] was made using ranked SI data from this study with SRI from the previous tests.

RESULTS

The sample for this study was made up of eight subjects. The mean age for the sample was 19.9 years; mean education level in years for the group was 13.7 years; 100% were students; 75% were single and 25% married; and 75% were female and 25% male. The CAIN[39] scores obtained for this sample of students ranged from a high of 69 to a low of 28. The CAIN has a possible high score of 155 and a possible low score of 26, with a higher score indicating a higher level of computer anxiety. The mean for college students on the CAIN is 62.3. A score of 116 or higher was designated as a score too high to be a participant in this study. The mean of 45 for this sample was below the reported mean for a group of college students. The question of equivalence was addressed by comparing the percentage of items matching between test sessions in two broad categories of SI and SRI. With a further break down by symptoms, stressors, and coping activities, the range of percentage matching SI for symptoms was found to be 80.9% PP to 86.5% CP. Stressors ranged from 78.7% (PC) to 86.5% (CP). Coping activities ranged from 86.5% (PC) to 88.3% (CP). For all items, percentages were 83.3% (PC), 87% (CP), and 82.8% (PP). Most matching items came from comparing paper to computer and computer to paper. The lowest was paper to paper.

The range of percentage matching SRI, for symptoms was found to be 50.0% PP to 56.3% CPR, stressors 57.6% (PPR) to 67.6% (CPR), and coping activities 65.0% (CPR) to 67.5% (PCR). The percentages for all items were 61.3% (PCR), 62.9% (CPR), and 57.1% (PP). The two highest scores again were in comparing paper to computer, computer to paper, with the lowest paper to paper.

Results are consistent for each category of symptoms, stressors, and activity copers. All SI show a test retest of 84%. SRI also show consistent numbers in the range of 50% to 67%, with an overall of 60.4%. Given these results, further analysis was done comparing SRI from previous studies. The frequency of SI in the symptoms section of the SMQ was compared with two previous studies of the SMQ by Stein[2] and Bentley and Stein.[11] The frequency of symptoms of stress in the SI for this study was found to be in concordance with 91% of subject-ranked symptoms, 66% of stressors, and 83% of coping activities.

SMQ Self-Evaluation Results

Comparisons were made with the evaluation results (ER) from the third test session of the SMQ from this study and compared with the results obtained from previous studies by Stein[2] and Bentley and Stein.[11] In general the results were consistent with the previous studies. All of the subjects felt that the test was not too long—91.7% felt that the instructions were clear; 100% felt that the questionnaire was interesting; 87.5% felt that the list of items accurately reflected their feelings; 87.5% thought that the SMQ helped them become more aware of the stressors in their everyday life; 87.5% thought that they had identified a new method of dealing with stress from taking the questionnaire; and 87.5% felt that they might benefit from an individualized stress management program.

Conclusions of the Natz Study

The purpose of this study was to develop a computerized version of the SMQ, with printed reports of the test results and a stored database of scores obtained by subject. This software was used to examine the equivalence to the SMQ in a paper and pencil form. The results positively supported the equivalence of the paper and pencil form to the computerized version. In the comparison of all selected items, subjects selected the same items over three test sessions 84% of the time, which is comparable with reported test retest results of the SMQ in paper form of 85% to 89%. The comparison of symptoms that most frequently are selected by subjects using the SMQ is in agreement with previous studies—91% of those items selected in this study were also ranked highest in frequency in previous studies; stressors showed a 66% concordance; and activities showed a 83% concordance. Comparison of paper to computer (PC) and computer to paper (CP) was higher in both selection items (SI) and subject ranked items (SRI) for this study then the paper to paper (PP) comparison.

SUGGESTIONS FOR FUTURE RESEARCH

Future study of the computer version of the SMQ should include computer to computer (CC) data. This would provide additional evidence of test-retest equivalency. This study while supporting the equivalency of the computerized version of the SMQ also provides evidence of the impact of test "form" changes on test-retest results. A study to enumerate which elements of test "form" can cause converted tests not to be equivalent and possible solutions might be useful to test designers and to the software designers of converting tests. Further research is needed to determine which elements of computerized assessments, such as screen changes, have an impact on the test taker, and what effects they have on the results.

SUMMARY

The SMQ appears to be a valid and reliable test instrument that can be used for profiling an individual's stress reactions and coping mechanisms. It has the potential for a wide use in clinical practice and in health-promotion programs. In a pilot study a computerized version of the SMQ was shown to be highly reliable and equivalent to the paper and pencil form. Further research is needed to establish homogeneous norms and to validate the computerized version of the SMQ.

REFERENCES

1. Selye H. *Stress Without Distress.* Philadelphia, Pa: JB Lippincott Co; 1974.
2. Stein F. *Reliability and Validity of the Stress Management Questionnaire.* Unpublished manuscript. University of Wisconsin-Milwaukee; 1986.
3. Stein F, Neville SA. *Biofeedback, locus of control and reduction of anxiety in alcohol dependent adults.* Unpublished manuscript. University of Wisconsin-Milwaukee; 1987.
4. Stein F, Nikolic S. Teaching stress management techniques to a schizophrenic patient. *Am J Occup Ther.* 1989a;43:162-169.
5. Stein F, Smith J. Short-term stress management programme with acutely depressed in-patients. *Canadian Journal of Occupational Therapy.* 1989b;56:185-192.
6. Cannon WB. *The Wisdom of the Body.* New York, NY: Norton; 1939.
7. Selye H. A syndrome produced by diverse nocuous agents. *Nature.* 1936;138:32.
8. Holmes TH, Rahe RH. The Social Readjustment Rating Scale. *J Psychosom Res.* 1967;11:213-218.
9. Kanner AD, Coyne JC, Schaefer C, Lazarus RS Comparison of two modes of stress measurement: Daily hassles and uplifts versus major life events. *J Behav Med.* 1981;4:1-39.
10. Lazarus R, Folkman S. *Stress, Appraisal and Coping.* New York, NY: Springer; 1984.

11. Bentley DE, Stein F. *The Stress Management Questionnaire:Development and Work in Progress.* Paper presented at NATCOM, Ottowa, Ontario;1994.

12. Walker SN, Sechrist KR, Pender NJ. The Health-Promoting Lifestyle Profile: Development and Psychometric characteristics. *Nursing Research.* 1987;36:76-81.

13. Kohn PM, MacDonald JE. The survey of recent life experiences: A decontaminated hassles scale for adults. *J Behav Med.* 1992;15:221-236.

14. Natz M. *Comparing computer based and traditional versions of the Stress Management Questionnaire in a general population sample.* Unpublished manuscript. University of South Dakota at Vermillion; 1995.

15. Simmons Market Research Bureau Inc. *Study of Media and Markets.* New York, NY: Author; 1991:28, 163.

16. Frankenfeld FM. Trends in computer hardware and software. *Am J of Hospital Pharmacy.* 1993; 50(4):707-711.

17. Hammel JM, Van-der-Loos HFM, Perkash I. Evaluation of a vocational robot with a quadriplegic employee. *Arch Phys Med Rehab.* 1992;71:683-93.

18. Matarazzo JD. Computerized psychological testing (Editorial). *Science.* 1983; 221:323.

19. Matarazzo JD. Clinical psychological test interpretations by computer: Hardware outpaces software. Special Issue: Computer Assessment and Interpretation: Prospects, Promise and Pitfalls. *Computers in Human Behavior.* 1985;1(3-4):235-253.

20. Smith RO. Computer assisted functional assessment and documentation. *Am J Occup Ther.* 1993;47:988-991.

21. Lau C, O'Leary S. Comparison of computer interface devices for persons with severe physical disabilities. *Am J Occup Ther.* 1993;47:1022-1029.

22. Farrell WJ, Muik EA. Computer applications that streamline test scoring and other procedures in occupational Therapy. *Am J Occup Ther.* 1993;47:462-465.

23. King TI. Hand strengthening with a computer for purposeful activity. *Am J Occup Ther.* 1993;47:635-637.

24. Buning ME, Hanzlik JR. Adaptive computer use for a person with visual impairment. *Am J Occup Ther.* 1993;47:998-1008.

25. Taylor B, Cupo ME, Sheredos SJ. Workstation robotics: A pilot study of a desktop vocational assistant robot. *Am J Occup Ther.* 1993;47:1009-1014.

26. Angelo J, Smith RO. An analysis of computer-related articles in occupational therapy periodicals. *Am J Occup Ther.* 1993;47:25-29.

27. Ross FL. The use of computers in occupational therapy for visual-scanning training. *Am J Occup Ther.* 1992;46:314-322.

28. Matarazzo JD. Psychological testing and assessment in the twenty-first century. *American Psychologist.* 1992;47:1007-1018.

29. Lukin, et al. Comparing computerized versus traditional psychological assessment. *Computers in Human Behavior.* 1985;2:49-58.

30. Kennedy RS, Wilkes RL, Dunlap WP, Kuntz LA. Development of an automated performance test system for environmental and behavioral toxicology studies. *Perceptual and Motor Skills.* 1987;65:947-962.

31. Kobak KA, Reynolds WM, Rosenfeld R, Greist JH. Development and validation of a computer-administered version of the Hamilton Depression Rating Scale. *Psychological Assessment.* 1990;2:56-63.

32. Booth-Kewley S, Edwards JE, Rosenfeld P. Impression management, social desirability, and computer administration of attitude questionnaires: Does the computer make a difference? *J Appl Psychol.* 1992;77(4):562-566.

33. Sanitioso R., Reynolds JH. Comparability of standard and computerized administration of two personality questionnaires. *Personality and Individual Differences.* 1992;12:899-907.

34. George CE, Lankford JS, Wilson SE. The effects of computerized versus paper-and-pencil administration on measures of negative affect. *Computers in Human Behavior.* 1992;8:203-209.

35. Brauer GW. Telehealth: the delayed revolution in health care. *Medical Progress and Technology.* 1992;18(3):151-63.

36. Kern J, Dezelic G, Durrigl, Vuletic S. Medical decision making based on inductive learning method. *Artificial Intelligence-Med.* 1993;5(3):213-23.

37. Berney B. Round and round it goes: the epidemiology of childhood lead poisoning, 1950-1990. *Milbank-Q.* 1993;71(1):3-39.

38. Groth-Marnat G, Schumaker J. Computer-based psychological testing: Issues and guidelines. *Am J Orthopsychiatry.* 1989;59:257-263.

39. Matarazzo JD. Computerized clinical psychological test interpretations: Unvalidated plus all mean and no sigma. *American Psychologist.* 1986;41:14-24.

40. Simola SK, Holden RR. Equivalence of computerized and standard administration of the Piers-Harris Children's Self-Concept Scale. *J Pers Assess.* 1992;61:287-294.

41. Simonson M, Montage M, Maurer M, Oviatt L, Whitaker M. *Computer Anxiety Index (CAIN).* Ames, Iowa: Iowa State University Foundation, Inc; 1992.

PART IX:
RESEARCH CONCEPTS USED IN THE DEVELOPMENT OF ASSESSMENTS

22

Research Principles Used in Developing Assessments in Occupational Therapy

Nancy J. Powell, PhD, OTR, FAOTA

Occupational therapy assessments are vital to the survival of the profession. If occupational therapy is going to take its unique place among health care providers, therapists must provide valuable evaluation information to the treatment team and be accountable for the outcomes of their intervention. The past two decades have seen an emphasis on the development and use of valid, reliable instruments to assess occupation and related domains of function. Occupational therapists at all levels need to be involved in developing, improving, and evaluating assessment tools.

The purposes of this chapter are twofold. The first is to guide potential assessment developers with an overview of the basic information needed. It is hoped that graduate students, practicing therapists, and beginning faculty will find this chapter helpful in learning basic concepts and selected techniques for evaluation tool development. The second is to assist students and therapists in developing a deeper understanding of the research principles underlying the construction of evaluation instruments, so they can examine more critically the tools they choose to use in practice.

BASICS OF ASSESSMENT

Definitions

It is important to have consistent definitions of assessment, evaluation, and measurement in any research effort. First, assessment, according to the *Uniform Terminology for Occupational Therapy*, Second Edition, is "… the planned process of obtaining, interpreting, and documenting the functional status of the individual."[1] It is a holistic data-gathering process that includes obtaining patient information from records, such as a chart, observing the patient and family, interviewing family members, and administering one or more testing procedures or evaluation tools. By engaging in this process, dysfunction or risk for dysfunction can be identified, and appropriate occupational therapy can be planned.

Evaluation in this chapter refers to gathering data on performance, such as activities of daily living or observation, using a specific tool or tools in one or more areas.

Tools used as part of the assessment process will be identified as evaluation instruments in this chapter.

Measurement is "...quantifying or assigning a number to express the degree to which a characteristic is present."[2] In occupational therapy, the phenomena of interest are behaviors or performance of patients and families. Therapists are searching for the true, accurate amount of some characteristic related to function. A therapist might be evaluating the amount of independence a patient has, the degree to which a patient is oriented, or the number of leisure skills in which a patient participates. Classical measurement theory states that any measurement consists of a person's true score on a test, plus an error component.

Types of Evaluation in Occupational Therapy

Criterion-referenced tests are those which present predetermined standards or criteria that a patient is expected to achieve. This is most commonly performed occupational therapy evaluation. Developers of these kinds of evaluation instruments first choose an area or domain that they want to assess, for example, daily living skills. Then skills are selected, such as face washing, hair combing, or shirt buttoning. These may be scored on a nominal scale of satisfactory or not satisfactory.

Norm-referenced evaluation instruments are those where an individual's performance is compared to the performance of others or normative data. These are the least common in mental health assessment in occupational therapy, probably because these are the most time-consuming and costly to develop. Developers of this kind of tool decide which performance areas or characteristics they wish to assess. Then, they construct test items to assess the characteristics. The norming process consists of administering the instrument to large numbers of the target population for whom the instrument was developed. Procedures in administering and scoring the instrument are standardized. Specifically, testing equipment, instructions to the patient, and contextual elements are all kept the same to ensure that the assessment is always given the same way.

VALIDITY IN EVALUATION DEVELOPMENT

Validity is defined as the extent to which an evaluation measures what it is supposed to measure. In mental health assessment, validity represents the truthfulness of the instrument about a trait or behavior. For example, a therapist might wish to evaluate how oriented a mentally impaired patient is to his or her environment. The tested trait is orientation. The evaluation tool used needs to accurately measure orientation. The Mini-Mental State Examination (MMSE) is one such evaluation.[3]

Types of Validity

Validity can be broken down into several types. The first type is content validity. If an evaluation tool has content validity, the content of the test covers aspects of the area being assessed as completely as possible. For example, with reality orientation, the tool must cover orientation to at least person, place, and time, or it would not be comprehensive enough. A test developer is concerned with how many test items are necessary to cover all the major aspects of the behavior or trait being measured, as well as if the format of the test is suited to gathering information relevant to the trait or behavior.

Construct validity refers to ensuring that a test remains true to the domain it purports to assess. For example, one would not include items about dressing performance on a test of orientation; these would be better suited to a test that assessed occupational performance.

Groth-Marnat explains criterion validity as being "...determined by comparing the test scores with some sort of performance on an outside measure."[4] He divides criterion validity into two kinds—concurrent and predictive. Concurrent occurs when a test is compared to another similar tool that is taken at approximately the same time. For example, the MMSE[3] could be compared to another test of orientation, or scores on two measures of functional performance might be compared.

The second type of validity discussed by Groth-Marnat is predictive validity.[4] This kind of validity is established when a test is compared to another similar test taken after a period of time. For example, a patient might be tested on a vocational evaluation, then tested 2 years later on a work performance evaluation at a job site. Groth-Marnat states that predictive validity is best sought for tests of selection and classification of personnel.[4] Occupational therapists possibly could use this sort of validation of tests used for work placement of patients. He concludes that concurrent validity might be of most concern to those developing tests that measures a patient's current status on some trait. In occupational therapy, such a trait might be functional performance in self-care.

Aiken[5] states that factors affecting validity include heterogeneity and length of the test. Generally, the shorter and more homogeneous the group taking the test, the less the variability will affect validity.

Methods to Establish Content and Construct Validity

There are a variety of ways that evaluation developers can check the validity of the tools they develop. Content and construct validity can be verified by having a panel of experts examine the test. In relation to content validity, Brown suggests using scales on which judges can rate coverage of the area being tested, the appropriateness of the format of the items, and the emphasis of important points.[6] When using this method, he points out that interrater reliability can be calculated and then serve as an index of content validity. Aiken also points out that experts can analyze the processes the patients have to go through to respond to the test items.[5] He also urges test developers to use experts to help establish validity as the tool is being developed. He suggests another specific method to use early on, which is comparing test content to an outline from written works on the subject or to a table of contents of a published work of the domain being tested.

Aiken suggests several methods to use to establish construct validity.[5] Specifically, these are using experts' judgments, analyzing the internal consistency of the test, correlating the test with other related tests and factor analyses of these intercorrelations, and the querying of testees and raters about the mental processes they go through completing the evaluation. Groth-Marnat reports the method for examining the internal consistency of a test is to correlate subtests within the tool to the test's total score.[4] For example, in occupational therapy, a subtest of items related to dressing might be correlated to the full scale of items on a functional performance evaluation.

RELIABILITY IN EVALUATION DEVELOPMENT

After validity, next in importance is the establishment of reliability. Validity cannot ensure reliability; a test can be reliable without being valid.

Definition of Reliability

Reliability is the stability of an evaluation tool over time. It means that barring any intervening factors, a patient will perform in a consistent manner on a test, ie, the test items will produce the same responses. Lack of reliability can result from errors in measurement which are produced by changes in the patient, such as fatigue or pain, or problems in the environment, such as distractions or temperature. The therapist using the evaluation must try to eliminate these sources of unreliability. Lack of reliability can also result from problems in test-item construction, such as the lack of clarity of an item, making interpretation of the item difficult.

Methods of Estimating Reliability

The first method of estimating reliability of any evaluation instrument is test-retest reliability. In this method, a test is given once, then repeated. The two test scores are correlated. Groth-Marnat states that the length of the interval between the two administrations of the test can affect reliability due to a practice effect.[4] In general, he recommends this kind of reliability assessment for relatively stable traits, such as problem-solving ability, not for traits that are likely to vary due to outside influences, such as work skills.

There are two types of test-retest reliability—alternate and parallel. The alternate form has two methods. In the first method, the order of the items is rearranged, for example, making item No. 1 on the initial test item No. 10 on the retest. This may prevent the test taker from remembering the test items. The second method involves using a different form of the same question, for example, by turning the question around.

The second type of test-retest reliability is the parallel form. Here the test writer writes two similar items on the same content. Then puts one of the items on the first test and one on the retest. For example, on a test of adaptive behavior, one item could be making change for a 75-cent item from a dollar in quarters. The similar item put on the retest could be making change for a 50-cent item from a dollar in quarters. In contrast to the alternate form, this method eliminates the memory effect. Drawbacks to this method are expense and uncertainty whether the two tests are parallel.

Another area of testing the reliability of evaluations involves measures of internal consistency. These measurements include split-half reliability, Kuder-Richardson method, and Cronbach's alpha. Aiken states that these measures of internal consistency do not reflect errors in measurement caused by different conditions and times of measurement, so they are not equivalent to the test-retest methods.[5] The split-half method involves dividing the items in the evaluation into two parts arbitrarily; for example, a test may be divided into Part A, items 1-20, and Part B, items 21-40. A statistical test of correlation can then be run between the scores on Part A and the scores on Part B. Also, the items on an evaluation could be split by odd- and even-numbered items. This is similar to the parallel form above, except the correlation is between items on a single test, given at one time.

Carey described the Kuder-Richardson internal consistency reliability index.[2] He states that this method is to be used for objective-style tests that have items that are scored correct or incorrect. The index compares the sum of the item variances with the total test variance. Factors that affect the score on the index are content homogeneity, group homogeneity, test length, and item difficulty. Kuder-Richardson indices are typically generated by computer-scored tests and range from .00 to 1.00. Carey states that values at about .80 indicate good internal consistency for classroom-type tests.[2]

Cronbach's alpha extends the Kuder-Richardson index in that it can be used for measures other than that of ability.[7] Thorndike explains that this internal consistency measure "...is based on the idea that each item is a parallel form 'minitest,' and the overall reliability is an average of all interitem correlations, corrected to the length of the total test."[7] Carey states that the Kuder-Richardson and Cronbach's alpha give support for the homogeneity of the test. These two measures can be accessed on computerized statistical programs.[2]

DESIGNING AN EVALUATION

The concepts of validity and reliability are fundamental to evaluation instrument development. Once these concepts are understood by the would-be evaluation developer, then the process of construction can begin. Because this is not a textbook of test construction, the instrument development process has been condensed to a set of 10 steps that will serve as guidelines for the development of the kinds of evaluations used in mental health. The steps that will be described below are expanded from the work on test construction by Kline[8] and listed below. A brief description of each step follows the list.

1. Identify the domain or area to be evaluated.
2. Formulate a comprehensive outline of the content or behaviors related to the domain.
3. Select the type of evaluation format best suited to the domain.
4. Write the test items.
5. Perform validity checks.
6. Field-test the instrument.
7. Analyze the instrument.
8. Standardize the evaluation.
9. Write the evaluation manual.
10. Seek a publisher!

Identify a Domain or Area to Evaluate

An idea for an evaluation may come from three different sources—a need in one's clinical practice, a needs assessment, or a need written about by experts or other test developers in the mental health occupational therapy literature. Once the area is selected, the literature on assessment of that area or domain should be thoroughly reviewed. Also, a survey of experts or a focused needs assessment for an evaluation instrument can also be done. At this point, funding for evaluation instrument development can be sought. For example, some foundations, such as the AOTF, might fund the development of a needed evaluation. One might also try a publishing house (see step 10) or government agencies, such as state developmental disabilities councils or departments of mental health to obtain funding for instrument development.

Formulate a Comprehensive Outline

This step will help ensure content validity. The developer should write a comprehensive outline of areas to be evaluated that are related to the construct of interest. For example, in constructing an assessment of work aptitude, the items related to attendance, punctuality, attitude toward work, ability to relate to people, manual dexterity, and other related areas must be identified.

Select a Type of Evaluation

In this step, the developer needs to decide which kind of evaluation format best fits the kind of behavior or trait that is being examined. Examples of formats are observation checklists, Likert scales, objective tests, or behavioral rating scales. In the above example of a work aptitude evaluation, perhaps an observation checklist would be best. The evaluator would check off items related to performing the occupation of work. On punctuality, the patient might be given a check for an item stating "usually on time."

Write the Test Items

Now, the evaluation developer is finally ready to do what some people try to do first, write the test items. Clarity and understandability of the items to patients and evaluators is the key to making the test reliable and valid. The language should be at the reading level of the patients to be tested if reading by them is involved. Professional terminology that is current and accepted in occupational therapy should be used, so that an occupational therapist using the instrument can understand what is involved. Two traits or behaviors should not be included in one item. For example, in the work aptitude evaluation discussed above, an item should not state both punctuality and attendance. As these are two different behaviors, interpretation of the item will be difficult. If appropriate, it is also a good idea to include some filler items that everyone can answer correctly, so as not to discourage the test taker (EM Hockman, PhD; personal communication, May 1, 1998).

Perform Validity Checks

Once the evaluation is written, the real work begins. At this point, the developer usually needs to seek help from experts to see if the evaluation instrument completely measures what it is intended to measure. The evaluation should be reviewed by no fewer than three experts.

Field-Test the Instrument

Finally, the valid instrument is ready to try out on real live people. It is best to choose people who have similar traits to the patients for which the evaluation is intended; Kline stresses that the field-test sample must be similar to the one for which the test is intended.[8] For example, if developing a measure of work aptitude for patients with mental impairment, then field-test the instrument on people with this impairment. Limiting the size of the field-test population to less than 40 is not recommended.[8] This number will enable the developer to use more powerful statistics to analyze the field-test results.

Analyze the Instrument

In this step, the developer will analyze the results of the field-test. It is beyond the scope of this chapter to instruct in depth in test analysis, but two methods will be briefly discussed. Kline has described the item analytic method as the best, and most simple way to construct a homogeneous test, ie, one containing items measuring the same characteristic.[8] After field-testing the pool of items, the developer can run a statistical analysis to determine the item difficulty (p) or the item mean for each item, such as an attitude evaluation item, by asking for a response on a scale of 1 to 5 (EM Hockman, PhD; personal communication, May 1, 1998). P is the proportion who answered the item correctly on a test such as a multiple-choice test. On a test with dichotomous answers, eg, this trait is like me or this trait is not like me, it is the proportion who answered in the scored direction, who chose the answer representing the trait being measured. For attitude scales, it is the item mean (EM Hockman, PhD; personal communication, May 1, 1998).

Next, a corrected correlation, the Pearson product moment correlation or r, can be calculated for each item, which is a correlation between the item response and the sum of the responses to all the other test items minus the item whose correlation is being computed. For example, if on a 10-item test, the developer is trying to correlate item No. 6, this item is correlated with the sum of items 1 through 5, plus 7 through 10 (EM Hockman, PhD; personal communication, May 1, 1998). The correlation should be positive; in Kline's opinion, the correlation should be >0.30.[8] Filler items—the easy items discussed in the Write the Test Items section—are expected to show a very low correlation. Negative item correlations are not acceptable and should be discarded (EM Hockman, PhD; personal communication, May 1, 1998).

If the evaluation is an attitude scale, examine an item receiving a strong negative correlation to determine if the polarity of the response to the item is correct. For example, does the scored response need to be flip-flopped, with the low score on the scale now representing the attitude being evaluated, not the high score on that item? If a scoring problem is apparent, the scoring must be corrected and recomputed (EM Hockman, PhD; personal communication, May 1, 1998).

Also, in Kline's opinion, a p value for an item should be between .20 and .80; but, if the r is high, then it is acceptable to keep the item.[8] He states that the aim of the test is to discriminate those with a certain characteristic such as anxiety from those who do not have this trait. An item with a p of .50, therefore, is maximally discriminating.

After checking that all items reach the recommended p and r values, items can be discarded or rewritten. Then, it is recommended that a second field test be performed, and the p and r values for rewritten items be rechecked.

The second step in instrument analysis is to compute the Cronbach's alpha. This is the final reliability check. If all items survive, then a reliable and homogeneous evaluation tool has been devised.

Although some measures of validity were initially done in the construction of the evaluation, now as the final part of this step, the developer may want to perform concurrent validity checks. If another test is available that assesses the same characteristic as the newly developed test, an analysis can be performed to see if scores on the old test and the new test correlate. If the scores correlate, this adds validity to the newly developed instrument.

Standardize the Evaluation

Tallent describes three criteria that evaluations must exhibit to become widely accepted, standardized tools: 1) demonstrate adequate validity; 2) have precise instructions that administrators must follow including strict time limits, if applicable; and 3) be normed correctly.[9]

Norming a test involves giving the test to the non-disabled population in, for example, a similar age range. This will enable the scores of persons with suspected disability to be compared to the scores of those without disability. Kline has stated that the two most crucial characteristics of normal samples are that they be large and representative.[8] How large the sample should be is dependent on the heterogeneity of the sample. His recommendations are from 5000 for a heterogeneous group, to 300 if special subgroup norms are formed. In addition, the sample must represent the population as a whole and not be biased by the variable studied. For example, on a test for work aptitude, it must include equal numbers of males and females. Lastly, Kline recommends that the instrument developer decide how best to describe the norms and score the test.[8] For example, would stanines or percentile ranks be best?

Write the Evaluation Manual

Well-written, complete, and clear user manuals need to accompany all evaluations that are developed. The contents of a manual are described by Kline.[8] His ideas are expanded and applied to occupational therapy evaluation instruments below in the approximate order in which they might best appear.

Introduction and Description

The need for the evaluation, the occupational therapy theory relating to the instrument, and the background of the development of the tool can be described here to orient the user. The domains or areas of human performance should be described in sufficient detail. The aims and purposes of the instrument need to be clearly described. An overview of the contents is designated in this section, as is the length of time needed to administer the instrument.

Population

Describe for whom the test is devised, ie, the parents of children with autism or the adult with schizophrenia, and to whom it should not be given. It is hoped that this latter information will help dissuade misuse of the instrument.

Standardization and Analysis Sections

Give detailed information to the users on the methods used to standardize the test. Include a description of the population used to norm the test. Identify the validity and reliability checks done and report the related statistical results.

Administration Qualifications

Cite the professionals who, by tradition, may be qualified to give the evaluation. Identify if special training is necessary to administer the instrument and where that training is available.

Materials and Environmental Requirements

List and describe any materials needed to give the test, eg, stopwatch, paper, and pencil. Specify where the evaluation is to be given, eg, in a testing room, with a group of patients in a classroom.

Precautions

Point out to the user which precautions need to be taken into account, if any, during the testing. These precautions can be related to the performance required on test items, test materials used, or physical and mental disabilities the patient may have.

Protocol

Clearly describe the instructions for administering the test. For example, describe what the administrator specifically says and does item by item.

Scoring Instructions

Detail how the evaluation is scored, and include methods and forms that have been developed to help report the outcomes clearly.

Seek a Publisher

Once you have an idea for developing an evaluation, do a needs assessment to see what has been published. At this time, note which publishers publish the type of instrument you wish to develop. Write to secure the author guidelines, if available, from those publishers you decide are the best. To get the best results, work from the beginning with a representative of the company you choose.

Ethics in Evaluation Development

There are three major ethical considerations in evaluation tool development. The first is the unauthorized use of test items from someone else's evaluation. Whenever a test developer "borrows" items from an instrument developed by another author, credit in the form of a citation must be given to the original author of the item or items, and permission from the publisher obtained. In the past, it has been observed that personnel at clinical sites developed and adapted forms of published tests for which no permission had been sought or the original authors cited.

The second ethical issue is the development of evaluation tools that are culturally biased.[4] Developers need to make sure that the language in test items does not disadvantage any group of patients from responding in a truthful and complete way. When devising scoring procedures, developers need to take into consideration various responses related to culture. In the evaluation manual, developers need to point out any limitations, including the lack of generalizability of the instrument to ethnic and other groups.[10]

The third issue is developing an evaluation that is in another professional's turf. For example, an occupational therapist might attempt to develop an intelligence evaluation, which traditionally is in the area of psychology. Occupational therapy has had an especially difficult time in this area due to perceived or actual lack of definition of the profession and its boundaries. Scholars are ever expanding the theory of occupational therapy, and we need to keep pace with new, updated assessment and concomitant evaluation instrument development. We need to remain vigilant about the development of instruments in areas that are traditionally occupational therapy areas by others who are less qualified. Function suddenly appears to be every professional's area in the '90s, possibly resulting in more multidisciplinary evaluation tools.

SUMMARY

Future assessment studies in occupational therapy would do well to investigate treatment utility. Hayes et al have defined this as "...the degree to which assessment is shown to contribute to beneficial treatment outcome."[11] As Silva has stated, evaluators need to move from looking at whether assessment versus no assessment is desirable to improve treatment outcomes, to which specific assessment is most useful.[12] This calls for refinement and updating of existing evaluation tools and the assessment process in occupational therapy. More patient-centered, functional evaluation instruments are needed to provide better usefulness and guidance for therapists to design effective treatment procedures.

As occupational therapists, we need to move away from the medical model of developing evaluation tools and move toward community-based types of evaluation that enable or empower patients and their families. Evaluation can enable patients to obtain proper treatment, demonstrate when improvement has occurred, and capitalize on abilities. Evaluations must lead to clear treatment goals and objectives from which clearly discernable outcomes can be derived. In this age of cost containment, the benefits and outcomes of treatment are of utmost importance. Therefore, evaluation developers and users alike need to work with their professional organizations on outcomes research to ensure quality development and the appropriate use of evaluations.

REFERENCES

1.   American Occupational Therapy Association, Uniform Terminology Task Force and the Commission on Practice, Uniform Terminology for Occupational Therapy, 2nd ed. In Hopkins HL, Smith H, eds. *Willard and Spackman's Occupational Therapy*, 8th ed. Philadelphia, Pa: JB Lippincott Co; 1993.

2.   Carey L. *Measuring and Evaluating School Learning*, 2nd ed. Boston, Mass: Allyn and Bacon Inc; 1994:76.

3.   Folstein MF, Folstein S, McHugh PR. Mini-mental state: A practical method of grading the cognitive state of patients for the clinician. *J Psychiatr Res.* 1975;12:189

4.   Groth-Marnat G. *Handbook of Psychological Assessment.* New York, NY: Van Norstrand Rheinhold Co Inc; 1984:15.

5.   Aiken LR. *Psychological Testing and Assessment*, 8th ed. Needham Heights, Mass: Allyn and Bacon Inc; 1994.

6.   Brown, FG. *Principles of Educational and Psychological Testing*, 3rd ed. New York, NY: Holt, Reinhart and Winston; 1983.

7.   Thorndike RM. Reliability. In Bolton B. *Handbook of Measurement and Evaluation in Rehabilitation*, 2nd ed. Baltimore, Md: Paul Brookes Publishing Co; 1987:31.

8.   Kline P. How tests are constructed. In Beech JR, Harding L. *Testing People: A Practical Guide to Psychometrics.* Windsor, England: The Neer-Nelson Publishing Co Ltd; 1990.

9.   Tallent N. *The Practice of Psychological Assessment.* Englewood Cliffs, NJ: Prentice Hall; 1992.

10.   Canter MB, Bennett BE, Jones SE, Nagy TF. *Ethics for Psychologists: A Commentary on the APA Ethics Code.* Washington, DC: American Psychological Association; 1994.

11.   Hayes SC, Nelson RO, Jarrett, RB. The treatment utility of assessment: a functional approach to evaluating assessment quality. *American Psychologist.* 1987;42:963-974.

12.   Silva F. *Psychometric Foundations and Behavioral Assessment.* Thousand Oaks, Calif: Sage Publications; 1993.

The author wishes to thank Elaine M. Hockman, PhD, director of the Research Support Lab at Wayne State University, for her assistance with sections of this chapter.

APPENDICES

A

Comprehensive Occupational Therapy Evaluation Scale (COTE Scale)

	Initial	Week 1	Week 2	Week 3	Week 4
I. General Behavior **Date**					
A. Appearance					
B. Non-Productive Behavior					
C. Activity Level (a or b)					
D. Expression					
E. Responsibility					
F. Punctuality/Attendance					
G. Reality Orientation					
H. Conceptualization					
Sub-Total					
II. Interpersonal Behavior					
A. Independence					
B. Cooperation					
C. Self Assertion (a or b)					
D. Sociability					
E. Attention Getting Behavior					
F. Negative Response From Others					
Sub-Total					
III. Task Behavior					
A. Engagement					
B. Concentration					
C. Coordination					
D. Follow Directions					
E. Activity Neatness/Attention to Detail*					
F. Problem Solving					
G. Complexity and Organization of Task					
H. Initial Learning					
I. Interest in Activity					
J. Interest in Accomplishment					
K. Decision Making					
L. Frustration Tolerance					
Sub-Total					
Total					

Scale: 0=Normal; 1= Minimal; 2= Mild; 3=Moderate; 4=Severe
*Rate either Activity Neatness or Attention to Detail, not both
Comments:_____

_____Therapist   _____Date

Definitions of Terms for the
COTE Scale

I. General Behavior

A. Appearance
   The following six factors are involved: 1) clean skin, 2)clean hair, 3) hair combed, 4) clean clothes, 5) clothes neat, and 6) clothes suitable for occasion
   - 0- No problems in any area
   - 1- Problem in 1 area
   - 2- Problems in 2 areas
   - 3- Problems in 3 or 4 areas
   - 4- Problems in 5 or 6 areas

B. Non-Productive Behavior
   (Rocking, playing with hands, repetitive statements, appears to be talking to self, preoccupied with own thoughts, etc)
   - 0- No non-productive behavior during session
   - 1- Nonproductive behavior occasionally during session
   - 2- Nonproductive behavior for half of session
   - 3- Nonproductive behavior for three-fourths of session
   - 4- Nonproductive behavior for the entire session

C. Activity Level (A or B)
   (a)
   - 0-No Hyperactivity
   - 1- Occasional hyperactivity
   - 2- Hyperactivity attracts the attention of other patients and therapists, but participates
   - 3- Hyperactivity level such that can participate but with great difficulty
   - 4- So hypoactive that patient cannot participate in activity
   (b)
   - 0- No hyperactivity
   - 1- Occasional hyperactivity.
   - 2- Hyperactivity attracts the attention of other patients and therapists, but participates
   - 3- Hyperactivity level such that can participate but with great difficulty
   - 4- So hyperactive that patient cannot cannot participate in activity

D. Depression
   - 0- Expression consistent with situation and setting
   - 1- Communicates with expression, occasional inappropriate
   - 2- Shows inappropriate expression several times during session
   - 3- Show of expression but inconsistent with situation
   - 4- Extremes of expression-bizarre, uncontrolled or no expression

E. Responsibility
>   0- Takes responsibility for own actions
>   1- Denies responsibility for 1 or 2 actions
>   2- Denies responsibility for several actions
>   3- Denies responsibility for most actions.
>   4- Denial of all responsibility—messes up project and blames therapist or others

F. Attendance/Punctuality
>   0- Consistently ready for therapy
>   1- Needs encouragement 20% of time
>   2- Needs encouragement 50% of the time
>   3- Refuses up to 50 % of the time
>   4- Refuses more than 50% of the time

G. Reality Orientation
>   0- Complete awareness of person, place, time and situation
>   1- General awareness but inconsistency in 1 area
>   2- Awareness of 2 areas
>   3- Awareness in 1 area
>   4- Lack of awareness of person, place, time and situation

H. Conceptualization
>   0- Demonstrates abstract thinking
>   1- Responds abstractly 1 + times
>   2- Relevant concrete responses.
>   3- Responds concretely 1+ times
>   4- Responses unrelated to situation

II. Interpersonal

A. Independence
>   0- Independent functioning
>   1- Only 1 of 2 dependent actions
>   2- Half independent and half dependent actions
>   3- Only 1 of 2 independent actions
>   4- No independent actions

B. Cooperation
>   0- Cooperates with program
>   1- Follows most directions, opposes less than one half
>   2- Follows half/opposes half
>   3- Opposes three fourths
>   4- Opposes all directions/suggestions

C. Self-Assertion
>   (a)
>   0- Assertive when necessary
>   1- Passive < 50% of session
>   2- Passive 50% of session
>   3- Passive >50% of session
>   4- Passive entire session
>   (b)
>   0-Assertive when necessary
>   1- Dominant< 50% of session
>   2- Dominant 50% of session
>   3- Dominant >50% of session
>   4- Dominates aggressively

D. Sociability

    0- Socializes with staff and patients

    1- Socializes with staff and occasionally with other patients or vice versa

    2- Socializes only with staff or only with patients

    3- Socializes only if approached

    4- Does not join others in activities, unable to carry on casual conversation even if approached.

E. Attention-Getting Behavior

    0- No unreasonable attention-getting behavior

    1- Less than 50% of time spent in attention getting behavior

    2- 50% of time spent in attention-getting behavior

    3- 75% of time spent in attention-getting behavior

    4- Verbally or non-verbally demands constant attention

F. Negative Response from Others

    0- Evokes no negative responses

    1- Evokes 1 negative response

    2- Evokes 2 negative responses

    3- Evokes 3 or more negative responses during session

    4- Evokes numerous negative responses from others and therapist must take some action

III. Task Behavior

A. Engagement

    0- Needs no encouragement to begin task

    1- Encourage once to begin activity

    2- Encourage 2 or 3 times to engage in activity

    3- Engages in activity only after much encouragement

    4- Does not engage in activity

B. Concentration

    0- No difficulty concentrating during session

    1- Off task less than 25% of time

    2- Off task 50 % of time

    3- Off task 75% of time

    4- Loss of concentration on task in less than 1 minute

C. Coordination

    0- No problems with coordination

    1- Occasionally has trouble with fine detail, manipulating tools and material

    2- Occasionally trouble manipulating tools and materials but has frequent trouble with fine detail

    3- Some difficulty in gross movement—unable to manipulate some tools and materials

    4- Has great difficulty in movement (gross motor), virtually unable to manipulate tools and materials.

D. Follow Directions

    0- Carries out directions without problems

    1- Carries out simple directions; has trouble with 2 step directions

    2- Carries out single directions, has trouble with two

    3- Can carry out only very simple one step directions (demonstrated, written, or oral)

    4- Unable to carry out any directions

E. Activity Neatness

    0- Activity neatly done

    1- Occasionally ignores fine detail

    2- Often ignores fine detail and materials are scattered

    3- Ignores fine detail and work habits disturbing to those around

    4- Unaware of fine detail, so sloppy that therapist has to intervene

F. Attention to Detail
  0- Pays attention to detail appropriately
  1- Occasionally too concise
  2- More attention to several details than is required
  3- So concise that project will take twice as long as expected
  4- So concerned that project will never get finished

G. Problem Solving
  0- Solves problems without assistance
  1- Solves problems after assistance is given once
  2- Can solve only after repeated instructions
  3- Recognizes a problem but cannot solve it
  4- Unable to recognize or solve a problem

H. Complexity and Organization of Task
  0- Organizes and performs task given
  1- Occasionally has trouble with organization of complex activities that should be able to do
  2- Can organize simple but not complex activities
  3- Can do only very simple activities with organization imposed by therapist
  4- Unable to organize or carry out an activity when all tools, materials, and directions are available

I. Initial Learning
  0- Learns a new activity quickly and without difficulty
  1- Occasionally has difficulty learning a complex activity
  2- Has frequent difficulty learning a complex activity
  3- Unable to learn complex activities; occasionally difficulty learning simple activities
  4- Unable to learn a new activity

J. Interest in Activities
  0- Interested in a variety of activities
  1- Occasionally not interested in a new activity
  2- Shows occasional interest in a part of an activity
  3- Engages in activities but shows no interest
  4- Does not participate

K. Interest in Accomplishment
  0- Interested in finishing activities
  1- Occasional lack of interest or pleasure in finishing a long term activity
  2- Interest or pleasure in accomplishment of a short term activity—lack of interest in a long term activity.
  3- Only occasional interest in finishing any activity
  4- No interest or pleasure in finishing an activity

L. Decision Making
  0- Makes own decisions
  1- Makes decisions but occasionally seeks therapist's approval
  2- Make decisions but often seeks therapist's approval
  3- Makes decisions when given only 2 choices
  4- Cannot make any decisions or refuses to make a decision

M. Frustration Tolerance
  0- Handles all tasks without becoming overly frustrated
  1- Occasionally becomes frustrated with one or more complex tasks; can handle simple tasks
  2- Often becomes frustrated with more complex tasks, but is able to handle simple tasks
  3- Often becomes frustrated with any tasks, but attempts to continue
  4- Becomes so frustrated with simple tasks that refuses or is unable to function

Occupational Therapy Evaluation
(KidCOTE)

Demographic _____

Patient Goal _____

Evaluation Procedures Administered: __ Chart Review __ Task Evaluation __Clinical Observation

__Piers Harris __ Bruininks-Oseretsky __TVPS __ TVMS __Gessell

__ Other _____

General Behavior	ADM	D/C	Cognitive Behavior	ADM	D/C
Activities of Daily Living			Attention Span/Concentration		
Responsibility			Memory		
Reality Orientation			Sequencing and Categorization		
Attendance/Punctuality			Concept Formation		
			Problem Solving/Judgment		
Psychosocial Behaviors			Follows Directions		
Self-Concept			Organizational Skills		
Social Conduct			Decision Making		
Self-Expression			Initial Learning		
Coping Skills			Interest in Activity		
Time Management			Interest in Accomplishment		
Insight			Frustration Tolerance		

Scale:
  0 = WNL—Functions to satisfaction of self and environment; independent
  1 = MIN—Requires assist/cueing 1-2 times per session; occasional difficulties
  2 = MOD—Frequently needs assist 3+ times per session; requires supervision; frequent difficulties
  3 = SEVERE—Requires constant supervision or is completely unable to perform

Assets: _____ **Problems:** _____
          _____   _____
          _____   _____

Sensorimotor Performance:
Sensory Awareness/Processing _____
Neuromuscular
  Fine Motor
_____

  Gross Motor
_____

EXPECTED OUTCOMES:
_____
_____

SHORT TERM OBJECTIVES:
_____
_____
_____

TREATMENT PLAN:
_____

_____ Therapist _____ Date

Evaluation Results/Standardized Tests
Bruininks-Oseretsky Tests/Complete Battery

Gross Motor Composite	Sum	Standard Score	Percentile Rank	Stanine	Age Equivalent	Standard Deviation
Upper Limb Coordination Fine Motor Composite Battery Composite						

Short Form   Point Score ___   Standard Score ___   Percentile Rank ___   Stanine ___

Test of Visual Perception: Sum of Scaled Scores _____ Percentile Rank _____
                                  Perceptual Quotient _____ Median Perceptual Age _____
Test of Visual Motor Skills: Total Raw Scores _____ Motor Age _____
                                  Standard Scores _____ Percentile Rank _____
                                  Stanine _____
Piers Harris Self-Concept Scale: Raw Score _____ Percentile _____ Stanine _____
Clusters: Behavior _____ Intellectual _____ Physical Appearance _____
             Anxiety _____ Popularity _____ Happiness and Satisfaction _____

Other: _____

REPORT_____
_____
_____
_____
_____
_____
_____
_____
_____
_____
_____

RECOMMENDATIONS:
Consult Outpatient Occupational Therapy appointments for the following:
___ Social Skills Training
___ Developmental Assessment/Treatment
___ Sensory Motor

_____ Therapist _____ Date

D
Cognitive Adaptive Skills Evaluation: Protocol Sheet

Examinee Information:

Name: _____ Birth Date/Age: _____ Sex: _____
Floor/Unit: _____ Admitting and Discharge Diagnosis: _____
Test Date: _____ Indicate Day of Week Tested: _____
Examiner: _____ Length of Test Time: _____

Evaluation Materials:

12 inch ruler with numbers
One sheet each of 8 ½ x 11 paper
    (yellow, blue, pink, white)
#2 pencil with eraser
Three pens (one blue, one red, one black)
Box of eight assorted wax crayons
A sample calendar
Written directions, typed on an index card

Presentation of Materials:

All materials with the exception of the sample
calendar listed above are to be laid out directly
in front of the examinee. Writing tools and crayons
are to be placed in the same general area, in a group.
All sheets of paper are to be in a loose pile with
each sheet being exposed or visible to some degree;
in the following order: yellow, blue, pink, white.

General introduction to be given to examinee:
Examiner States: "I am interested in how you go about doing a task. I need this information in order
    to help plan a program with you. We will discuss what you have done after you have completed
    the activity."

Turn the page and go on to specific directions and interview questions. Check behaviors as observed;
    note additional behaviors and comments in the Comments column.

Directions	Behaviors and Categories	Checks	Comments/Examinee's Responses

Present written directions to the examinee.

(Allow silent reading time.)

Examiner states: "Please read the directions aloud and begin when you are ready."

(If the examinee begins to work and completes the task, note and record behaviors and proceed with first set of interview questions and direction #2.)

(If the examinee reads directions but does not begin to work, read direction #1 to the examinee.)

Examiner states:
#1. "Here are supplies. Use what you want to make a calendar for one week."

(If the examinee is unable to begin working after directions are read to him or her, read directions again and proceed to direction #3.)

(If the examinee can complete the task with no further directions, observe and record comments and behaviors.)

Proceed with interview questions.

Language
• Follows written directions
• Understands directions as given by "authority figure" (9)
• Attempts to perceive others' viewpoint; seems to know what is expected/being asked of him or her; seeks validation (8)

Cause and Effect
• Seems to have a plan, works rapidly, efficiently, systematically (10)
• Trial and Error behavior noted with objects, but works independently (9)
• Process seems inflexible; deliberate manipulation of objects (7-8)
• Tries to work with objects and process, seeks validation (5-6)

Images
• Seems to understand "calendar" and the steps involved in making one (9)
• Seeks validation about "what kind" of calendar (6)
• Seeks validation about own perception of "calendar" (6)

Judgement/Moral Behavior
• Knows the rules and agrees to follow them; engages in activity as presented (does not ask for extra materials or try to make something else) (9)
• Believes he or she knows the rules but tries to alter or refuse task (8)

Classification
• Can form classes and consider objects in several classes simultaneously (S to S=1 week; 7 days=1 week) (9)

Relations
• Has one to one correspondence; sees connection and knows S to S=7 days=1 week
• Equivalence unstable, confused by space; counting doesn't help (confuses days of week or number of days) (8)

Numbers
• Can arrange figures along some quantities dimension; seriation; can construct group of equal number and knows they are equal when spatial relations are changed or are counted in a different order (9)
• Counts repeatedly; changes size of figures to make them equal (7-8)

Directions	Behaviors and Categories	Checks	Comments/ Examinee's Responses

Interview questions: First set

Examiner asks: (One question at a time)

A. "What does the word calendar mean to you?"

Language
• Meanings are discussed in the abstract, hypothetical (10)
• Can discuss several meanings from different perspectives (9)
• Meanings deal with the present, here and now (8)
• Word has personal meaning based on own perception, intuition, experience (7)

B. "How did you decide what materials to use?"

Judgement/Decision Making
• Seems to have inner value system and a sense of moral judgement about use of materials (10)
• Choice seems to be part of a systematic plan (10)
• Past experience and desires influence behavior (7)
• Random selection; no thought

C. "Did you have a plan for making the calendar?"

(If response is yes, ask question C1; if no, skip to C2.)

C1. "Can you describe the plan to me?"

Cause and Effect (Problem Solving)
• Has a work plan; is rational, systematic flexible (10)
• Operations are concrete; apply only to objects physically present (9)
• Plan based on past experience (7-8)
• Convert trial and error; problem solved as they developed (6)
• Overt trial and error; concretely tested out solutions (5)
• Establish a goal; one scheme to deal with each goal (4)

C2. "Were you taught to make calendars in that way or did you think of it yourself?"

D. "What came to your mind when you saw or heard the word calendar?"

Images
• Transformational; can change shape and position, and the intermediary steps involved (9)
• Static; lacks reversibility (7-8)
• Images used to test solutions (5)
• Trial and error variations (5)

D1. "Does the calendar you made look like others you have seen?"

D2. "Does your calendar look the way you had hoped it would?"

Directions	Behaviors and Categories	Checks	Comments/ Examinee's Responses
Examiner states: # 2. "Make another calendar for one week."	**Language** • Seems to plan work steps; rational, systematic (10) • Understands directions as given by "authority figure," verbal directions (9) • Seems to know what is expected/being asked of him or her (8)		
(Observe and record behaviors while the examinee is working on second calendar.) (If the examinee does not begin to make second calendar, repeat direction # 2.)	**Judgement** • Willingly responds to directions (9) • Ignores rules; testing, resistive (6) • Past experience influence behavior; disinterest expressed (7)		
(If there is still no response, the examiner asks: "Are there other ways to make a calendar?") (If the response is yes, the examiner states: "Please show me or tell me how.")	**Cause and Effect** • Transformational images used; able to change shape, size, direction of new calendar (9) • Static; calendar identical to first; product and process (7-8) • Overt trial and error; seeking novelty, tries to make calendar different, tries possibilities; expanding schemes (5-6)		
(Note in comments section if responses are verbal only, and check appropriate boxes.)	**Classification** • Can form classes; days of week and number of days (9) • Can place into class but not rearrange; days and number of days identical to first calendar (8) • Starts to form class and becomes confused or distracted (7)		
(If response is no, go on to interview questions.) On completion of second calendar, proceed with second set of interview questions.	**Relations** • Plans how to establish equivalence; concept of week remains even if calendar is different in shape or size or made differently (9) • Equivalence is unstable, confused by space; counting doesn't help; overtly tries to pattern second calendar after first (8) • Centers; focuses on one part or aspect of an object, ignoring the rest (7)		

Directions	Behaviors and Categories	Checks	Comments/ Examinee's Responses

Interview questions: Second set

E. "What does the word another mean to you?"

F. "How is your calendar like or different from a monthly calendar?"

G. "How can these calendars be used?"

(Pointing to or indicating calendars examinee has made.)

H. "How is your first calendar the same or different from your second calendar?"

If the examinee is able to follow directions above and answer interview questions with no further clarification from the examiner...

Evaluation is complete—STOP.

Language
• Can discuss several meanings from different perspectives (9)
• Meanings deal with the present, here and now (8)
• Concrete reasoning based on past experience (7)

Relations
• Has correspondence; establishes equivalence (weeks to month) (9)
• Equivalence unstable, confused by space (8)
• Focuses on one part only and ignores other possibilities (7)

Classification
• Can form classes and consider objects in several classes simultaneously; (month/weeks) (9)
• Cannot rearrange or place in other relationships; (weeks to month)
• Starts to form a class and becomes confused or distracted (7)

Cause and Effect
• Can think about abstract, hypothetical; thought is flexible, rational (10)
• Use according to previous operations performed physically by individual (9)
• Static use; stated only as individual currently uses (7-8)
• Delayed imitation; indicates he or she has seen or heard of uses in past (6)

Relations
• Can establish equivalence (9)
• Equivalence unstable; confused by space; counting doesn't help (8)

Number
• Can identify equal number and knows they are equal (9)
• Does not understand they are equal even if they are equal in number (8)

Classification
• Can consider objects simultaneously; discusses similarities and differences (9)
• Alternates discussion of similarities and/or differences; one calendar to another (7-8)
• Discusses calendars separately; does not do comparative analysis (7)

Directions	Behaviors and Categories	Checks	Comments/ Examinee's Responses

Directions

Examiner states:
3. "Please repeat the directions to me."

(If the examinee is able to proceed after he or she states directions or after the examiner restates directions, allow to complete task and then proceed with interview questions.)

(If the examinee cannot repeat direction and/or does not engage in task even after the directions have been restated, proceed with the following.)

Examiner states:
"Do you understand what I mean by a calendar for one week?"

Examiner states:
"Can you tell me how to make one?"

(A positive response to both questions may indicate no problems with language or problem solving; restate reason for task to address moral judgement.)

(In the case of a negative response to either question, proceed to direction # 4.)

Examiner states:
4. "Make a calendar that looks like this."

Present sample calendar and continue to show it until the examinee stops examining it (looks away), then remove.

Behaviors and Categories

Language
• Is able to repeat directions (9)
• Can auditorily focus and understand the viewpoint of others including authority figures
• Is unable to repeat directions (questions written and/or auditory memory, ability to auditorily focus and/or use language)
• Words have personal meaning; own definition of words. repeats directions in own words (7)
• Understands the viewpoint of others; including authority figures (9)
• Attempts to perceive viewpoint of others (8)
• Words have personal meaning (7)

Circular Reactions (Cause and Effect)
• Covert trial and error problem solving; images used to test solution (describing procedure) (6)
• Perceived actions, varied, repeated varied another way, repeated (5)
• Uses 2 familiar schemes to establish a goal (4)
• Chance movement; magical thinking (3)
• No attempt to reach out (2)

Imitation
• Uses delayed imitation (6)
• Serial imitation; new scheme imitated and assimilated into own scheme (5)
• Action expands his or her familiar scheme (4)

		Checks	Comments/
Directions	Behaviors and Categories		Examinee's Responses

(If after reviewing sample, the examinee begins to work and complete task, return to direction # 2. Make another calendar and interview questions following it.)

(If the examinee asks to see sample again, or to have sample continuously visible, present sample and note behaviors.)

(If the examinee completes task using sample, return to direction # 2. If unable to do second calendar, go on to interview questions. If unable to do second calendar, break down activity and attempt a second calendar.)

(If unable to begin task even with sample visible, break activity down and proceed with structured direction # 5.)

Examiner states:
5. "First draw the lines, then write in the days."

(If the examinee is able to begin work and complete the calendar, go back to direction # 2 and interview questions.)

(If the examinee is unable to begin working, go on to direction # 6.)

Circular Reaction (Cause and Effect)
• Images used to test solution to problem (6)
• Seeking novelty; variations in own actions (6)
• Utilizes two schemes to establish a goal (4)
• Magical thinking

Object Permanence
• Explores potential of other objects and people (5)
• Object visually perceived as different from self; object has own movement, causing own effect (4)
• Objects understood in terms of own actions; action can be stopped and then resumed (3)

Time Concept
• Attention focused until bored with activity (5)
• Can focus for 30-45 minutes; can anticipate future events based on interpreting signs, utilizing actions of others (4)
• Attention is action oriented (3)

Circular Reaction
• Utilizes two familiar schemes to establish goal (4)

Imitation
• New learning based on old schemes (4)

Object Permanence
• Object perceived as different from self; has own movement and cause (4)
• Object is permanent; action stopped and resumed (3)

Time Concept
• Can focus attention 30-45 minutes (4)

Directions	Behaviors and Categories	Checks	Comments/ Examinee's Responses

Examiner states:
6. "Do as I do..."

a. "Draw a line like this." (Line 1) (Permit the examinee to draw line.)
b. "Now draw a line like this." (Line 2)
c. "Now write Sunday over the first square."

(If the examinee seems to have difficulty with the days of the week, use abbreviations: S, M, T, W, Th, F, S.)

Continue to label the days of the week.

(If the examinee is able to complete the calendar, attempt direction # 2 and/or interview questions.)

(If the examinee is unable to complete the calendar, attempt interview questions.)

End of evaluation procedure. Review and analyze results.

Imitation
• Patient can imitate therapist when own familiar schemes are used (3)
• Able to use direct imitation (3)

Circular Reactions
• Own actions are the cause of everything (3)
• Chance body movements, attempts to repeat (2)

Object Permanence
• Patient can stop an action and then resume (3)

Time Concept
• Focused attention for repetitive actions. Can remember events based on own action (3)
• Can focus attention for 2 minutes before he or she gets distracted (2)

References
Allen C. *Thought Process and Activity Analysis Chart*. Unpublished. 1972.
Ginsburg H, Opper S. *Piaget's Theory of Intellectual Development*. Englewood Cliffs, NJ: Prentice-Hall; 1969.
Mosey AC. *Three Frames of Reference for Mental Health*. Thorofare, NJ: Charles B. Slack; 1970.
Singer D, Reverson T. *A Piaget Primer: How a Child Thinks*. NY: A Plume Book, New American Library; 1978.

	Sunday	Monday	Tuesday	Wednesday	Thursday	Friday	Saturday

Sample for Direction # 6 Only

	(11)	(12)	(13)	(14)	(15)	(16)	(17)
Line #1	Sunday	Monday	Tuesday	Wednesday	Thursday	Friday	Saturday

Line #3	Line #5	Line #6	Line #7	Line #8	Line #9	Line #10	Line #4

Line #2

For examiner use only; not to be presented to the examinee.

Cognitive Adaptive Skills Evaluation Summary Sheet

Frequency and Distribution of Behaviors:

	Time Concept	Language	Judgement & Moral Behavior	Images	Classifica-tion	Relations	Numbers	Imitation	Circular Reactions	Object Permanence
Level 3										
Level 4										
Level 5										
Level 6										
Level 7										
Level 8										
Level 9										
Level 10										

Problem Identification:

Summary of Assets:

Goals:

Possible Learning Approaches:

E

Excerpts of OT FACT Psychosocial Categories and Definitions

I. Role Integration

Functions appropriately in all life roles and balances roles in unified life activity. Does not demonstrate overemphasis or skill in some roles to the deficit of others.

  A. Role Performance

Functions adequately in each applicable life role, encompassing all aspects of each role.

    1. Personal Maintainer

Takes care of self (self-care and health management).

    2. Student

Performs all functions required of a student.

    3. Worker / Volunteer

Contributes time and skills to complete tasks toward vocational / volunteer goals.

    4. Caregiver

Provides necessary nuturance and support to those requiring care.

    5. Employer

Responsibly recruits and maintains employees to secure short- and long-term needs for self and employees.

    6. Citizen / Neighbor

Participates in societal activities and interacts respectfully as next door and world neighbor.

    7. Player / Recreator

Initiates, develops, and participates in individual and social leisure activities to self-satisfaction.

    8. Friend / Companion

Develops, maintains, and participates in non-family social relationships.

    9. Significant Other

Participates effectively in an intimate relationship with another.

10. Family Member	Participates constructively in family. Interacts with parents, siblings, in-laws, etc as appropriate.
11. Consumer	Makes knowledgable purchases to meet needs and interests.
B. Integrates Self/External Roles	Coordinates physical, social, and cultural expectations with internal role expectations.
C. Balances Roles	Balances number and time allocation among life roles to prevent role overload, role conflict, or role deprivation.
1. Role Overload	Limits number of roles to maintain quality of life and effective role functioning.
2. Role Conflict	Roles coexist without interference among them.
3. Role Deprivation	Effectively assumes an adequate number of roles.
D. Integrates Role Over Time	Experiences no disruption among past, present, and future roles.

II. Activities of Performance

  A. Personal Care Activities

1. Cleanliness, Hygiene, and Appearance	Bathes, performs, toilet and oral hygiene activities, and dresses as needed.
a. Bathing	Obtains and uses supplies; doffs clothing; achieves bathing position; maintains bathing position; soaps, rinses, and dries all body parts; leaves bathing position.
b. Toilet Hygiene	Position.
c. Hand Washing	Obtains and uses supplies; regulates water; soaps, scrubs, and rinses, shuts water off; dries hands.
d. Oral Hygiene	Obtains and uses supplies; cleans mouth and teeth; rinses pertinent to natural teeth or dentures.
e. Grooming	Obtains and uses supplies; shaves; applies and removes cosmetics; combs and brushes hair.
1) Cares for hair	Obtains needed tools and supplies; combs/brushes; styles hair.

2) Fingernails	Obtains needed tools and supplies; cares for fingernails.
3) Toenails	Obtains needed tools and supplies; cares for toenails.
4) Shaves	Obtains supplies; shaves face, legs, axilla, as needed.
5) Cosmetics	Applies and removes cosmetics (obtains materials, applies appropriate amount in an acceptable fashion).
6) Deodorant	Obtains and applies deodorant.
f. Dressing	Selects appropriate clothing; obtains clothing from storage area; sequentially dons and doffs all items including appliances (eg, glasses, prostheses, orthoses), underwear, shoes, outerwear, and accessories; adjusts clothing; and fastens and unfastens.
g. Nose Blowing	Grasps tissue or handkerchief; blows and wipes nose.
2. Medical and Health Mgmt. Act.	Performs exercise programs, uses medication, manages unhealthy behavior, and communicates in emergencies as needed.
a. Health Maintenance & Improvement	Manages healthy routines to maintain or improve status; avoids unhealthy practices.
1) Exercise program / Routine	Performs prescribed physical and psychosocial health promotion routines, eg, functional exercise program, pressure relief activities, splint wearing schedules.
2) Manages unhealthy behaviors	Health and welfare.
a) Smoking	Regulates smoking.
b) Alcohol and drug use	Regulates alcohol and drug use.
c) Food consumption	Regulates quantities of food consumption.
d) Sexual practices	Avoids sexual activities that ignore self-health and welfare, including infectious disease and unwanted pregnancy.
b. Medication Routine	Effects and precautions.
1) Schedule	Uses correct schedule.
2) Obtains medication	Obtains medication from storage location.

3) Containers	Opens and closes containers.
4) Selects / Measures	Selects / measures appropriate amount of medication.
5) Administers / Takes	Administers / takes medication in available form (manipulates pills, swallows, places under tongue, IM, etc).
6) Stores medication	Stores medication properly.
7) Manages side effects	Takes action as necessary when dosage problems arise.
c. Emergency Communication	Performs steps required to obtain appropriate help at all times of the day or night.
3. Nutrition Activities	Prepares, cleans-up meals, and eats as needed.
4. Sleep and Rest Activities	Plans and takes sleeping and rest breaks, relaxes; sleeps in appropriate locations and positions; has established cycle and sufficient amount of sleep and rest for normal daily routine.
5. Mobility Activities	Moves indoor, outdoor, with private transportation, and outdoor with public transportation as needed.
6. Communication Activities	Speaks, writes, reads, uses the telephone, and expresses oneself sexually as needed.
a. Speaking	Intelligibly expresses basic needs orally, gesturally, or symbolically without documentation including identifying need and obtaining equipment when needed.
b. Writing	Legibly writes, prints, or types appropriate person, place, and time information and short message.
c. Reading	Comprehends public signs, messages, and follows simple step-by-step written directions including identifying need to read and obtaining equipment when needed.
d. Telephone	When appropriate.
e. Sexual Expression	Recognizes, communicates, and performs sexual behaviors appropriate for individual and environment.
7. Assistive Device Repair & Maintenance	Cares for assistive technology devices such as wheelchair or communication aid to avoid damage; replaces and fixes broken devices; cleans devices as needed; or obtains appropriate assistance for these functions.

B. Occupational Role Related Activities

    1. Home Management Activities   Acquire home, plans meals, cares for clothing, cleans the home, repairs and maintains the facility and contents, keeps the home safe, and manages the yard as needed.

        a. Home Acquisition   Finds an apartment/home that is suited to one's geographic, economic, mobility, and personal preferences; uses newspaper ads or agencies as needed; and appropriately interacts with potential landlords and banks.

        b. Menu Planning   Plans nutritional meals within one's own budget; coordinates grocery needs with food required; plans meals over an extended period of time (ie, more than just one meal at a time).

        c. Care of Clothing/Launderables   Launders, stores, and mends clothing and other launderables. Arranges for dry cleaning.

        d. Cleaning   Picks up; dusts; removes garbage; maintains sinks, tub, shower, and toilet; vacuums; sweeps; scrubs/mops; and makes bed.

        e. Household Repair & Maintenance   Repairs and maintains items in the living environment as needed, eg, replaces lightbulbs and fuses; fixes broken appliances, furniture, and other household items; paints/weatherizes, and/or obtains appropriate assistance for these functions.

        f. Household Safety   Doors and windows.

           1) Safe building/facility   Recognizes and prevents damage to home (eg, fires, fire hazards, water damage, intruders, etc).

           2) Safe contents   Recognizes and prevents loss of material goods (secures/locks doors and windows, turns off equipment).

           3) Safe for people   (Etc).

        g. Yard Work   Picks up; mows; trims; shovels; and gardens.

    2. Consumer Activities   Purchase items and manages money as needed.

a. Purchasing Activities	Shops for food, clothing, and supplies; handles money transactions; finds; obtains and transports needed items in store; negotiates store geography; uses catalogs as needed.
b. Money Management Activities	Budgets, uses bank, buys within one's means; allocates money for all necessary areas of expenses; uses credit prudently; and conserves money before next income arrives.
1) Banking	Uses bank (eg, checking, savings accounts, loans, balances accounts).
2) Budgeting	Budgets (buys within one's means, conserves money, allocates money for all necessary areas of expense).
3. Educational Activities	Participates in a school/campus environment and school sponsored activities; attends educational activities regularly and on time; studies; performs homework; physically negotiates campus.
4. Employment & Volunteer Activities	Functions in appropriate work-related activities: determines interests; selects and locates job opportunities; develops appropriate skills; performs tasks of jobs.
5. Caregiving activities	Functions in appropriate nurturance activities: provides both necessary physical care and emotional support.
a. Physical Nurturance	Feeds, bathes, and provides other necessary physical care for a child, sibling, or adult (if appropriate), and/or pet.
b. Emotional Nurturance	Provides love, security; meets realistic psychological needs of a child, sibling, adult, and/or pet.
6. Community Activities	Participates and functions as citizen and in local organizations as needed.
7. Avocational Activities/Play	Participates and functions in solitary and social leisure activities/play as needed.
a. Solitary Leisure Activities	Productively uses free time alone; may include hobbies, reading, television, etc; person considers it consistent with abilities; leisure is not likely to conflict with the environment or to create maladaptation within individual.

1) Explores activities	Explores objects, space, places, new experiences as appropriate.
2) Chooses	Chooses satisfying activities.
3) Gets materials	Obtains needed materials and resources for activities.
4) Performs	Performs play or leisure activities alone, both sedentary and non-sedentary.
5) Puts away	Returns materials to appropriate storage.
b. Social Leisure Activities	Productively engages in leisure/play with other people. Person considers it consistent with abilities; leisure is not likely to conflict with the environment or to create maladaptation within the individual.
8. Employer Activities	Recruits, selects, and retains employees as needed.

III. Integrated Skills of Performance

A. Motor Integration Skills	Moves body parts effectively in activities.
B. Sensory-Motor Integration Skills	Incorporates sensory information effectively into coordinated mental and motor processes.
C. Cognitive Integration Skills	Comprehends, synthesizes, evaluates environmental information and incorporates results into behavior.
D. Social Integration Skills	Skills that enable successful interaction in peer relationships, work, and family; includes one-to-one relationships as well as group interaction; involves ability to give and take in social situations.
1. Peer Interactions	Negotiates, compromises, competes, and cooperates with peers (eg, other children, coworkers, neighbors).
a. Initiates Interaction	Starts a peer interaction or joins an existing one.
b. Manages Own Behavior	Manages own behavior and displays no inappropriate aggressive behaviors during peer interactions independently.
c. Follows Rules	Follows documented or undocumented rules of activities involving peers.

d. Provides Positive Feedback	Provides positive feedback and reinforcement to other peers, eg, smiles, helps out, compliments.
e. Provides Negative Feedback	Alternate opinions.
f. Obtains and Integrates Cues	Obtains and responds to relevant situational cues in the social environment.
g. Offers Information/Assistance	Provides information and assistance to other peers.
h. Obtains Information/Assistance	Solicits and accepts assistance from other peers when needed.
i. Adjusts to Negative Situations	Exhibits alternative strategies to cope with negative peer social situations.
j. Terminates Interaction	Terminates or withdraws from a peer interaction.
2. Authority/Subord Interactions	Negotiates, compromises, competes, and cooperates with individuals in authority and with individuals under one's authority.
3. Family Interactions	Negotiates, compromises, competes, and cooperates with family members; maintains satisfactory relationships with family members; recognizes own role in contributing to family dynamics; achieves individualization from family if appropriate.
4. Pet and Animal Interactions	Approaches and interacts with pets and animals.
E. Psychological Integration Skills	Includes ability to respond to environmental demands in a personally and socially satisfying manner.
1. Coping/Stress Management	Can modulate responses to environmental demands such that problem solving skills remain evident; has identified and uses mechanisms for reducing stress; is able to function under a range of environmental conditions.
2. Time Use/Planning	Develops plans to accomplish tasks; meets obligations on time; is generally on time for appointments.
a. Plans	Develops plans to accomplish tasks.
b. Timely	Is generally on time for appointments.
c. Meets obligations	Meets obligations on time. Delivers by due date.

3. Initiation & Termination of Activities	Starts and stops activities when necessary. (Inability in this area is not to be confused with components such as perseveration or motivation. Cause is not defined.)
4. Maintains Physical Integrity	Acts in ways that will not cause physical harm to own body.

IV. Components of Performance

A. Neuromuscular Components	Effective musculoskeletal and neuromuscular functioning.
B. Sensory Awareness Components	Gustatory.
C. Cognitive Components	Fundamental intellectual processes.
D. Social Components	Includes oral and gestural communication; nonverbal communication; includes component skills for group and dyadic roles.
1. Group Interaction	Takes on a variety of roles as necessary for maintenance of a group; cooperates with others; shares in responsibility for decision making and task completion; uses appropriate verbal and nonverbal communication.
a. Environment Interactions	Respects property and objects including things belonging to self, neighbors, community, or general environment (eg, does not unwarrantedly destroy or break things in the environment).
b. Personal Behaviors	Manages personal behaviors in social situations in an acceptable manner (eg, avoids behaviors that are socially or culturally offensive such as picking one's nose, expelling gas, touching genitals, talking too loud).
2. Dyadic Interaction	Interacts in one-to-one relationships with peers, authority, etc, uses appropriate verbal and nonverbal communication; modulates behavior to reflect changing dynamics in relationships.
E. Psychological Components	Ability to establish a positive self-concept and take action.
1. Personal Responsibility	Accountable for one's actions and contributing accomplishments.

2. Self-Image | Realistic appraisal of self; accepts own personal qualities and limitations.

3. Value Identification | Identifies values that one regards as important, admirable, or worthy of emulating.

4. Interest Identification | Situation.

5. Goal Setting | Possibility.

V. Environment

A. Social/Cultural Environment | Appropriate and sufficient resources and organizational structures required for personal care and occupational role-related environments are available.

1. Resources | Appropriate social support, financial, and medical resources for adequate performance in personal care and occupational role-related activities are available.

a. Social Support System | Appropriate family, friends, community, service providers, and advocates are available, share values and support goals; reliable people are available to help out when things go wrong or for emergencies.

b. Financial Resources | Has adequate funds (wages, supplemental income, insurance) to engage in valued activities including emergency resources (ie, parent, friend, insurance) and basic necessities of life, medical, educational, and recreational needs.

c. Medical Resources | Has access to needed medical care. Adequate emergency, primary care, specialty, rehabilitative, and long-term care, including therapy, is available within reasonable distance.

d. Educational Resources | Adequate formal and informal regular educational and special educational and training programs are available to meet the particular needs of this individual.

2. Organizational System | Organizational structures required to support individual in personal care and occupational role-related activities are available.

B. Physical Environment | Appropriate and sufficient accessibility, accommodation and access to tools and technologies meet individual needs of user.

OT FACT Profile for an Individual with Early Alzheimer's Behavior

BACKGROUND

An 82-year-old woman named "Grandmother" was living in a supported retirement efficiency apartment in a facility called "Pleasant Manor." Her family lived in several nearby states, and also included a daughter who lived in the same town as Grandmother. The family became concerned about Grandmother's decreased involvement in many of the social activities she had performed regularly for decades. Initially, this included performance changes, such as not making regular phone calls to family, failing to write weekly letters, showing disinterest in family members' visits, forgetting appointments and scheduled social events, offering empty descriptions of recent social activities, and confabulating to fill in the gaps in her recollection of recent social activities. Later, the memory difficulties shifted to major personality changes, such as a shift from being fastidious in self-care, highly inhibited and controlling of social behavior, to not bathing and publicly exhibiting expressions of intimate social interaction. These functional changes became major sources of frustration for her children, who increasingly related being aggravated by interpersonal interactions with their mother, being unprepared to help a family member with these behaviors, and feeling totally helpless in keeping Mom like Mom. This resulted in the suggestion of an overall occupational performance assessment to quantify Grandmother's current performance, and to highlight possible interventions to improve the quality of life of Grandmother and her concerned children.

INTERESTS AND OCCUPATIONS

Grandmother has a master's degree in music education and once was a proficient keyboard player (piano and organ). She has been an avid reader, music listener, knitter, cook, and companion. Recently, knitting and cooking became too complex, and using a radio or television was also too complicated. She attended events in the senior center when possible, and continued to actively participate in group activities. She remains fully ambulatory and physically able to perform all daily activities appropriate for an individual in her eighth decade. However, independent attendance at social activities or the initiation of solitary activities was extremely limited or totally absent. She was widowed a number of years ago, but since then had been easily able to renew old friendships and develop new casual relationships, including one intimate relationship. She continued to actively participate effectively in one-to-one social interactions. Her participation in social activities continued to be appropriate, with the exception of recent uninhibited behaviors—social hugging and kissing in environments in which more conservative social behaviors were expected. She ate meals in a common dining room with other residents in her facility, who eat at assigned seats and have individualized menus. The mealtimes provided a scheduled structure both for her day and that of the other residents in her facility.

THE OT FACT QUANTIFIED PROFILE

Some of her children collected data for OT FACT. The discussion during the data collection process showed a mix of frustration with Grandmother's inability to perform activities, and her ability to physically perform virtually all categories of tasks in OT FACT. Her general profile, seen in Graph 1, reveals severe disability across all areas of all domains of function. More careful examination of the activities of performance reveals that Grandmother exhibits significant functional performance deficits across most activities in personal care and occupational-role-related activities. These performance deficits are further explained by examining the skills and components of performance. In the skills level, it is apparent that Grandmother's assets include most areas of neuromotor and musculoskeletal performance, while her most significant deficits are in the psychological and cognitive areas. Further scrutiny of OT FACT details in the psychosocial area indicate a high degree of skill in some social areas, yet very low skill in others (Graph 2). This comparison of social skills also highlights the psychometric characteristics of OT FACT, in which scoring is contextual. While Grandmother's social skills are considered a strength in most social situations, within a more conservative social environment, her more intimate behaviors are considered inappropriate. An examination of the components or performance level again illustrates the contrasting abilities between various areas of underlying pathology (Graph 3).

RECOMMENDATIONS

This administration of OT FACT resulted in specific discoveries that led to a set of recommendations. The recommendations included:

1. Design an intervention to help coach Grandmother and her new intimate friend to recognize which behaviors are appropriate in which social environments.
2. Discuss these findings with the facility staff to increase their support in achieving these recommended goals.
3. Administer OT FACT, using three covariates to obtain a focused baseline of performance that isolates and quantifies the contribution of: a) memory, b) social skill deficits, and c) family support to her overall functional performance deficits. The rationale for performing these covariate assessments is to:
   - obtain a baseline for comparing the rate and extent of Alzheimer's-related problems.
   - specifically quantify social skills to monitor any progress in the social intervention area.
   - identify the contribution of family support to Grandmother's functional performance to demonstrate that Alzheimer's symptoms are not a result of or the "fault" of Grandmother's family support.

4. Incorporate specific social intervention strategies, which could include increasing family, facility staff, and friends' discussions with Grandmother about the inappropriateness of her uninhibited social behaviors in public situations. Additionally, increase the external stimuli for Grandmother that relate to her past social behaviors, such as memorabilia of her family, activities with her deceased husband, church activities in line with her conservative religious background, and previous lifestyle and personality characteristics. As Grandmother seems to forget who she was, external and more frequent information may assist the linkage of past behaviors to the present.

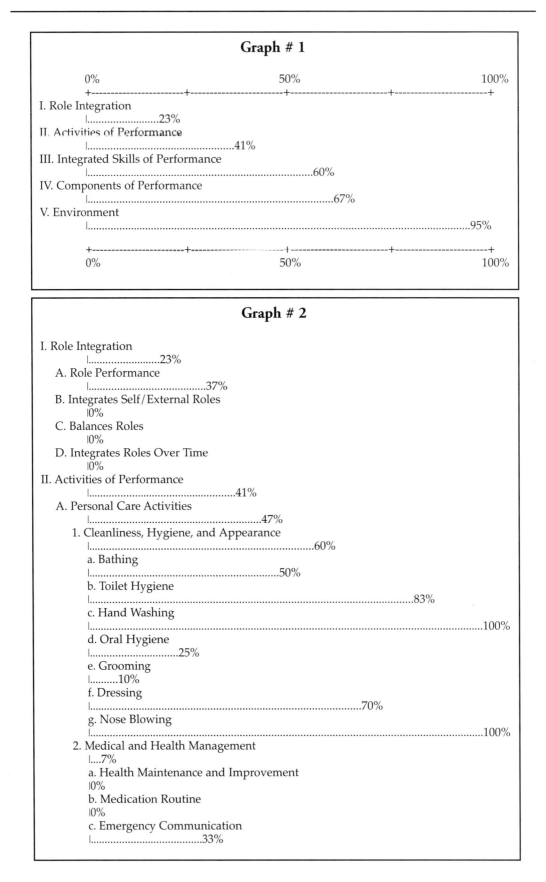

Graph # 1

```
        0%                        50%                        100%
        +----------------+----------------+----------------+----------------+
I. Role Integration
        |................23%
II. Activities of Performance
        |..........................41%
III. Integrated Skills of Performance
        |........................................60%
IV. Components of Performance
        |..............................................67%
V. Environment
        |..................................................................................95%

        +----------------+----------------+----------------+----------------+
        0%                        50%                        100%
```

Graph # 2

```
I. Role Integration
        |................23%
   A. Role Performance
        |.........................37%
   B. Integrates Self/External Roles
        |0%
   C. Balances Roles
        |0%
   D. Integrates Roles Over Time
        |0%
II. Activities of Performance
        |...........................41%
   A. Personal Care Activities
        |...............................47%
      1. Cleanliness, Hygiene, and Appearance
        |.....................................60%
         a. Bathing
        |.............................50%
         b. Toilet Hygiene
        |...............................................83%
         c. Hand Washing
        |..................................................................100%
         d. Oral Hygiene
        |...................25%
         e. Grooming
        |........10%
         f. Dressing
        |...................................70%
         g. Nose Blowing
        |..................................................................100%
      2. Medical and Health Management
        |....7%
         a. Health Maintenance and Improvement
        |0%
         b. Medication Routine
        |0%
         c. Emergency Communication
        |......................33%
```

Graph # 2 (continued)

3. Nutrition Activities
   a. Feeding/Eating
   |...100%
   b. Meal Preparation and Cleaning
   |0%
4. Sleep and Rest Activities
   |...50%
   a. Plans/Takes Sleep/Early
   |...50%
   b. Relaxes/Quiets Self
   |...50%
   c. Uses Appropriate Locations
   |...50%
   d. Uses Appropriate Positions
   |...50%
   e. Regular Sleep-Wake
   |...50%
   f. Sufficient Sleep/Relaxation
   |...50%
5. Mobility Activities
   |...75%
   a. Indoor
   |...100%
   b. Outdoor/Community (Private)
   |0%
   c. Outdoor/Community (Public)
   |0%
6. Communication Activities
   |.............14%
   a. Speaking
   |...50%
   b. Writing
   |...50%
   c. Reading
   |...50%
   d. Telephone
   |0%
   e. Sexual Expression
   |0%
7. Assistive Device Repair
   |0%
B. Occupational Role Related Activities
   |...6%
   1. Home Management Activities
   |0%
   2. Consumer Activities
   |0%
   3. Educational Activities
   | n/a
   4. Employment and Volunteer Activities
   | n/a
   5. Caregiving Activities
   |0%
   6. Community Activities
   |...............................25%
   a. Citizenship Activities
   |...50%

Graph # 2 (continued)

        b. Civic/Religious Activities
        |0%
     7. Avocational Activities
        |................................25%
        a. Solitary Leisure Activities
        |0%
        b. Social Leisure Activities
        |...50%
     8. Employer Activities
        |0%
III. Integrated Skills of Performance
        |...60%
  A. Motor Integration Skills
        |..75%
     1. Functional Motor Skills
        |..75%
        a. Gross Motor Coordination
        |..50%
        b. Fine Motor Coordination/Dexterity
        |..50%
        c. Oral-Phalangeal Function
        |...100%
        d. Facial Movement
        |...100%
        e. Ocular Movement
        |...100%
        f. Bowel and Bladder Control
        |..50%
     2. Postural Control
        |...100%
     3. Activity Tolerance
        |..50%
  B. Sensory-Motor Integration Skills
        |...100%
     1. Perceptual
        |...100%
     2. Perceptual-Motor
        |...100%
        a. Motor Planning (praxes)
        |...100%
        b. Bilateral Motor Coordination
        |...100%
        c. Crossing-the-Midline
        |...100%
        d. Laterality
        |...100%
        e. Visual-Motor Integration
        |...100%
  C. Cognitive Integration Skills
        |................................28%
     1. Problem Solving
        |...50%
     2. Generalizes Learning
        |0%
     3. Sequencing
        |0%
     4. Concept Formation
        |...50%

Graph # 2 (continued)

5. Categorization
|0%

6. Intellectual Operations
|...100%

7. Learning Style Breadth
|0%

D. Social Integration Skills
|...50%

1. Peer Interactions
|...50%

2. Authority/Subordinate Interactions
|...50%

3. Family Interactions
|...50%

4. Pet and Animal Interactions
|...50%

E. Psychological Integration
|.................................41%

1. Coping/Stress Management
|0%

2. Time Use/Planning
|0%

3. Initiation and Termination
|...50%

a. Takes Initiative
|...50%

b. Terminates Behavior
|...50%

4. Maintains Physical Integrity
|...100%

IV. Components of Performance
|..67%

A. Neuromuscular Components
|...92%

1. Muscle Tone
|...100%

2. Reflexes (including synergies)
|...100%

3. Range of Motion
|...100%

4. Strength (pinch, hand, muscle)
|...100%

5. General Endurance
|...50%

6. Soft Tissue Integrity
|...100%

7. Skeletal Integrity
|...100%

B. Sensory Awareness Component
|...81%

1. Tactile
|...100%

2. Proprioceptive
|...100%

3. Kinesthesia
|...100%

4. Ocular Control and Visual
|...100%

Graph # 2 (continued)

5. Vestibular
|...100%
6. Auditory
|...50%
7. Olfactory
|...50%
8. Gustatory
|...50%
C. Cognitive Components
|..57%
   1. Level of Arousal
|...100%
   2. Processing Flow
|...50%
   3. Memory
|...50%
   4. Orientation
|...50%
   5. Attention Span
|...50%
   6. Recognition
|...50%
   7. Thought Processes (formations of thought)
|...50%
D. Social Components
|...50%
   1. Group Interaction
|...50%
   2. Dyadic Interaction
|...50%
E. Psychological Components
|.......................................30%
   1. Personal Responsibilities
|...50%
   2. Self-Image
|...50%
   3. Value Identification
|...50%
   4. Interest Identification
|0%
   5. Goal Setting
|0%
V. Environment
|...95%
A. Social/Cultural Environment
|...90%
   1. Resources
|...100%
   2. Organizational System
|...50%
B. Physical Environment
|...100%

Graph # 3

II. Activities of Performance
  |..41%
  A. Personal Care Activities
    |..47%
    1. Cleanliness, Hygiene, and Appearance
      |...60%
      a. Bathing
        |...50%
      b. Toilet Hygiene
        |...83%
      c. Hand Washing
        |...100%
      d. Oral Hygiene
        |.............................25%
      e. Grooming
        |..........10%
      f. Dressing
        |..70%
      g. Nose Blowing
        |...100%
    2. Medical and Health Management
      |....7%
      a. Health Maintenance and Improvement
        |0%
      b. Medication Routine
        |0%
      c. Emergency Communication
        |.....................................33%
    3. Nutrition Activities
      a. Feeding/Eating
        |...100%
      b. Meal Preparation and Cleaning
        |0%
    4. Sleep and Rest Activities
      |...50%
      a. Plans/Takes Sleep/Early
        |...50%
      b. Relaxes/Quiets Self
        |...50%
      c. Uses Appropriate Locations
        |...50%
      d. Uses Appropriate Positions
        |...50%
      e. Regular Sleep-Wake
        |...50%
      f. Sufficient Sleep/Relaxation
        |...50%
    5. Mobility Activities
      |..75%
      a. Indoor
        |...100%
      b. Outdoor/Community (Private)
        |0%
      c. Outdoor/Community (Public)
        |0%
    6. Communication Activities
      |.............14%

Graph # 3 (continued)

a. Speaking
|...50%
b. Writing
|...50%
c. Reading
|...50%
d. Telephone
|0%
e. Sexual Expression
|0%
7. Assistive Device Repair and Maintenance
|0%
B. Occupational Role Related Activities
|...6%
1. Home Management Activities
|0%
2. Consumer Activities
|0%
3. Educational Activities
|n/a
4. Employment and Volunteer Activities
|n/a
5. Caregiving Activities
|0%
6. Community Activities
|...............................25%
a. Citizenship Activities
|...50%
b. Civic/Religious Activities
|0%
7. Avocational Activities
|...............................25%
a. Solitary Leisure Activities
|0%
b. Social Leisure Activities
|...50%
8. Employer Activities
|n/a
III. Integrated Skills of Performance
|...60%
A. Motor Integration Skills
|..75%
1. Functional Motor Skills
|..75%
a. Gross Motor Coordination
|...50%
b. Fine Motor Coordination/Dexterity
|...50%
c. Oral-Phalangeal Function
|...100%
d. Facial Movement
|...100%
e. Ocular Movement
|...100%
f. Bowel and Bladder Control
|...50%
2. Postural Control
|...100%

Graph # 3 (continued)

3. Activity Tolerance
|...50%

B. Sensory-Motor Integration Skills
|..100%

C. Cognitive Integration Skills
|.................................28%

  1. Problem Solving
  |...50%

  2. Generalizes Learning
  |0%

  3. Sequencing
  |0%

  4. Concept Formation
  |...50%

  5. Categorization
  |0%

  6. Intellectual Operations
  |..100%

  7. Learning Style Breadth
  |0%

D. Social Integration Skills
|...50%

E. Psychological Integration Skills
|..40%

  1. Coping/Stress Management
  |0%

  2. Time Use/Planning
  |0%

  3. Initiation and Termination
  |...50%

  4. Maintains Physical Integrity
  |..100%

IV. Components of Performance
|...67%

A. Neuromuscular Components
|...92%

B. Sensory Awareness Component
|...81%

  1. Tactile
  |..100%

  2. Proprioceptive
  |..100%

  3. Kinesthesia
  |..100%

  4. Ocular Control and Visual
  |..100%

  5. Vestibular
  |..100%

  6. Auditory
  |...50%

  7. Olfactory
  |...50%

  8. Gustatory
  |...50%

C. Cognitive Components
|..57%

  1. Level of Arousal
  |..100%

Graph # 3 (continued)

2. Processing Flow
   |..50%
3. Memory
   |..50%
4. Orientation
   |..50%
5. Attention Span
   |..50%
6. Recognition
   |..50%
7. Thought Processes (form and content)
   |..50%
D. Social Components
   |..50%
   1. Group Interaction
      |..50%
   2. Dyadic Interaction
      |..50%
E. Psychological Components
   |..30%
   1. Personal Responsibilities
      |..50%
   2. Self-Image
      |..50%
   3. Value Identification
      |..50%
   4. Interest Identification
      |0%
   5. Goal Setting
      |0%
V. Environment
   |..95%
A. Social/Cultural Environment
   |..90%
   1. Resources
      |..100%
   2. Organizational System
      |..50%
B. Physical Environment
   |..100%

INDICES

Assessment Index

Author Index

Word Index

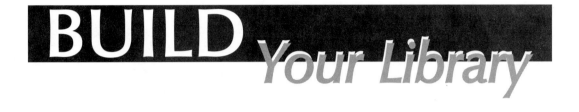

BUILD *Your Library*

This book and many others on numerous different topics are available from SLACK Incorporated. For further information or a copy of our latest catalog, contact us at:

Professional Book Division
SLACK Incorporated
6900 Grove Road
Thorofare, NJ 08086 USA
Telephone: 1-856-848-1000
1-800-257-8290
Fax: 1-856-853-5991
E-mail: orders@slackinc.com
www.slackbooks.com

We accept most major credit cards and checks or money orders in US dollars drawn on a US bank. Most orders are shipped within 72 hours.

Contact us for information on recent releases, forthcoming titles, and bestsellers. If you have a comment about this title or see a need for a new book, direct your correspondence to the Editorial Director at the above address.

Thank you for your interest and we hope you found this work beneficial.

DATE DUE